HEMATOPOIESIS

HEMATOLOGY

Series Editor

Kenneth M. Brinkhous, M.D.
Department of Pathology
University of North Carolina
School of Medicine
Chapel Hill, North Carolina

Volume 7 Hemostasis and Animal Venoms, *edited by Hubert Pirkle and Francis S. Markland, Jr.*

Volume 8 Hematopoiesis: Long-Term Effects of Chemotherapy and Radiation, *edited by Nydia G. Testa and Robert Peter Gale*

Additional Volumes in Preparation

Disorders of the Spleen, *edited by Carl Pochedly, Richard H. Sills, and Allen D. Schwartz*

HEMATOPOIESIS

Long-Term Effects of Chemotherapy and Radiation

edited by

NYDIA G. TESTA
Paterson Institute for Cancer Research
Christie Hospital and Holt Radium Institute
Manchester, England

ROBERT PETER GALE
University of California—Los Angeles
School of Medicine
Los Angeles, California

MARCEL DEKKER, INC. New York and Basel

Library of Congress Cataloging in Publication Data

Hematopoiesis

(Hematology ; v. 8)
Includes bibliographies and index.
1. Bone marrow–Effect of drugs on. 2. Bone marrow–Effect of radiation on. 3. Antineoplastic agents–Toxicology. 4. Cancer–Chemotherapy–Complications and sequelae. 5. Cancer–Radiotherapy–Complications and sequelae. I. Testa, Nydia G. . II. Gale, Robert Peter. III. Series: Hematology (New York, N.Y.) ; v. 8.
RC645.7.B66 1988 616.4'1 88-3572
ISBN 0-8247-7938-X

MARCEL DEKKER, INC.
270 Madison Avenue, New York, New York 10016

Current printing (last digit):
10 9 8 7 6 5 4 3 2 1

PRINTED IN THE UNITED STATES OF AMERICA

Series Introduction

For most of this century hematology has followed a pattern of major scientific discoveries, improved understanding of disease, and rapid application of new knowledge in the clinic. The rate of advance continues at an accelerating pace, so that all but the most zealous have difficulty in keeping up with the literature in even a limited area of specialized interest. As the explosive development of knowledge continues apace, it is a continuing challenge to keep abreast of significant new developments as they impact on clinical and laboratory hematology. The Hematology series is designed to help in this respect, by providing up-to-date, expert presentations on important subject areas in our field. It is hoped that these works, both individually and collectively, will become important volumes for updating information and for reference for the clinician, investigator, teacher, and student, and in this manner contribute to the advancement of hematology.

This volume of the series is devoted to the detection and nature of the chronic adverse effects of radiotherapy and chemotherapy. The success of these modalities in the treatment of many malignant states has resulted in the long-term survival of a large number of patients with associated abnormalities, sometimes subtle, of their hemopoietic and immune systems. The publication of this volume is most timely, since the recent advances in the basic understanding of both these systems provide the means for a rational analysis of these adverse effects. Attention is given to those organs and tissues with rapidly proliferating cells, in particular the bone marrow. The importance of the stroma of the marrow, which creates the microenvironment for blood cell formation, has only recently been fully documented. The role of the stroma is a central one, providing as it does the tissue base for "homing" of stem cells in marrow transplantation, a source of hemopoietic growth factors, and mechanisms for the regulation of hemopoietic cell growth, both proliferation and suppression. Taking advantage of the many recent advances, this volume throws new light on the problem of the late or delayed effects of radiotherapy and chemotherapy. Promise of amelioration or control of these adverse effects is evident. The editors, Nydia G. Testa and Robert Peter Gale, are pioneers in the field. They have enlisted an outstanding group of contributors who have made many of the advances described.

Kenneth M. Brinkhous
Series Editor

Preface

Chemotherapy and radiation are increasingly used to treat cancer. The probability of cure of many malignancies is also increasing. As a consequence, there is heightened awareness of the long-term effects of cytotoxic treatment on hemopoiesis. Although the acute effects of such treatment on bone marrow have been well studied, precise information on long-term bone marrow damage is lacking.

This volume presents experimental and clinical data on the delayed effects of cytotoxic agents (drugs, chemicals, and radiation) on hemopoietic cells and regulatory cells that comprise the inductive microenvironment. These effects are analyzed from the perspective of mechanisms of myelosuppression, mutagenesis, chromosome abnormalities, and effects on the immune system and on other tissues. The book includes authoritative reviews of clinical and experimental hemopoietic damage placed within a framework of basic cell biology with emphasis on the control of cell proliferation and differentiation.

The increased awareness of the potential long-term problems posed by chemotherapy and radiation occurs at a time when advances in cell and molecular biology have led to increased understanding of hemopoiesis. Developments in these areas will likely lead to new therapeutic approaches such as trials with recombinant hemopoietic growth factors.

We hope this book will interest hematologists, oncologists, immunologists, and scientists working in cancer research, as well as biologists interested in the basic problems of regulation of cell proliferation and differentiation.

Nydia G. Testa
Robert Peter Gale

Contributors

Manju Bhavnani* Department of Haematology/Oncology, Royal Manchester Children's Hospital, Manchester, England

Mary K. Conner Department of Biostatistics and Industrial Environmental Health Sciences, Graduate School of Public Health, University of Pittsburgh, Pittsburgh, Pennsylvania

T. Michael Dexter Department of Experimental Haematology, Paterson Institute for Cancer Research, Christie Hospital and Holt Radium Institute, Manchester, England

Stephen G. Emerson Hematology/Oncology Division, Department of Medicine, University of Michigan Medical Center, Ann Arbor, Michigan

Robert Peter Gale Department of Medicine, Division of Hematology/Oncology, University of California–Los Angeles School of Medicine, Los Angeles, California

Jolyon H. Hendry Department of Radiobiology, Paterson Institute for Cancer Research, Christie Hospital and Holt Radium Institute, Manchester, England

William H. Knospe Section of Hematology, Department of Medicine, Rush-Presbyterian-St. Luke's Medical Center and Rush Medical College, Chicago, Illinois

Hans-Peter E. Lohrmann II. Medizinische Abteilung, Kreiskrankenhaus, Lemgo, Federal Republic of Germany

---

**Present affiliation*: Department of Haematology, Royal Albert Edward Infirmary, Lancaster, England.

Brian I. Lord Department of Experimental Haematology, Paterson Institute for Cancer Research, Christie Hospital and Holt Radium Institute, Manchester, England

Hans A. Messner Department of Medicine, Ontario Cancer Institute, University of Toronto, Toronto, Ontario, Canada

Alan M. Miller Division of Medical Oncology, Department of Medicine, University of Florida, College of Medicine, Gainesville, Florida

Graham Molineux Department of Experimental Haematology, Paterson Institute for Cancer Research, Christie Hospital and Holt Radium Institute, Manchester, England

N. Morardet Institut Gustave Roussy and INSERM, Villejuif, France

Alexander A. Morley Department of Haematology, Flinders University and Medical Centre, Adelaide, South Australia, Australia

Patricia H. Morris Jones Department of Haematology/Oncology, Royal Manchester Children's Hospital, Manchester, England

Elizabeth Naparstek Department of Bone Marrow Transplantation and Cancer/Immunobiology Research Laboratory, Hadassah University Hospital, Jerusalem, Israel

Claude Parmentier Institut Gustave Roussy and INSERM, Villejuif, France

Donna Przepiorka* Fred Hutchinson Cancer Research Center, and Division of Oncology, Department of Medicine, University of Washington, Seattle, Washington

Wolfgang Schreml Department of Internal Medicine, Kreiskrankenhaus, Günzburg, Federal Republic of Germany

Paul J. Simmons Transplantation Biology, Fred Hutchinson Cancer Research Center, Seattle, Washington

Shimon Slavin Department of Bone Marrow Transplantation and Cancer/Immunobiology Research Laboratory, Hadassah University Hospital, Jerusalem, Israel

Nydia G. Testa Department of Experimental Haematology, Paterson Institute for Cancer Research, Christie Hospital and Holt Radium Institute, Manchester, England

---

**Present affiliation*: Hematology/Oncology Unit, Department of Medicine, University of Pittsburgh, and Montefiore Hospital, Pittsburgh, Pennsylvania.

Beverly Torok-Storb Transplantation Biology, Fred Hutchinson Cancer Research Center, and Division of Oncology, Department of Medicine, University of Washington, Seattle, Washington

Maurice Tubiana Institut Gustave Roussy and INSERM, Villejuif, France

Niel Wald Department of Radiation Health, Graduate School of Public Health, University of Pittsburgh, Pittsburgh, Pennsylvania

Roy Samuel Weiner Division of Medical Oncology, Department of Medicine, University of Florida, College of Medicine, Gainesville, Florida

Andrew Will Department of Haematology/Oncology, Royal Manchester Children's Hospital, Manchester, England

Kazuo Yamasaki Department of Medicine, Ontario Cancer Institute, University of Toronto, Toronto, Ontario, Canada

Neal S. Young Cell Biology Section, Clinical Hematology Branch, National Heart, Lung, and Blood Institute, National Institutes of Health, Bethesda, Maryland

Dov Zipori Department of Cell Biology, Weizmann Institute of Science, Rehovot, Israel, and DNAX Research Institute of Molecular and Cellular Biology, Palo Alto, California

Contents

HEMATOPOIESIS

1

The Hemopoietic System
Structure and Regulation

BRIAN I. LORD and NYDIA G. TESTA
Paterson Institute for Cancer Research, Christie Hospital and Holt Radium Institute, Manchester, England

I. INTRODUCTION

The diagnosis and prognosis of hematological disease and the assessment of hemopoietic damage and recovery have traditionally been made on the basis of morphological examinations of smears prepared from bone marrow cell aspirates. From such preparations, no structure is discernible. Neither do histological sections give any idea of structure apart from indicating blood-filled sinusoids dotted about the marrow spaces. It is only at the level of electron microscopy that any sort of structure becomes apparent in the bone marrow, and even there it is limited to the location of marrow in relation to the stromal elements of its environment (1,2). It comes as no surprise, therefore, to find that hemopoietic tissue has largely been regarded as a collection of "free-living cells, not constrained by organ-defining structures, such as basement membranes, required where specific anatomical relationships underline function" (3).

Bone marrow, however, is an extremely complex tissue, the hemopoietic stem cells giving rise to many developing functional cell lineages within the marrow spaces. It will be seen later that it is regulated by an equally complex set of factors: factors that are products of the determinative microenvironment enveloping the hemopoietic marrow. For the proper functioning of such a tissue, it is not unreasonable to expect that the various cell types will be suitably organized in relation to their appropriate environments: that the right cells will be in the right place at the right time.

In this introductory chapter, we first define the types of cell populations constituting the hemopoietic development processes. We then discuss the factors involved in regulating the maintenance, proliferation, and differentiation of the

STEM CELLS

0.4% of total hemopoietic cells
Population self-maintained by proliferation
Multilineage differentiation potential
Not morphologically recognizable
Measured by functional clonal assays in vivo and in vitro

↓

COMMITTED PRECURSOR CELLS

3% of total hemopoietic cells
Transit population with restricted self-renewal
Population amplified by proliferation
Committed to one or, at most, two lines of cellular development
Not morphologically recognizable
Measured by clonal assays in vitro

↓

MATURING CELLS

>95% of total hemopoietic cells
Transit population, numerically amplified by proliferation
Morphologically recognizable as belonging to one of several lines of cellular development
Proliferative sequence completed before full maturity

Figure 1 Properties and proportions of the three categories of cell populations found in hemopoietic tissue.

various cell populations, and finally we consider the evidence for, and significance of, a strictly organized spatial distribution of the cells in the tissue.

II. THE STRUCTURE OF HEMOPOIESIS

The salient details of hemopoiesis are summarized in Figure 1. The developmental sequence is seen to progress through a three-tiered hierarchy of cell populations, from the stem cells, through a stage committed to one or other blood cell line, to full maturational cell development.

A. Stem Cells

The stem cell population is the fundamental base from which all the major blood lines are derived. It is thus considered pluripotent in its differentiation potential, giving rise to erythroid, granulocytic, macrophagic, megakaryocytic, and lymphoid cell lines (Fig. 2). In addition, it now seems clear that osteoclasts (4,5), epidermal Langerhans cells (6), and tissue mast cells (7,8) are also derived from the bone marrow stem cell. However, stem cells comprise only about 1 in 250 of the bone marrow cells and are not morphologically distinguishable. In fact, primitive stem cells, isolated by fluorescence-activated cell sorting, show a morphology very similar to that of the small lymphocytes (Fig. 3; Ref. 9) which account for a significant proportion of the bone marrow cells (~20% or more).

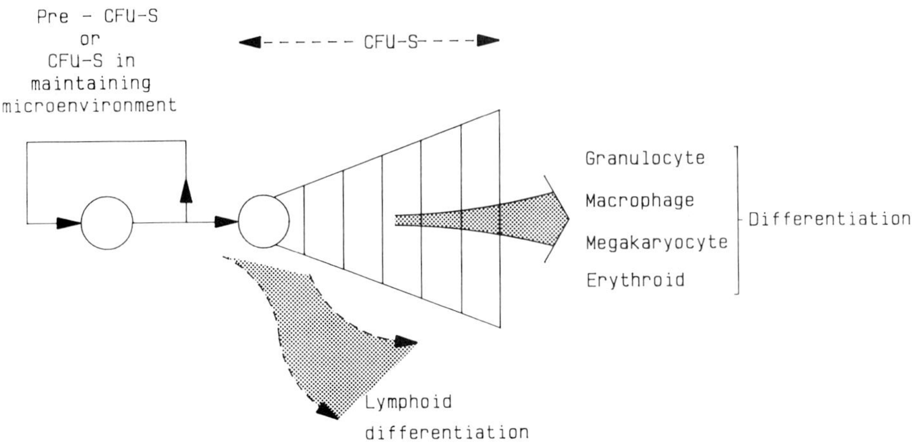

Figure 2 Development of hemopoietic tissue from the primary stem cell or pre-CFU-S (spleen colony-forming unit) and through the pluripotent CFU-S compartment from which differentiation into the various blood cell lineages arises.

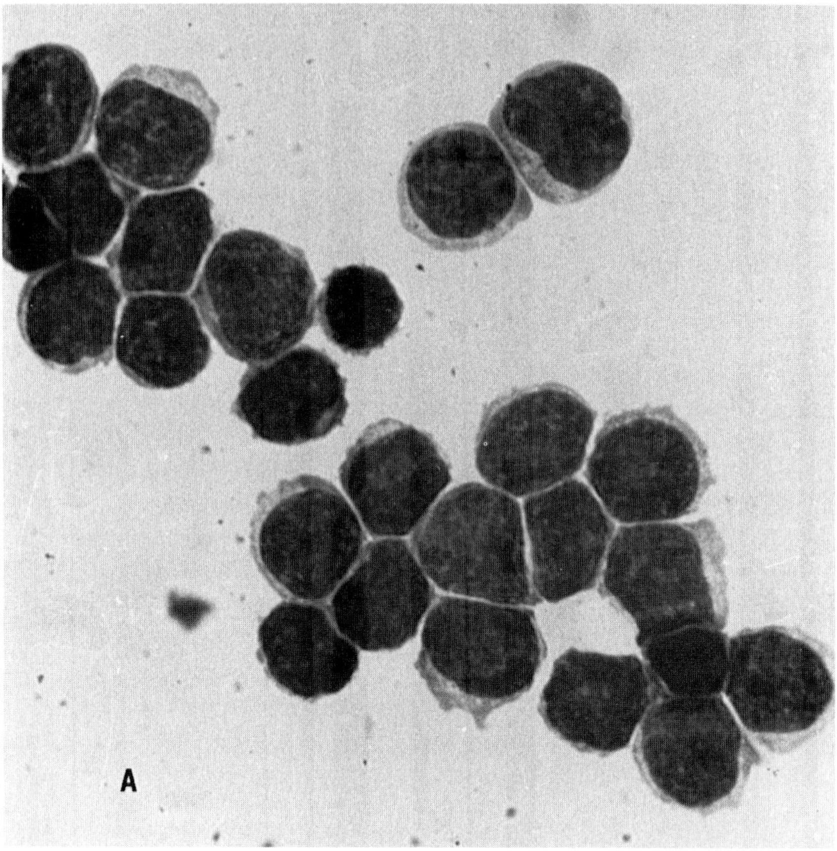

Figure 3 Cells obtained from normal bone marrow by fluorescence-activated cell sorting (FACS), demonstrating approximately 90% purity for the primitive pluripotent spleen colony-forming cell. (A) ~1800X magnification; (B) ~3000X magnification. Reprinted with permission from Ref. 9, *Lymphokine Research 5*, 66 (1986).

The stem cell's most characteristic property distinguishing it from the other cell populations is its ability to maintain its own numbers—it is a self-renewing population. Nevertheless, its proliferation rate is low. In the normal steady state, less than about 10% of the population is in a proliferation cycle. It is its self-renewal property that allows it to remain a small population while giving rise to the necessarily large numbers of functional blood cells over the normal life span of the individual and, when necessary, responding adequately to severe and prolonged hemopoietic stress.

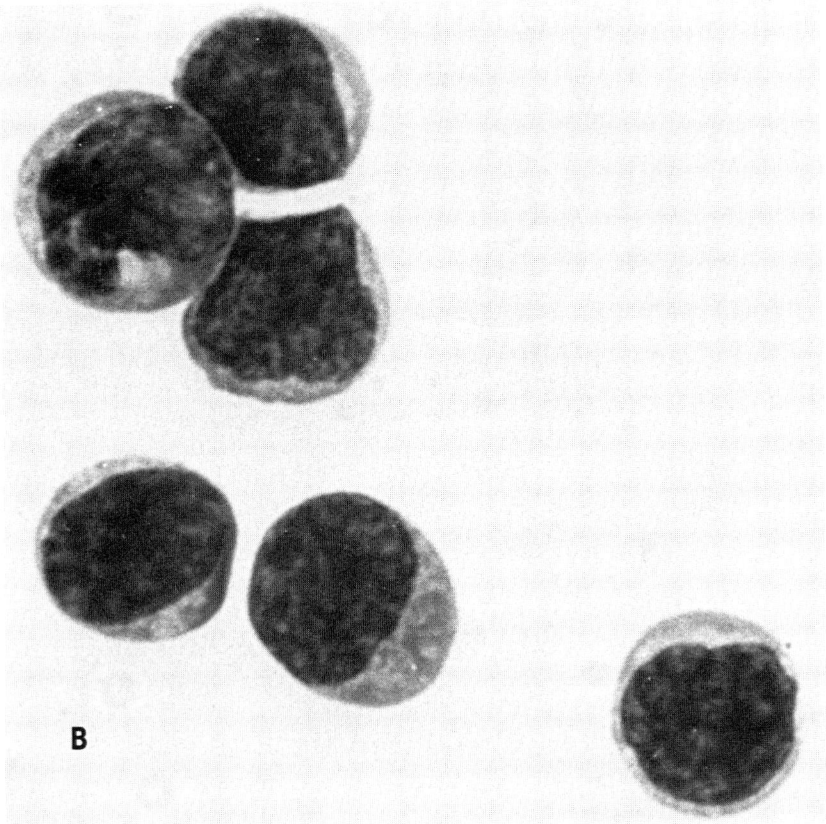

Since the stem cells are not morphologically identifiable, it is necessary to measure them by means of a functional assay. In the mouse, this is the spleen colony-forming test (10) in which hemopoietic cells are injected into lethally irradiated mice and the colonies that develop on the spleen are counted about 9 days later (for details see Ref. 11). Unfortunately, this test is applicable only to the mouse. Cells of mixed differentiation potential can, however, be grown as colonies in vitro from a variety of animal species, from mouse to human (12). These mixed colony-forming cells have a more limited self-renewal potential as measured in vitro but may also contain CFU-S and are probably a subpopulation of stem cells.

B. Committed Progenitor Cells

Committed progenitor cells are derived directly from the stem cells and, as their name implies, are committed to a particular line of cell development, presumably by some specific differentiation trigger. They are already transit cells on a suicide maturation pathway, and although they have some residual self-replicative capacity, this serves only to amplify the population prior to its entering the functional maturation stages.

As can be seen from Figure 4 (see also Figs. 7 and 8), the development of the individual cell lineages is dependent on a large family of growth factors, mainly known as colony-stimulating factors (CSFs) by virtue of their requirement in the various assay procedures. In most cases, their physiological relevance is still unclear, but several of them are now available in pure recombinant form and are being found to be active in vivo (13-17).

As with the pluripotent stem cell population, the number of committed precursor cells is still small, and they remain morphologically undefined. A variety of in vitro colony techniques using appropriate colony-stimulating factors has therefore been developed for their assay (12).

C. Maturing Cells

After a series of amplifying divisions, the committed precursor undergoes a further change when the cell takes on the morphological characteristics of its cell type. This may be the result of a further differentiation step, such as the switching on of hemoglobin synthesis by erythropoietin, or it may be a prolongation of the proliferation sequence throughout the maturation phase by the appropriate growth factor. In either case, proliferation boosts these populations to over 95% of the total cells, and it is on the basis of their number and conditions that, traditionally, the physician has made the diagnosis of disease.

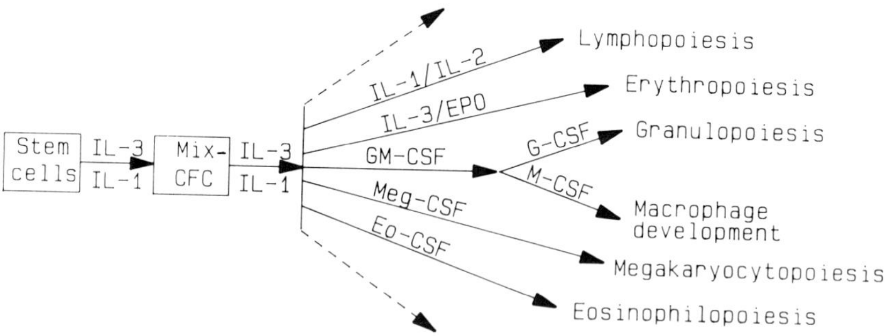

Figure 4 Growth factors involved in the development of the various blood cell lineages. IL = interleukin; EPO = erythropoietin; G = granulocyte; M = macrophage; Meg = megakaryocyte; Eo = eosinophil; CSF = colony-stimulating factor.

In normal circumstances, proliferation ceases by the time a cell is fully mature and it migrates to the periphery to carry out its function and final senescence.

III. STRUCTURE OF THE STEM CELL POPULATION

Before considering the regulation of these cell populations, it is necessary to pay a little more attention to the stem cell compartment. In experiments involving the retransplantation of regenerating spleen colony-forming units (CFU-S) it was observed that between the individual cells in the population there is an extremely heterogeneous capacity for self-renewal (18,19). This led to the idea that the CFU-S population also has an age structure; that some CFU-S are more mature than others (20) and that the more primitive ones take longer (perhaps 12-14 days) to develop as spleen colonies than the more mature ones, which may develop in 7-10 days (21). The implication of this is that the CFU-S population, although pluripotent and having extensive self-renewal capacity, is, like its daughter populations, a transit population in which the individual cells lose their residual proliferative or self-renewal capacity as they proliferate—that is, they age.

A further implication of this principle is that the population should eventually run out. But it does not. The old mouse has a normal number of CFU-S which have exactly the same self-renewal capacity as those in the young mouse (22,23) and it has also been demonstrated that the CFU-S population has enough reserve capacity to generate hemopoietic tissue for at least five, and probably many more, normal life spans (24). As a result, Schofield (20) postulated that the CFU-S population must be anchored by certain stem cells, possibly also CFU-S and generally the most primitive, in which the maturational element is arrested so that any proliferation is geared solely to self-renewal. In this way, a constant supply of pluripotent daughter CFU-S can be maintained.

IV. REGULATION OF STEM CELLS

A. Molecular Regulation

In any stable kinetic system, regulation seems likely always to be effected by negative feedback whereby the products of a process act as a governor to determine the degree of activity of the process. In a cellular system, the greater the number of daughter cells produced, the bigger is the feedback signal generated by the daughter cells. This signal then acts on the parent cells, either by direct inhibition or indirectly by suppression of a stimulatory process, thus limiting further production. Figure 5 illustrates this principle. Class A cells give rise to class B cells, which elaborate an inhibitor of the process. This either acts directly on A cells (Fig. 5a) or blocks the production of the process' driving stimulator (Fig. 5b). In a self-renewing system, B cells may be identical to A cells, but this does not alter the principle. It

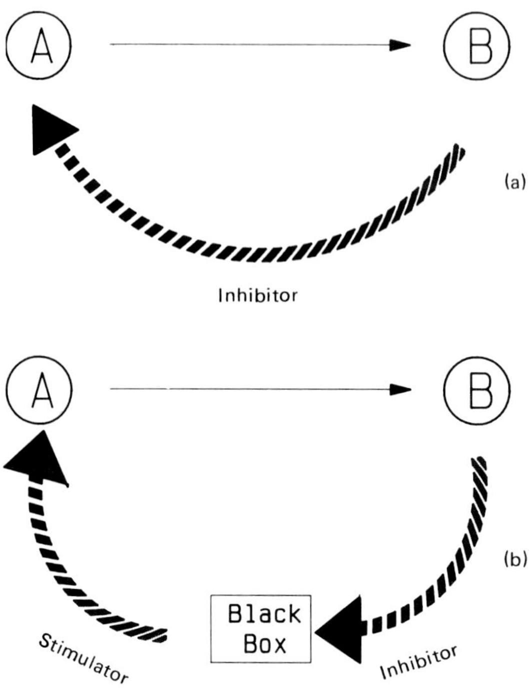

Figure 5 Regulation by negative feedback. The production of cells B from cells A is limited by an inhibitor elaborated by B acting either (*a*) directly on A to suppress its activity or (*b*) via an intermediary structure (the black box) to suppress the production of a stimulator that promotes the activity of A.

should be noted that positive feedback is not a viable alternative. Such a system is inherently unstable and could lead to conditions equivalent to those in certain neoplasms.

The independent proliferative behavior of stem cells in localized sites following partial body irradiation (25) or following a hemolytic shock due to injections of phenylhydrazine (26) suggested that this population is controlled at a local level; that is, regulation is determined within the vicinity of the stem cells. It was natural, therefore, to look first in the bone marrow itself for endogenous physiological regulators of cell proliferation.

Since bone marrow CFU-S have a low overall rate of turnover and proliferatively are almost totally quiescent, the possibility of a direct inhibitor was considered first and duly reported by two main groups, but there remain some differences of opinion with regard to its nature. Frindel and Guigon (27) (who consider their inhibitor to act humorally rather than locally) took a dialyzable extract of low molecular weight from frozen fetal bovine bone marrow. Lord et al. (28), on the other hand, reported that a rather larger molecule (>50,000 daltons), locally active and obtained from fresh, viable adult marrow cells, had proliferation-inhibiting properties. The relationship between these factors is not yet known, but both appear to be specific for the CFU-S population. The inhibitor reported by Lord et al. (28), for example, has no effect on GM-CFC, BFU-E, or Mix-CFC (28,29). In fact, its main sensitivity lies with the early, more primitive CFU-S (29,30). It is, however, species-independent, in that inhibitor obtained from several species (rat, rabbit, pig, and human marrow) act on mouse CFU-S.

It therefore appeared that stem cell proliferation is controlled by one or more negative feedback proliferation inhibitors. In carrying out control experiments, however, it was observed that in regenerating marrow, when the CFU-S population is growing and proliferating rapidly, not only is the inhibitor missing, but it is replaced by a stimulator (31) that is also specific for the CFU-S population (29). This is in accord with the French group who reported that damaged bone marrow is stimulatory to CFU-S (32). Thus, CFU-S proliferation appears to be under the control of competing inhibitory and stimulatory factors, the one blocking entry to DNA synthesis and accumulating cells in the stationary G_0 phase while the other triggers cells from G_0 rapidly into DNA synthesis. By alternating the application of stimulator and inhibitor, it is possible to switch CFU-S into and out of the cell cycle via a $G_0 \rightarrow S$ phase switch (31).

Furthermore, this appears to be a general phenomenon. In most hemopoietic tissues studied, where the size of the CFU-S population is normal or supranormal, the cells are not proliferating and inhibitor is present. When the CFU-S population is depleted and proliferating to regenerate the population, however, stimulator is present (33).

B. Microenvironmental Regulation

Having seen that the inhibitor and stimulator, both naturally occurring (physiological) molecules, appear to regulate specifically the proliferative activity of the CFU-S, it is pertinent next to ask what their origin is. We have already suggested that they act locally, and in addition we have endorsed the principle of a stem cell regulatory microenvironment, the "niche" hypothesis. Furthermore, the importance of microenvironment can be seen in long-term bone marrow culture (34) when an intact adherent layer of macrophages, endothelial cells, fibroblastoid reticular cells, and adipocytes is essential for the maintenance of active hemopoiesis. It is this adherent layer that houses the primitive CFU-S and generates the bulk of hemopoietic cells that grow into the overlying medium. It has also been shown that both inhibitor and stimulator are produced in this adherent layer (35,36), and from a variety of studies it has been shown that the producer cells are subpopulations of macrophages (37-39). Studying the localization and growth of CFU-S in genetically anemic W/W^v mice, Maloney and her colleagues (40) came to the conclusion that there are "stem cell regulatory domains" (niches?)

and that "the partitioning of bone marrow into highly localised functional units is consistent with the putative regulatory role of short-range interactions between stem cells and essential stromal elements." It is possible, therefore, that the macrophages responsible for generating the proliferation inhibitor and stimulator form an integral part of these microenvironmental regulatory units.

Another feature of the microenvironment appears to be the fibroblastoid colony-forming unit (CFU-F). This cell, first described by Friedenstein et al. (41), is grown and assayed in vitro. Its progeny are fibroblastoid in appearance and it seems to be the cell responsible for establishing the appropriate stroma necessary to support the development of hemopoiesis in a bone capsule when marrow is implanted under the kidney capsule (42).

An extensive analysis of the marrow environment is given in Chapter 2.

C. Stem Cell Feedback

In terms of a negative feedback process, as illustrated in Figure 5, the presence of stimulator and inhibitor suggests the indirect regulation method (fig. 5b) whereby the latter blocks production of the former. This has been verified experimentally. However, so has the opposite effect; the stimulator also blocks production of the inhibitor (43). This situation is illustrated in Figure 6*a*. The stem cell population, in a regulatory microenvironment including inhibitor- and stimulator-producing cells, is acted upon by one or the other of these factors depending on the strength of the interaction within the microenvironment. This is not the exact equivalent of Figure 5, however. It is the size of the stem cell population that is to be regulated, and it is therefore those cells that must provide the feedback signal (Fig. 6*b*), the strength of which depends on the size of the population.

The inhibitor and stimulator are not themselves the feedback signals, only its mediators. A study of purified CFU-S populations collected by fluorescence-activated cell sorting (FACS) (9) showed that such a feedback factor exists and that it acts by blocking stimulator production, thereby permitting inhibitor production, which limits further proliferation of the stem cells—a classical negative feedback loop (44).

D. Interleukin-3

Interleukin-3 (IL-3) is one of the large family of factors that have been found to stimulate the growth of hemopoietic cells in vitro. It is a T-lymphocyte product, being generated by those cells under mitogenic stimulation. Another major experimental source of IL-3 is a mouse leukemic cell line (WEHI-3B) that appears to grow primarily because of its endogenous synthesis of IL-3.

Used as an in vitro colony-stimulating factor, IL-3 is capable of generating colonies with a variety of morphologies, so its major function may be one of

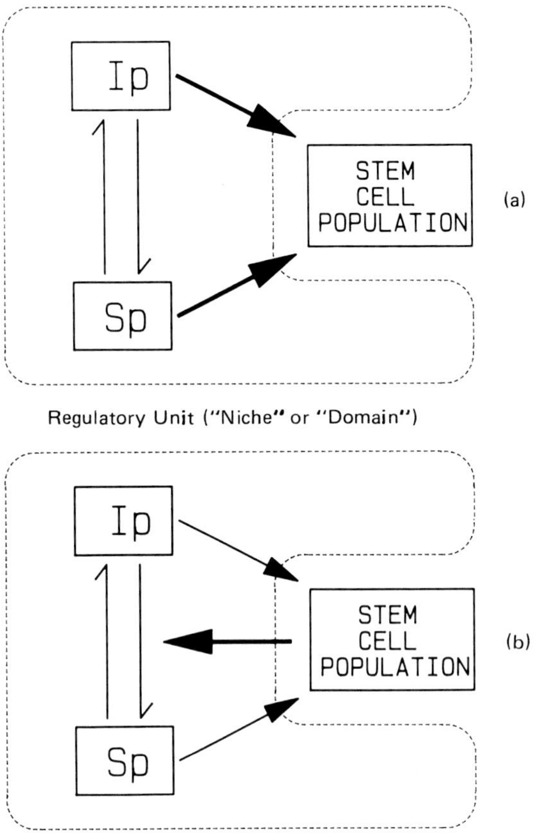

Figure 6 Regulation of the stem cell (or CFU-S) population by negative feedback. Ip, inhibitor-producing cells; Sp, stimulator-producing cells. (*a*) Ip and Sp act on the stem cell population. (*b*) The stem cell returns a feedback signal to the regulatory unit.

initiating stem cell differentiation. On the other hand, CFU-S proliferation is also stimulated by IL-3, although this could be an indirect consequence of differentiation loss.

IL-3 is now available in pure recombinant form, and used in vivo it mobilizes and stimulates CFU-S proliferation but fails to increase their total number, probably due to increased differentiation (14). While IL-3 remains an interesting and potentially useful molecule, its precise role in the regulation and maintenance of the stem cell population remains obscure. However, its effects over a wide spectrum of hemopoietic cells (i.e., its lack of cell lineage specificity) detracts from its major participation in the regulatory processes of the stem cells.

The maintenance of a balance between self-renewal, proliferation, and differentiation of the stem cell population and between proliferation and maturation of the differentiated populations is clearly a question of tight regulatory processes. While all cell lineages have a common origin, each must be regulated independently by processes that are specific for it. Many of the factors involved, some of which are indicated in Figure 4, have been extensively studied, giving us a reasonable picture of the functional aspects of hemopoietic tissue. Indeed, in recent years this field has been the subject of a good number of extensive reviews (e.g., see Ref. 45), and in these pages we propose only to present a brief catalog and outline of their function.

V. REGULATION OF PROGENITOR CELLS

A. In Vitro Action of Colony-Stimulating Factors

The growth of progenitor cells in clonal cultures requires the continuous presence of the growth factors originally described as colony-stimulating factors or CSFs. In the recent past we have progressed from discussing what relevance, if any, those factors detected and assayed in vitro have in the physiological regulation of hemopoiesis to purifying them and cloning the relevant genes (Table 1). The expression of such genes in mammalian cells or bacteria has led to the availability of sufficient amounts of material to investigate their effects in vivo.

In vitro, this family of growth factors is needed for survival and proliferation, and they are required continuously throughout the processes that lead to the production of mature functional cells from multipotential cells. If the relevant factors are withdrawn, the cells die within hours (52). As seen in Figure 7, CSFs differ in their window of action: IL-3 acts on multipotential cells as well as on progenitor cells that are restricted to differentiate along any of the myeloid

Table 1 Recombinant Human Hemopoietic Growth Factors

Growth factor	Synonym	Molecular weight	Ref. (cloned)	% Homology (mouse)
IL-3	Multi-CSF HCGF	25,000	46	29
GM-CSF	Pluripoietin	22,000	47	54
G-CSF	Pluripoietin	19,600	48	69
M-CSF	CSF-1	45,000	49 50	80
Erythropoietin	–	18,400	51	?

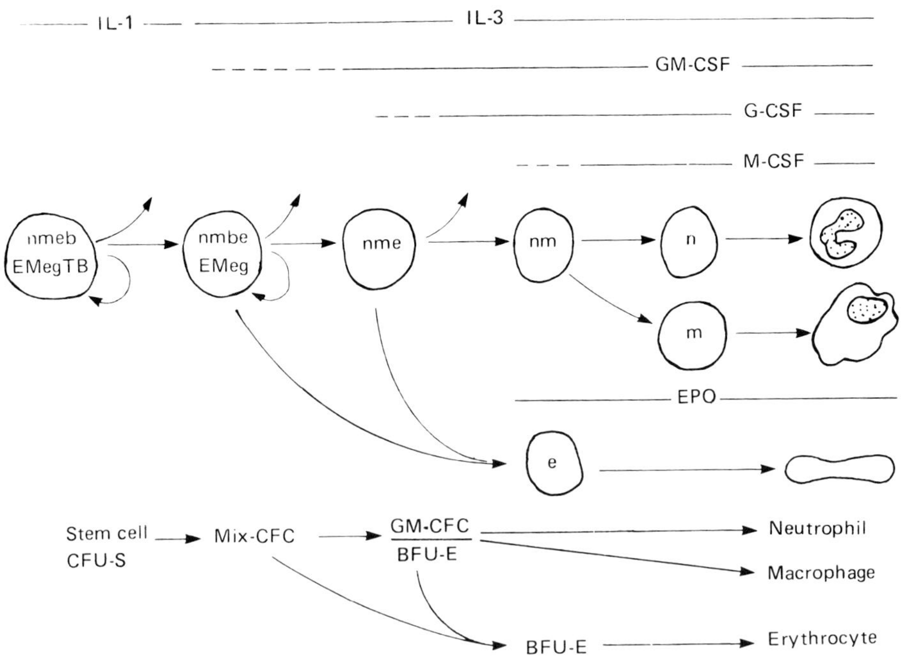

Figure 7 Ranges of action of hemopoietic growth factors. IL = interleukin; EPO = erythropoietin; G = granulocyte; CSF = colony stimulating factor; M,m = macrophage; CFC = colony-forming cell; BFU-E = erythroid burst-forming unit; n = neutrophilic lineage; e = erythroid lineage; Meg = megakaryocytic lineage; E = eosinophilic lineage; b = basophilic lineage; T,B = lymphoid lineages.

lineages (granulocyte-macrophage, eosinophil, erythroid, megakaryocyte, or mast cells). Thus, IL-3 is probably the least restricted of the CSFs with regard to cell lineage and is also the factor with the widest window of action with regard to target cells. Granulocyte-macrophage colony-stimulating factor (GM-CSF) acts on progenitors of granulocytes and macrophages, but at higher concentrations it can influence the early development of megakaryocyte, early erythroid, and eosinophilic progenitor cells (53,54).

This overlap of target cells for different growth factors is a striking feature of the regulation of hemopoiesis. In some cases, however, a given CSF may not be acting directly on the progenitor cells stimulated to proliferate, but indirectly through regulatory cellular networks, action that will result in the production of other growth factors. A prime example is the action of granulocyte colony-stimulating factor (G-CSF), which, when added to bone marrow cultures, will stimulate the formation of fully developed colonies of granulocytes and macrophages and, at high concentrations, the development of mixed and erythroid colonies (55).

However, if the target bone marrow has been highly purified to remove accessory cells [themselves able to produce growth factors (56)], only granulocytic colonies will develop. This indicates that G-CSF acts directly on GM-CFC but that its action on other colony-forming cells (Mix-CFC and BFU-E) is mediated through accessory regulatory cells, probably through the production of other growth factors (17).

Macrophage colony-stimulating factor (M-CSF) is lineage-restricted and acts on GM-CFC and M-CFC, inducing the development of colonies composed of macrophages and occasional granulocytes. It is also a powerful inducer of several functions of the mature cells.

In the erythroid system, proliferation of BFU-E can be initiated by several factors—IL-3, GM-CSF, and G-CSF—although, as seen above, in some cases it is through mediation of accessory regulatory cells. The descriptive term burst-promoting activity (BPA) used in early work (57) probably encompasses this family of growth factors that are able to initiate the development of erythroid colonies. Full development of those colonies and hemoglobinization of the erythroid cells, however, requires the presence of erythropoietin (Fig. 7). In contrast with the CSFs, erythropoietin was described, and its action first analyzed, with in vivo systems (for a review, see Ref. 58). Erythropoietin fulfills the classical requirements of a hormone regulator, with its production (mainly in the kidney) negatively regulated by the level of the oxygen-carrying capacity of the erythrocyte population.

B. Production of Colony-Stimulating Factors

Practically all tissues in the body contain measurable, if minute, amounts of one or more types of CSF (reviewed in Ref. 45). The types of cells that have been shown to be efficient producers are T lymphocytes, macrophages, and endothelial and fibroblastic cells, as well as a variety of tumor cells. The latter have been of great practical importance as sources of large amounts of material, which allowed purification of factors and eventual cloning of the relevant genes. Perhaps the best examples are murine IL-3 purified from supernatant of cultures of WEHI myelomonocytic leukemic cells (59) and human G-CSF purified from the medium conditioned by the human bladder carcinoma cell line 5637 (48).

A comprehensive review of the biology of CSFs can be found in Ref. 45. Other bioregulators that may act to modulate hemopoietic cell production (hormones, interferons, tumor necrosis factor, lactoferrin, and others) are outside the scope of this chapter. Microenvironmental regulation is discussed in Chapter 2.

Some of the complicated networks that regulate the production of CSFs are illustrated in Figure 8, which emphasizes the importance of cell interactions in achieving a normal steady state and a prompt and adequate response to hemopoietic stress. The importance of the right environment is stressed by the recent observation (60) that GM-CSF binds to glycosaminoglycans produced by bone

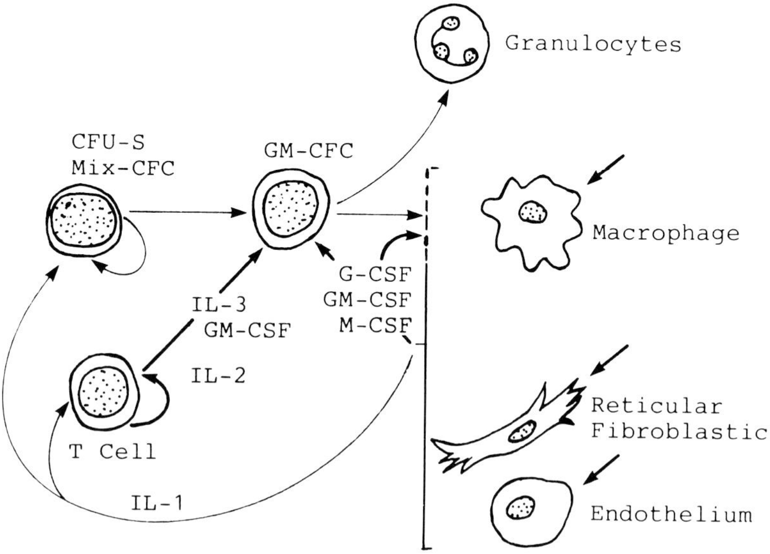

Figure 8 Interrelationships of hemopoietic growth factors. IL = interleukin; G = granulocyte; CSF = colony stimulating factor; M = macrophage, CFC = colony-forming cell; CFU-S = spleen colony-forming unit.

marrow stromal cells. This supports the concept that components of the extracellular matrix may be involved in concentrating the appropriate growth factors in the relevant regions of the bone marrow described below.

C. In Vivo Action of Colony-Stimulating Factors

The recent availability of relatively large amounts of recombinant growth factors has made it possible to assess their effect in vivo, both in normal animals and during recovery after hemopoietic stress. The available results are summarized in Table 2. As mentioned above (Section IV.D), a single dose of murine IL-3 induces stem cells to enter the cell cycle. Prolonged administration induces very active hemopoiesis in the spleen (14,15,61); this is a typical response to hemopoietic stress in the mouse and other mammals. In normal primates, administration of human recombinant GM-CSF results in a marked rise in the numbers of circulating neutrophils, to about 10 times control levels (13). Interestingly, the numbers of eosinophils and reticulocytes also increase. The latter response agrees with the stimulating effect seen in vitro on these cell lineages (Fig. 7). No toxic effects were noted, and the hematological parameters returned to normal following the cessation of treatment. A response similar to that of normal cells was seen

Table 2 In Vivo Effects of Recombinant Growth Factors

Factor	Species	Status	Effects measured	Ref.
Murine IL-3	Mouse	Normal	↑ Cycling of stem cells ↑ Numbers of progenitor cells ↑↗ Cellularity in spleen ↑ (moderate) Circulating granulocytes	14, 15, 61
Human GM-CSF	Monkey	Normal or pancytopenic	↑ Numbers of circulating granulocytes ↑ Reticulocytes	13
Human G-CSF	Monkey	Normal or myelosuppressed	↑ Numbers of circulating neutrophils Shortened recovery time after cytotoxic treatment	17
Human erythropoietin	Human	Anemia of renal disease	↑ Hemoglobin ↑ Sense of well being	16, 62

Where measured, the effects were found to be dose-dependent. There was no reported toxicity (except for some hypertension after erythropoietin). Phase I clinical trials with CSFs are presently taking place in several centers.

in a monkey that was pancytopenic following an infection with a type D retrovirus. The important clinical implications of their observations in the context of long-term bone marrow damage are discussed in Chapter 19.

VI. MICROARCHITECTURE OF HEMOPOIETIC TISSUE

A. Spatial Organization of Bone Marrow Cell Populations

Since approximately 95% of hemopoietic tissue is taken up by the morphologically identifiable maturing cell populations, it is understandable that the classification of hematological disorders has classically been based on their number, appearance, and relative distribution among the major cell lineages; for example, the erythroid/myeloid ratio. Good differential staining of hemopoietic cells is obtained only in smear preparations, and although a report in 1938 (63) that was largely ignored suggested a preponderance of relatively mature cells in the center of bone marrow spaces, it has always been assumed that the cells are randomly and uniformly distributed throughout those marrow spaces. This raises two questions.

First, since the production of maturing cells depends on the performance of stem and committed progenitor cell populations, do simple counts of the maturing cells adequately reflect the basic potential of the marrow? Very often, the answer is no. Because of the flexibility of cell kinetics under stress, the relationship of the progenitor cell populations to their more mature progeny can vary according to the nature of the stress. For example, under conditions of chronic irradiation, red cell output can remain normal while the precursors are reduced to as little as 2-3% of control (64,65). It is important, then, to measure changes in the precursor populations, and it will become evident in the following chapters that more consideration is now being given to these cells.

Second, when considering long-term damage from, for example, contamination with bone-seeking isotopes such as plutonium or radium, are susceptible target cells in the vicinity of the bone out of range of the high-LET α particles that irradiate only a narrow band of cells close to the bone? If cell populations are not uniformly distributed through the marrow spaces, then calculations based on classical models or measurements on whole bone marrow will not be valid.

It is, however, possible to estimate the location of various precursor and microenvironmental cell populations in relation to the bone surfaces. Using mouse femora, the marrow was fractionated longitundinally to give one population close to the longitudinal axis of the bone (axial cells) and a second population closer to the bone surface (marginal cells), and the two could be assayed separately for various cell types. Minor variations in the fractionation technique gave different ratios of marginal to axial cells and enabled a cross-sectional picture of the cell populations in the marrow to be built up.

It can be seen from Figure 9 that cells are not uniformly distributed throughout the bone. Spleen colony-forming units (Fig. 9*a*) are 2.5 times more concentrated close to the bone surface than along the central axis of the bone (66,67). More important, in some respects, is the fact that the CFU-S are not uniformly distributed within this distribution. Those shown in the shaded area of Figure 9*a* are CFU-S in DNA synthesis, showing that most of the CFU-S proliferation is taking place in the vicinity of the bone. This is consistent with the finding that the regions close to the bone contain the majority of the cells that produce the proliferation stimulator described above (Fig. 9*d*; 68), while inhibitor-producing cells are in greater abundance nearer the center (Fig. 9*c*; 68). A further feature of the CFU-S distribution is that the higher quality cells with large self-renewal capacity are found in the center, while the poorly self-renewing cells are close to the bone (69). The high quality stem cells are those that turn over very slowly so their coincidence with the greater concentrations of both inhibitor-producing cells and fibroblastoid colony-forming cells (Fig. 9*b*; 70) supports the suggestion that these latter cells form a part of the stem cell microenvironmental regulatory unit.

The committed GM-CFCs are most concentrated ~120 μm from the bone surface (Fig. 9*e*; 67), while the maturing granulocytic cells build up toward the center of the marrow space (Fig. 9*f*; 63). The changes in the distributions, from that of CFU-S, through differentiation and maturation, suggest a dynamic movement of cells away from the bone. CFU-S in the vicinity of the bone come under the influence of proliferation and differentiation factors that result in a buildup of committed precursors away from the bone. This wave of cells dies away as they mature and become replaced by the recognizable granulocytic cells in the center. From there, they pass into service via the central venous sinus.

Erythroid development follows a similar pattern (Fig. 9*g*, *h*; 71). Analysis of the BFU-E colonies suggested that the peak at ~40 μm from the bone contained the more primitive cells. It seems probable that these are in fact the Mix-CFC or late-stage CFU-S, while those in the peak ~180 μm from the bone are early erythroid progenitors.

Some investigators remain skeptical of these data, and one group (72) published a series of negative data leaving the principle as "an open question." Nevertheless, there is now a significant amount of information obtained from a wide variety of techniques and independent investigators that does suggest nonuniform distributions. Shackney and his colleagues (73,74), who used autoradiography, reported a high concentration of proliferating cells near the bone surfaces, falling off toward the center. Gong (75) found endosteal marrow to be a very rich source of CFU-S. Using ^{226}Ra to irradiate cells close to the bone, vertebral CFU-S with relatively large amounts of bone surface (see below) were depleted more than femoral CFU-S (76). An entirely different approach was taken by Lambertsen and Weiss (77), who, by stereomicroscopy, observed the zonal repopulation of marrow. They established a set of curves for undifferentiated

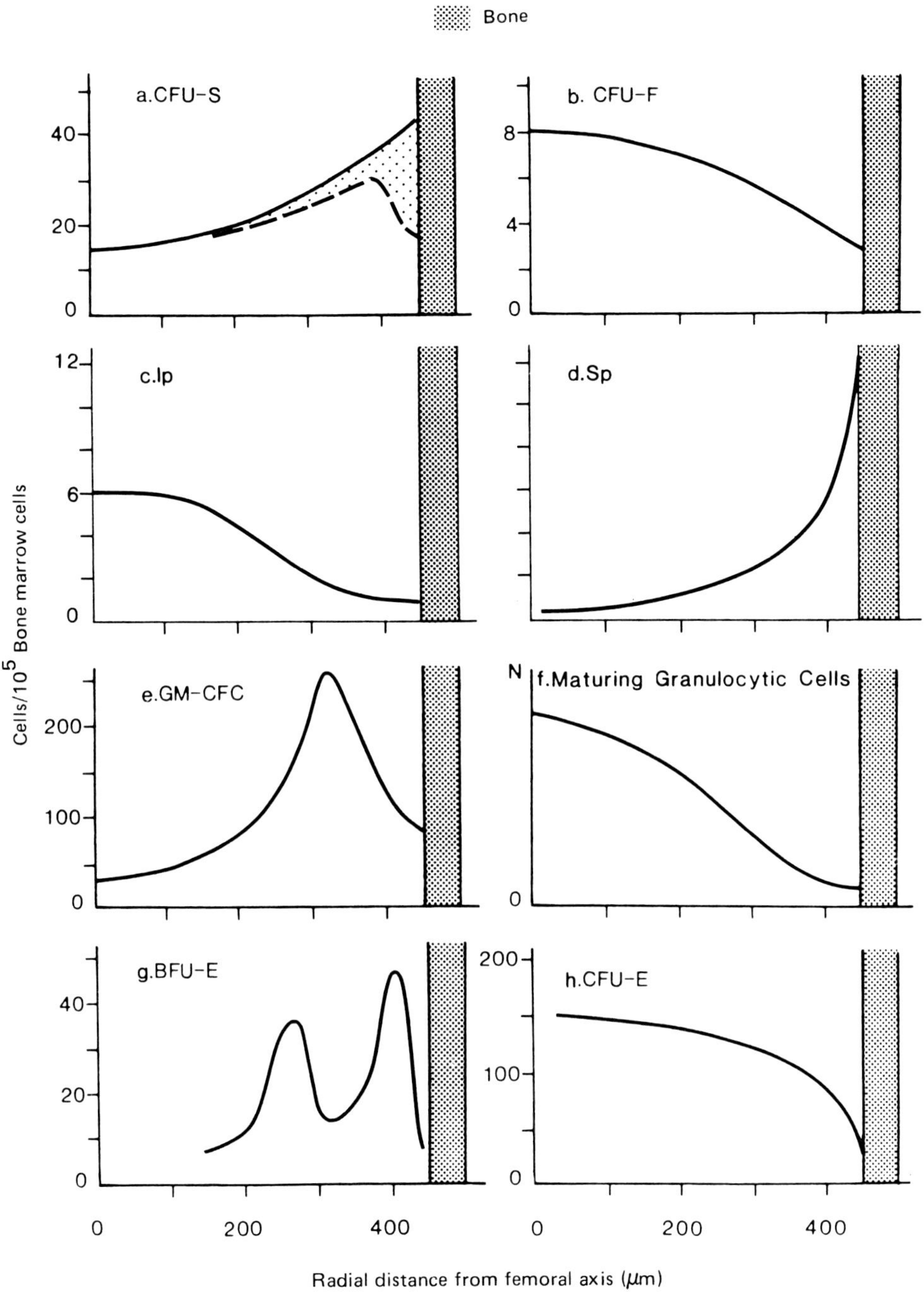

Figure 9 The distributions of bone marrow cells across a radial axis of the mouse femur. The ordinate represents the central longitudinal axis of the femoral shaft; the shaded area is bone.

granulocytic and erythroid committed colony-forming cells that were remarkably similar to those presented in Figure 9.

B. Relevance of Distributions in Mouse Compared to Human Bones

While mouse bones are small compared to human bones, a more relevant factor is the bone surface area relative to marrow volume enclosed. In the adult human, the long bones are devoid of hemopoietic marrow except in the small spaces of the trabecular regions (at the ends). The ribs, which are a major source of hemopoiesis in the human and contain red marrow, are very trabecular, and, seen in sections, they are not dissimilar to a bundle of mouse femora. In fact, the ratio of bone surface area to marrow volume enclosed in the rib is somewhat higher (9.4/mm) than for the mouse femur (4.5/mm) (78). This means that any effects relating to bone and cell distribution, such as those pertaining to different types of irradiation, will be at least as important in the human rib as they are in the mouse femur. The dimensions of other human marrow sites have not been measured, but from gross visual inspection they appear to be comparable to those in the rib.

It is difficult to establish that these distributions exist for all bones, particularly human bones. However, radiation survival experiments (76,78) show that it is probably so for the mouse. In addition, using a simple washing technique, a lower concentration of GM-CFCs close to the bone surfaces of the human rib was demonstrated (79) like that in Figure 9*e* for the mouse. It is probable, therefore, that all hemopoietic tissue has this spatially organized structure and that data from the mouse model are appropriate also for human studies.

VII. CONCLUSION

The developing use, in vivo and with human material, of the various hemopoietic growth-regulating factors is now making it imperative that their effects should be fully understood. Much work directed at unraveling the complex interrelationships of their mechanisms of action is currently underway in many centers worldwide. In situations such as bone marrow transplantation where lethal whole body irradiation combined with stroma-damaging drug treatments is essential, although almost inevitably causing longer-term effects, it will become particularly important to use such factors to their greatest effect.

The current concern over the potential hazards of nuclear accidents and other sources of uncontrolled release of radioactive isotopes into the environment, in particular those that are recognized as bone-seeking, is not easily or directly resolvable. Microdosimetry within the bones and marrow can be determined, but it is still not clear which of the progenitor cells are potentially the most probable targets for leukemogenesis or the development of osteosarcomas. Taking the classical approach to risk estimation, this in itself poses no particular problem since the target cells have been assumed to be distributed randomly throughout the bone and marrow spaces. However, the observation that the progenitor, and indeed the stromal (regulatory), populations are not randomly distributed seriously compromises those estimates. In addition to defining accurately the microdosimetry among the various progenitor populations, therefore, it is necessary also to develop a complete understanding of the proliferative, self-regenerative, and transformational potentials of those cells.

ACKNOWLEDGMENT

The authors are funded by a grant from the Cancer Research Campaign, Great Britain.

REFERENCES

1. Weiss, L. The histology of the bone marrow. In *Regulation of hematopoiesis*, Vol. 1. Gordon, A. S. (Ed.). Appleton-Century-Crofts, New York, pp. 79-92 (1970).
2. Weiss, L. The hematopoietic microenvironment of the bone marrow: an ultrastructural study of the stroma in rats. *Anat. Rec. 186*, 161-184 (1976).
3. McCulloch, E. A. Stem cell functions and the clonal haemopathies of man. In: *Stem cells and tissue homeostasis.* Lord, B. I., Potten, C. S., Cole, R. J. (Eds.). Brit. Soc. Cell Biology Symposium, Vol. 2. Cambridge University Press, p. 139 (1978).
4. Ash, P., Loutit, J. F., Townsend, K. M. S. Osteoclasts derived from haemopoietic stem cells. *Nature* (*London*) *283,* 669-670 (1980).
5. Marks, S. C., Jr., Walker, D. G. The hematogenous origin of osteoclasts: experimental evidence from osteopetrotic (microphthalmic) mice treated with spleen cells from beige mouse donors. *Amer. J. Anat. 161,* 1-10 (1981).
6. Katz, S. I., Tamaki, K., Sachs, D. H. Epidermal Langerhans cells are derived from cells originating in bone marrow. *Nature* (*London*) *282,* 324-325 (1979).
7. Kitamura, Y., Shimada, M., Hatanaka, K., Miyano, Y. Development of mast cells from grafted bone marrow cells in irradiated mice. *Nature* (*London*) *268,* 442-443 (1977).
8. Kitamura, Y., Yokoyama, M., Matsuda, H., Ohno, T., Mori, K. J. Spleen colony forming cell as common precursor for tissue mast cells and granulocytes. *Nature* (*London*) *291,* 159-160 (1981).
9. Lord, B. I., Spooncer, E. Isolation of haemopoietic spleen colony-forming cells. *Lymphokine Res. 5,* 59-72 (1986).
10. Till, J. E., McCulloch, E. A. A direct measurement of the radiation sensitivity of normal mouse bone marrow cells. *Radiat. Res. 14,* 213-222 (1961).
11. Lord, B. I., Schofield, R. Haemopoietic spleen colony-forming units. In: *Cell clones; manual of mammalian cell techniques.* Potten, C. S., Hendry, J. H. (Eds.). Churchill-Livingstone, New York, pp. 13-26 (1985).

12. Testa, N. G. Clonal assays for haemopoietic and lymphoid cells in vitro. In: *Cell clones; manual of mammalian cell techniques.* Potten, C. S., Hendry, J. H. (Eds.). Churchill-Livingstone, New York, pp. 27-43 (1985).
13. Donahue, R. E., Wang, E. A., Stone, D. K., Kamen, R., Wong, G. G., Sehgal, P. K., Natham, D. G., Clark, S. C. Stimulation of hematopoiesis in primates by continuous infusion of recombinant human GM-CSF. *Nature (London) 321,* 872-875 (1986).
14. Lord, B. I., Molineux, G., Testa, N. G., Kelly, M., Spooncer, E., Dexter, T. M. The kinetic response of haemopoietic precursor cells, in vivo, to highly purified recombinant interleukin-3. *Lymphokine Res. 5,* 97-104 (1986).
15. Metcalf, D., Begley, C. G., Nicola, N. A., Lopez, A. F., Williamson, D. J. Effects of purified bacterially synthesised multi-CSF (IL-3) on hematopoiesis in normal adult mice. *Blood 68,* 46-57 (1986).
16. Winearls, C. G., Oliver, D. O., Pippard, M. J., Reid, C., Downing, M. R., Cotes, P. M. Effect of human erythropoietin derived from recombinant DNA on the anaemia of patients maintained by chronic haemodialysis. *Lancet ii,* 1175-1178 (1986).
17. Welte, K., Bonilla, M. A., Gillio, A. P., Boone, T. C., Potter, G. K., Gabrilove, J. L., Moore, M. A. S., O'Reilly, R. J., Souza L. M. Recombinant human G-CSF: effect on hematopoiesis in normal and cyclophosphamide treated primates. *J. Exp. Med. 165,* 941-948 (1987).
18. Worton, R. G., McCulloch, E. A., Till, J. E. Physical separation of hemopoietic stem cells differing in their capacity for self-renewal. *J. Exp. Med. 130,* 91-102 (1975).
19. Schofield, R., Lord, B. I., Kyffin, S., Gilbert, C. W. Self-maintenance capacity of CFU-S. *J. Cell. Physiol. 103,* 355-362 (1980).
20. Schofield, R. The relationship between the spleen colony-forming cell and the haemopoietic stem cell. A hypothesis. *Blood Cells 4,* 7-25 (1978).
21. Magli, M. C., Iscove, N. N., Odartchenko, N. Transient nature of early haemopoietic spleen colonies. *Nature (London) 295,* 527-529 (1982).
22. Lajtha, L. G., Schofield, R. Regulation of stem cell renewal and differentiation: possible significance in ageing. In: *Advances in gerontological research.* Strehler, B. (Ed.). Academic Press, New York, pp. 131-146 (1971).
23. Schofield, R., Dexter, T. M., Lord, B. I., Testa, N. G. Comparison of haemopoiesis in young and old mice. *Mech. Ageing Develop. 34,* 1-12 (1986).
24. Harrison, D. E., Astle, C. M. Loss of stem cell repopulating ability upon transplantation. *J. Exp. Med. 156,* 1767-1779 (1982).
25. Gidali, J., Lajtha, L. G. Regulation of haemopoietic stem cell turnover in partially irradiated mice. *Cell Tissue Kinet. 5,* 147-157 (1972).
26. Rencricca, N. J., Rizzoli, V., Howard, D., Duffy, P., Stohlman, F., Jr. Stem cell proliferation and migration during severe anemia. *Blood 36,* 764-771 (1970).
27. Frindel, E., Guigon, M. Inhibition of CFU-entry into cycle by a bone marrow extract. *Exp. Hematol. 5,* 74-76 (1977).
28. Lord, B. I., Mori, K. J., Wright, E. G., Lajtha, L. G. An inhibitor of stem cell proliferation in normal bone marrow. *Brit. J. Haematol. 34,* 441-445 (1976).

29. Tejero, C., Testa, N. G., Lord, B. I. The cellular specificity of haemopoietic stem cell proliferation regulators. *Brit. J. Cancer 50,* 335-341 (1984).
30. Wright, E. G., Lorimore, S. A., Lord, B. I. Effect of haemopoietic stem cell proliferation regulators on early and late spleen colony-forming cells. *Cell Tissue Kinet. 18,* 193-199 (1985).
31. Lord, B. I., Mori, K. J., Wright, E. G. A stimulator of stem cell proliferation in regenerating bone marrow. *Biomed. Exp. 27,* 223-226 (1977).
32. Frindel, E., Croizat, H., Vassort, F. Stimulating factors liberated by treated bone marrow: in vitro effect of CFU kinetics. *Exp. Hematol. 4,* 56-61 (1976).
33. Wright, E. G., Lord, B. I. Production of stem cell proliferation regulators by fractionated haemopoietic cell suspensions. *Leuk. Res. 3,* 15-22 (1979).
34. Allen, T. D., Dexter, T. M. Long term bone marrow cultures: an ultrastructural review. *Scanning Electron Microsc. 4,* 1851-1866 (1983).
35. Töksoz, D., Dexter, T. M., Lord, B. I., Wright, E. G., Lajtha, L. G. The regulation of hemopoiesis in long-term bone marrow cultures. II. Stimulation and inhibition of stem cell proliferation. *Blood 55,* 931-936 (1980).
36. Cashman, J., Eaves, A. C., Eaves, C. J. Regulated proliferation of primitive hematopoietic progenitor cells in long-term human marrow cultures. *Blood 66,* 1002-1005 (1985).
37. Wright, E. G., Garland, J. M., Lord, B. I. Specific inhibition of haemopoietic stem cell proliferation: characteristics of the inhibitor producing cells. *Leuk. Res. 4,* 537-545 (1980).
38. Wright, E. G., Ali, A. M., Riches, A. C., Lord, B. I. Stimulation of haemopoietic stem cell proliferation: characteristics of the stimulator producing cells. *Leuk. Res. 6,* 531-539 (1982).
39. Simmons, P. J., Lord, B. I. Enrichment of CFU-S proliferation inhibitor-producing cells based on their identification by the monoclonal antibody F4/80. *J. Cell Sci. 78,* 117-131 (1985).
40. Maloney, M. A., Lamela, R. A., Banda, M. J., Patt, H. M. Partitioning of bone marrow into stem cell regulatory domains. *Proc. Natl. Acad. Sci. USA 79,* 840-844 (1982).
41. Friedenstein, A. J., Chailakhjan, R. K., Lalykina, K. S. The development of fibroblast colonies in monolayer cultures of guinea pig bone marrow and spleen cells. *Cell Tissue Kinet. 3,* 393-403 (1970).
42. Friedenstein, A. J., Chailakhjan, R. K., Latsinik, N. V., Panasynk, A. F., Keiliss-Borok, I. V. Stromal cells responsible for transferring the microenvironment of hemopoietic tissue. *Transplantation 17,* 331-340 (1974).
43. Lord, B. I., Wright, E. G. Interaction of inhibitor and stimulator in the regulation of CFU-S proliferation. *Leuk. Res. 6,* 541-551 (1982).
44. Lord, B. I. Interactions of regulatory factors in the control of haemopoietic stem cell proliferation. In: *Biological regulation of cell proliferation.* Baserga, B., Foa, P., Metcalf, D., Polli, E. E. (Eds.). Serono Symposia Publications, Raven Press, New York, Vol. 34, pp. 167-171 (1986).
45. Metcalf, D. *The hemopoietic colony stimulating factors.* Elsevier, New York (1984).
46. Yang, Y. C., Ciarletta, A. B., Temple, P. A., Chung, M. P., Kovacic, S., Witek-Gianotti, J. S., Leary, A. C., Kriz, R., Donahue, R. E., Wong, G. G., Clark, S. C.

Human IL-3 (multi-CSF): identification by expression cloning of a novel hematopoietic growth factor related to murine IL-3. *Cell 47,* 3-10 (1986).
47. Wong, G. G., Witek, J., Temple, P. A., Wilkens, K. M., Leary, A. C., Luxemberg, D. P., Jones, S. S., Brown, E. L., Kay, R. M., Orr, E. C., Shoemaker, C., Golde, D. W., Kaufman, R. J., Herrick, R. M., Wang, E. A., Clark, S. C. Human GM-CSF: molecular cloning of the complementary DNA and purification of the natural and recombinant proteins. *Science 228,* 810-815 (1985).
48. Souza, L. M., Boone, T. C., Gabrilove, J., Lai, P. H., Szebo, K. M., Murdock, D. C., Chazin, V. R., Bruszewski, J., Lu, H., Chen, K. K., Barendt, J. Platzer, E., Moore, M. A. S., Metelsmann, R., Welte, K. Recombinant human granulocyte colony stimulating factor: effects on normal and leukemic myeloid cells. *Science 232,* 61-65 (1986).
49. Kawasaki, E. S., Ladner, M. B., Wang, A. M., van Audell, J., Warren, M. K., Coyne, M. Y., Schweickart, V. L., Lee, M. T., Wilson, K. J., Boosman, A., Stanley, R., Ralph, P., Mark, D. F. Molecular cloning of a complementary DNA encoding human macrophage-specific colony-stimulating factor (CSF-1). *Science 230,* 291-296 (1985).
50. Wong, G. G., Temple, P. A., Leary, A. C., Witek-Giannotti, J. S., Yang, Y. C., Ciarletta, A. B., Chung, M., Murtha, P., King, R., et al. Human CSF-1: molecular cloning and expression of 4-kb cDNA encoding the human urinary protein. *Science 235,* 1504-1508 (1987).
51. Jacobs, K., Shoemaker, C., Rudersdorf, R., Neill, S. D., Kaufman, R. J., Meefson, A., Seehra, J., Jones, S. S., Henrick, R., Fritsch, E. F., Kawaita, M., Shimizu, T., Miyake, T. Isolation and characterisation of genomic and cDNA clones of human erythropoietin. *Nature 313,* 806-810 (1985).
52. Metcalf, D. *Hemopoietic colonies.* Springer Verlag, Berlin, pp. 1-227 (1977).
53. Metcalf, D., Johnson, G. R., Burgess, A. W. Direct stimulation by purified GM-CSF of the proliferation of multipotential and erythroid precursor cells. *Blood 55,* 138-147 (1980).
54. Metcalf, D., Burgess, A. W. Clonal analysis of progenitor cell commitment to granulocyte or macrophage production. *J. Cell. Physiol. 111,* 275-283 (1982).
55. Ottmann, O. G., Welte, K., Souza, L. M., Moore, M. A. S. Proliferative effects of a recombinant human granulocyte-colony stimulating factor (rG-CSF) on highly enriched hematopoietic progenitor cells. *Haemat. Blood Transf. 31* (in press) (1987).
56. Rennick, D., Yang, G., Gemmell, L., Lee, F. Control of hemopoiesis by a bone marrow stromal cell clones: lipopolysaccharide and interleukin-1-inducible production of colony-stimulating factors. *Blood 69,* 682-691 (1987).
57. Iscove, N. N. Erythropoietin independent stimulation of early erythropoiesis in adult marrow by conditioned media from lectin-stimulated spleen cells. In: *Hematopoietic cell differentiation.* Golde, D. W., Cline, M. J., Metcalf, D., Fox, C. F. (Eds.). Academic Press, New York, pp. 37-52 (1978).
58. Adamson, J. W., Brown, J. E. Aspects of erythroid differentiation and proliferation. In: *Molecular control of proliferation and differentiation.* Papacoustantinou, J., Rutta, W. J. (Eds.). Academic Press, London, pp. 161-179 (1978).

59. Ihle, J. V., Keller, J., Henderson, L., Klein, F., Palasynski, E. Procedures for the purification of interleukin-3 to homogeneity. *J. Immunol. 129,* 2431-2436 (1982).
60. Gordon, M. Y., Riley, G. P., Watt, S. M., Greaves, M. F. Compartmentalization of a haematopoietic growth factor (GM-CSF) by glycosaminoglycans in the bone marrow microenvironment. *Nature 326,* 403-405 (1987).
61. Kindler, V., Thorens, B., de Kossodo, S., Allet, B., Eliason, J. F. Stimulation of hematopoiesis *in vitro* by recombinant bacterial murine interleukin 3. *Proc. Natl. Acad. Sci. USA 83,* 1001-1005 (1986).
62. Eschbach, J. W., Egrie, J. C., Downing, M. R., Browne, J. K., Adamson, J. W. Correction of the anemia of end-stage renal disease with recombinant human erythropoietin: results of a combined phase I and II clinical trial. *New Engl. J. Med. 316,* 73-78 (1987).
63. Weinbeck, J. Die Granulopese des Kindlichen Knockenmarkes und ihre Reaktion auf Infectionen. *Brit. Pathol. Anat. Allgem. Pathol. 101,* 268-283 (1938).
64. Lamerton, L. F., Pontifex, A. H., Blackett, N. M., Adams, K. Effects of protracted irradiation on the blood forming organs of the rat. 1, Continuous exposure. *Brit. J. Radiol. 33,* 287-301 (1960).
65. Wu, C-T., Lajtha, L. G. Haemopoietic stem cell kinetics during continuous irradiation. *Int. J. Radiat. Biol. 27,* 41-50 (1975).
66. Lord, B. I., Hendry, J. H. The distribution of haemopoietic colony-forming units in the mouse femur and its modification by x-rays. *Brit. J. Radiol. 45,* 110-115 (1972).
67. Lord, B. I., Testa, N. G., Hendry, J. H. The relative spatial distribution of CFU-S and CFU-C in the normal mouse femur. *Blood 46,* 65-72 (1975).
68. Lord, B. I., Wright, E. G. Spatial organisation of CFU-S proliferation regulators in the mouse femur. *Leuk. Res. 8,* 1073-1083 (1984).
69. Lord, B. I., Schofield, R. Some observations on the kinetics of haemopoietic stem cells and their relationship to the spatial organisation of the tissue. In: *Biological growth and spread* (Lecture notes in biomathematics, Vol. 38). Jäger, W., Rost, H., Tautu, P. (Eds.). Springer-Verlag, Berlin, pp. 9-22 (1980).
70. Xu, C. X., Hendry, J. H. The radial distribution of fibroblastic colony-forming cells in mouse femoral marrow. *Biomed. Exp. 35,* 119-122 (1981).
71. Frassoni, F., Testa, N. G., Lord, B. I. The relative spatial distribution of erythroid progenitor cells (BFU-E and CFU-E) in the normal mouse femur. *Cell Tissue Kinet. 15,* 447-455 (1982).
72. Malony, M. A., Lamela, R. A., Dori, M. J., Patt, H. M. Concentration gradient of blood stem cells in mouse bone marrow—an open question. *Blood 51,* 521-529 (1978).
73. Shackney, S. E., Bunn, P. A., Ford, S. S. The effects of colcemid on mouse bone marrow. *Cell Tissue Kinet. 9,* 363-369 (1976).
74. Shackney, S. E., Ford, S. S., Whitting, A. B. Kinetic micro-architectural correlations in the bone marrow of the mouse. *Cell Tissue Kinet. 8,* 505-516 (1975).
75. Gong, J. K. Endostial marrow: a rich source of hematopoietic stem cells. *Science 199,* 1443-1445 (1978).

76. Svoboda, V., Kofránek, V. Response of femoral and vertebral colony-forming units to ^{226}Ra internal contamination in mice. *Radiat. Res. 64,* 467-474 (1975).
77. Lambertsen, R. H., Weiss, L. A model of intramedullary hematopoietic microenvironments based on stereologic study of the distribution of endocloned marrow colonies. *Blood 63,* 287-297 (1984).
78. Lord, B. I. Cellular and architectural factors influencing the proliferation of haemopoietic stem cells. In: *Differentiation of normal and neoplastic hematopoietic cells* (Cold Spring Harbor Conferences on Cell Proliferation, Vol. 5). Clarkson, B., Marks, P. A., Till, J. E. (Eds.). Cold Spring Harbor Laboratory, Cold Spring Harbor, New York, pp. 775-788 (1978).
79. Testa, N. G., Hendry, J. H., Molineux, G. Long-term bone marrow damage in experimental systems and in patients after radiation or chemotherapy. *Anticancer Res. 5,* 101-110 (1985).

2

Hemopoietic Microenvironments

DOV ZIPORI
Weizmann Institute of Science, Rehovot, Israel, and DNAX Research Institute of Molecular and Cellular Biology, Palo Alto, California

I. INTRODUCTION

A new research field is often established following the accumulation of data that support an initially controversial proposal. The type of questions asked and the subjects that are regarded as pertaining to it become thereafter traditional, and many important aspects are set aside. The purpose of this chapter is to discuss a variety of aspects of hemopoiesis that relate to the area of research referred to as the "hemopoietic microenvironment." J. J. Trentin made pioneering observations that formed the basis for the assumption that hemopoiesis may be regulated by signals originating within the hemopoietic organ, in the close vicinity of stem cells (1). Yet dramatic progress in the field of in vitro hemopoiesis attracted most of the research effort. The ability to study hemopoiesis in culture that followed the observations of Bradley and Metcalf (2) and Pluznik and Sachs (3) caused an overwhelming progress in the understanding of the regulation of hemopoietic cell growth and differentiation. Within two decades a series of regulatory glycoproteins (colony-stimulating factors, CSF) were identified, their biological activities were characterized, the factors were purified, and their genes were molecularly cloned (reviewed in Refs. 4-8). Most of these factors were secreted, and some were relatively easily detected in body fluids and in many tissues such as uterus and lung. Like many hormones, CSFs could affect their target cells in body sites remote from their place of production. Moreover, the presence of cells producing the various differentiation-stimulating glycoproteins within specific sites in the marrow was presumed to account for the entire regulation of blood cell formation. Indeed, all four types of CSFs (M, GM, G, and IL-3) induce terminal differentiation, and it was suggested that IL-3 affects stem cell renewal (9-57). As will be discussed below, I do not share this view. Rather, our experiments indicate that additional factors, some of which are associated with the cell surface, play a crucial role in the regulation of the stem cell pool and in the determination of pattern formation within the hemopoietic organs (reviewed in Refs. 7 and 58). Nevertheless, the focus of research was, for a long time, remote from "stromal cells." According to Friedenstein's observations, these cells could transfer the hemopoietic microenvironment specific for their tissue of origin (59). A new wave of interest in hemopoietic microenvironments was created following the development of long-term bone marrow cultures (reviewed in Refs. 60 and 61). This in vitro system opened the way for the study of stromal cell functions and led to the examination of the mechanisms by which hemopoietic stem cell renewal is regulated. In the last decade, much information on long-term cultures has accumulated and the term "hemopoietic microenvironment" has gradually been adopted in the study of stromal cells and their interactions with hemopoietic cells. It is evident, though, that for a given blood cell, "environment" may mean surrounding hemopoietic cells that may be either identical to it or quite different.

The tridimensional structure of the marrow and the interactions of cells relative to their spatial arrangement undoubtedly have important roles in the regulation of hemopoiesis (see Chapter 1). In the nematode *C. elegans*, the number of cells in the whole organism and the exact fate and spatial position of practically each and every cell are known (reviewed in Ref. 62). This made it possible to study the pattern of stem cell commitment in relation to the cell's position in the tissue; individual cells with a potential to induce differentiation and determine the fate of stem cells have been described. Evidence for a gradient of a commitment factor that accounts for the position-related differentiation pattern was obtained (62,63). These types of experiments seem at the moment out of reach in mammalian systems, where cells assume different positions in different individuals and cell traffic is far more extensive. Other strategies are therefore required to resolve the dynamic rules that govern the structure and functions of the hemopoietic tissue. In this chapter, the aspects of the hemopoietic microenvironment that relate to interactions among hemopoietic cells, along with studies on stromal cell associated hemopoiesis, are discussed.

II. EXCHANGE OF INFORMATION AMONG NEIGHBORING HEMOPOIETIC CELLS

A. Hemopoietic Tissue Has a Highly Ordered and Complex Structure

The complexity of hemopoietic organs is apparent upon morphological examination. In the long bones of the mouse, the central vein that travels through the longitudinal axis sends out radial extensions that form sinusoids. The latter form complex intercommunicating systems. Hemopoietic cells are found among the sinusoids (64,65). Some cells are capable of penetrating the sinusoid wall and entering the circulation. Others, such as megakaryocytes, are located adjacent to the sinusoid wall in the hemopoietic space and send cytoplasmic protrusions into the sinus. The sinusoid wall and the tissue that is associated with it and extends from it into the hemopoietic space are made of cells of a variety of types, including fat cells, endothelial cells, and adventitial cells, referred to by the collective name stroma. These and the hemopoietic nests that include the variety of cellular intermediates of the hemopoietic differentiation scheme make an ordered tridimensional structure.

It may appear almost hopeless to resolve the structure-function relationships in the bone marrow in its in vivo state, owing to the large number of different cell interactions that occur concomitantly. Some interesting attempts in this direction have been reported. Lambertsen and Weiss used a combination of x-ray irradiation and microhistology to follow the fine patterns of hemopoietic cell growth in various anatomical sites of bone and marrow sections (66). Their studies demonstrated the localization of "stem cell" areas adjacent to the bone and to the periarterial regions. Nonrandom spatial distribution of erythroid progenitors in the marrow was also observed using functional assays (67).

In *Drosophila*, much progress has been achieved in understanding of pattern formation by use of in situ hybridization of cDNA probes in the search for particular gene transcripts in embryo tissue sections (68,69). A variety of regulator genes of the hemopoietic system have recently been molecularly cloned. It is likely that the availability of molecular probes in combination with microhistology of the bone and marrow would add a new dimension to the study of hemopoietic cell development in situ. Recently a technique has been designed to examine anchorage-dependent cells in vitro without removing them from their substrate. The technique allows one to follow interactions between cells and the passage of molecules between cells. This could, in the future, be applied for stromal cell-hemopoietic cell interactions in vitro (70).

The approach taken in the early 1960s to the study of hemopoietic differentiation was based on in vitro cultures under conditions where clonal growth of isolated stem cells is observed. Later, in the mid-1970s, techniques were developed to culture hemopoietic cells in conjunction with connective-tissue-like stromal cells that grow out in dense hemopoietic cell suspensions and were believed to emerge from the hemopoietic stroma, that is, the sinusoid wall and associated tissues. This provided an approach that is closer to the in vivo situation. It is clear, though, that even these simplified models are extremely complex from the point of view of cell interactions. Apart from the contacts between the hemopoietic cells with the stromal cells (64,65), there are numerous contacts made among hemopoietic cells themselves both in vivo and in vitro (reviewed in 71) and among particular types of stromal cells.

B. Homologous Versus Heterologous Cell Interactions

Some of the interactions of hemopoietic cells are heterologous in nature, that is, they occur between cells of different phenotypes, while others are homologous, occurring among cells with an identical phenotype. For example, during induction of macrophage colonies in vitro by colony-stimulating factor 1 (CSF-1, M-CSF) (43,44), the majority of cells in the developing clone are macrophages. Thus, many of the cells in the colony are surrounded by phenotypically "identical twins." Similarly, in the proposed "niche" theory of Scofield (72), stem cells encounter, apart from stromal cells, only daughter stem cells that arise from their self-renewal divisions. Conversely, in the blood stream, the mixture of cells of various lineages creates conditions under which cells encounter mostly those of different lineages and differentiation stages.

C. Leukemias as a Simplified Model for the Study of Interactions Among Hemopoietic Cells

The heterogeneity of hemopoietic cell populations endows the tissue with some of its basic characteristics and is a deterministic factor in the regulation of cell growth and differentiation (73,74). This heterogeneity, however, makes it extremely difficult to obtain uniform cell populations with identical or even similar phenotype. Furthermore, normal hemopoietic cells are often in a transitory state and would change dramatically over a relatively short time period. Stem cells that in vivo are either quiescent (in the G_0 stage of the cell cycle), or at least have an extended cell cycle, go into a proliferative state and differentiate upon in vitro culture. A way to circumvent the heterogeneity problem is to utilize leukemia cell populations. These hemopoietic tumors represent relatively homogeneous populations belonging to specific lineages and stages of differentiation. Examples are lymphoma cell lines corresponding to the three major steps in the B cell lineage: pre-B, B, and plasma cells. Among the B lymphomas, some correspond to relatively immature and others to relatively mature B cells (75). These cell lines may therefore be used as a model to study interactions among cells of a homogeneous phenotype, a study that is almost out of reach with normal cell populations.

It is important to emphasize here that none of the in vitro growth requirements of tumor cells are unique to the neoplastic nature of these cells. A variety of cultured normal cells exhibit analogous requirements. This encouraged us to use leukemia cells for studies aimed eventually at understanding the behavior of complex normal cell populations.

D. Concentration-Dependent Growth of Cultured Leukemia Cells

The following is a description of experience accumulated in our laboratory using a variety of cultured leukemia cell lines. Figure 1 demonstrates a number of growth

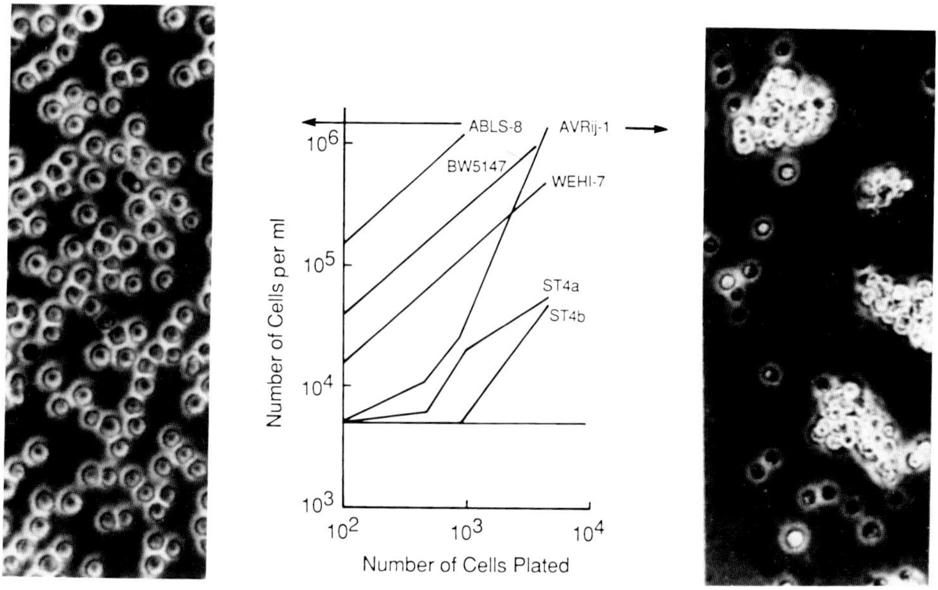

Figure 1 Leukemia cells are seeded in the various concentrations indicated, and their growth is determined following a few days of culture. The cell lines ABLS-8 (pre-B lymphoma), and BW5147 and WEHI-7 (T lymphomas) exhibit concentration-independent growth pattern. In contrast, the cell lines AVRij-1 (pre-B lymphoma) and ST4b and ST4a (T lymphoma) are concentration-dependent. The latter property frequently coincides with the formation of large cell aggregates (right) as opposed to growth in single-cell suspensions exhibited by concentration-independent cell lines (left).

features that a leukemia cell population may exhibit upon in vitro culture. Cells are seeded at various concentrations, and their growth is determined following a few days of culture. If the cells are completely concentration-independent, they exhibit a fixed doubling time irrespective of the concentration at which they were seeded. Plotting of cell growth as a function of number of cells seeded will yield a linear pattern with a slope of 1 (Fig. 1). This is indeed observed in many cell lines that have been cloned and maintained in vitro for prolonged periods of time. Figure 1 further demonstrates concentration-dependent growth patterns; primary tumors and newly derived cell lines show the latter pattern (76,77)—they do not proliferate at low concentrations, and they stimulate their own growth when seeded at high starting cell concentrations. They further tend to attach to one another and form large aggregates (Fig. 1, right). Concentration-independent cells tend to detach from each other shortly after mitosis and grow as unicellular suspensions (Fig. 1, left). Particular cells, such as many thiol-dependent B cell lymphomas, stop growing abruptly upon reaching a certain high concentration in vitro (about 10^6/ml). In some cell lines, death of the whole population occurs when the critical concentration is reached. Each of these growth patterns demonstrates the dependence of the individual cell upon the population. It is clearly the newly cultured cells that exhibit most of the above properties, rather than the established cell lines. The latter are usually selected vigorously by investigators to adapt to conditions that may be remote from those the cell would encounter in vivo. It is therefore desirable to keep in mind the flexibility of the cells' phenotype while designing in vitro experiments, so as to create as few selective conditions as possible and thus approach more reliable models for the study of cell growth control.

The requirement of cells for high density upon in vitro culture results partly from their deficiency in nonessential amino acids (78-80). Apparently cells tend to leak the amino acids they synthesize into the growth medium. It was proposed that cells that do not require external supplementation with nonessential amino acids are able to prevent the leakage of these acids (reviewed in 81). We found, though, that cell lines that are concentration-independent secrete into their growth medium a high titer of amino acids. They therefore appear to overcome the problem of leakage by producing high titers of the aminc acids. Consequently, they are able to condition their own medium. Ishii et al. suggested that mercaptoethanol enhances the transport of cystine into cells (82), implying that thiol dependence (82-89) and the requirement for nonessential amino acids may be one and the same phenomenon.

Supplementation of growth medium with both types of agents, however, is not sufficient to correct completely the growth deficiency of primary cells. Additional factors are required to allow optimal growth of primary tumors and newly derived cell lines. Some of these factors are produced by stromal cells (76,77). In addition, Nara and McCulloch (90) reported that acute myeloblastic leukemia blasts promote their own growth. Membrane fractions prepared from these blasts could substitute for intact cells, whereas fragments from lymphoblastic leukemia cells were inactive.

E. Autoinhibitors of Cell Growth: "Suicidines"?

Some thiol-dependent pre-B lymphoma cells exhibit concentration-independent growth capacity in the range of 1-1 $\times$ 10^6 cells/ml. Above these concentrations rapid death occurs. This is not due to a lack of nutrients. Alternatively, upon crowding, the lymphoma cells seem to produce some growth inhibitors. Tanapat et al. suggested that part of the autoinhibition is due to thiols or disulfides (91). Self-inhibition occurs also with cells that are not thiol-dependent. We found that thiol-dependent lymphoma cell lines seeded in coculture with dense cultures of stromal cells survive at high cell concentrations that would otherwise cause their death. The production or activity of a "death factor" can apparently be modulated. Recently, Horowitz et al. reported an autocrine growth inhibitor in a cloned line of helper T cells. The factor was estimated by gel filtration to be about 12 kD (92). Production of cell death signals have been reported also for nonhemopoietic cells such as primary rabbit endometrial cell cultures (93).

F. Cell Interactions During the Differentiation of Erythroleukemia Cells

An additional example of the effect of homologous cell interactions is provided by Friend erythroleukemia. This particular tumor differentiates in response to Me_2SO and a variety of other compounds. The final outcome of this differentiation is loss

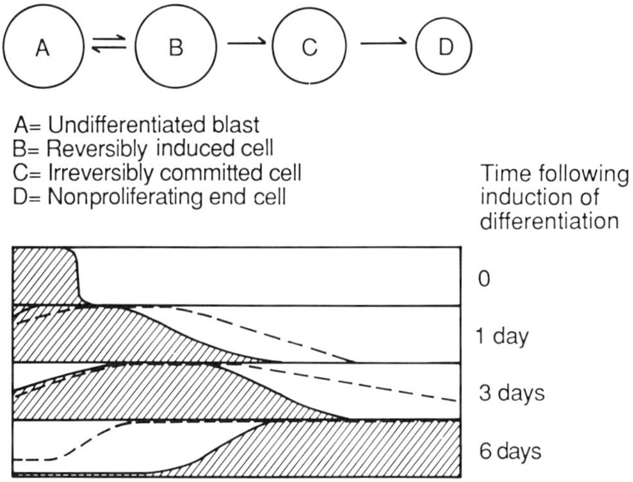

Figure 2 Four major steps in the differentiation pathway of Friend cells. The uninduced cell (A) has an unlimited capacity to proliferate without loss of cells through terminal differentiation. Following induction with Me_2SO, a chain of events occur, leading to irreversible commitment (stage C), hemoglobinization, and cell death (stage D). The figure shows schematically (cross hatching) that at day 1 after stimulation most of the cells are still at stage A, but some commence to stage B. At day 6 of culture, the entire population has passed the commitment stage. However, when dense populations of Friend cells are induced, an additional differentiation stage is revealed; following 6 days of induction, the dense population of Friend cells is seeded in sparse suspension, either without stromal cells or on top of confluent stromal cell layers. The result is that the former cells differentiate terminally whereas the latter continue to proliferate. The areas below the broken lines indicate that induced Friend cells seeded in the presence of stroma accumulate at stage B, which is reversibly induced and can revert to the proliferative stage A.

of clonal growth and cell death, similar to the fate of normal erythroid precursors. However, the inducer added in excess amounts is incapable of driving a large proportion of erythroleukemia cells into terminal differentiation, when the cells are seeded at high concentrations (94). Similar protection from differentiation is provided by stromal cells when they are added to induced erythroleukemia cells. The fraction of cells that does differentiate under these conditions is hemoglobinized faster than the normally stimulated population (94) (see also Fig. 2).

G. Some Thoughts on the Role of Homologous and Heterologous Interactions in the Regulation of Hemopoiesis

Hemopoietic organs are subject to dynamic changes due to extensive cell migration. Very little is known about the regulation of cell traffic from and to blood-producing tissues. It is, however, a highly selective process, as indicated by the tendency of stem cells and immature blood cell intermediates to remain in the bone marrow. Their fraction in the blood stream is far lower than that in their tissue of origin. Part of the selective traffic of cells from the bone marrow could be controlled by the endothelial lining of the sinus walls (64). However, there is no evidence to support the notion that stem cells are less effective in penetrating endothelial barriers than other hemopoietic cell types. An alternative mechanism would be that associations between cells in situ limit their motility. The tendency of primary tumors, especially those with a relatively immature phenotype, to form large cell aggregates may be an example of this occurrence. It is possible that the in vitro requirement of primary cells for crowding is an expression of their in vivo interdependence. Thus, a requirement for supply of a high titer of growth factors or nutrients is satisfied by cell packing that overcomes dilution problems. This in turn determines the position of the cells within the tissue and prevents their migration. One consequence of this is that the population remains homogeneous. The growth signals that cells produce at early differentiation stages support self-renewal. Conversely, as hemopoietic cells mature they appear to produce differentiation-potentiating factors. Interactions between cells of the same phenotype at an advanced differentiation stage would promote the maturation process (Fig. 3). The interplay of these activities is observed during the differentiation of Friend erythroleukemia cells (Fig. 2) (94).

Autocrine induction such as that occurring in macrophages by β-related interferon has an important role in the regulation of cell growth and differentiation (95). This phenomenon as well as the growth-inhibitory ability ascribed to tumor necrosis factor (TNF) and transforming growth factor β (TFG-β) (reviewed in 96) and the production of autoinhibitors that are toxic and induce rapid cell death may all serve as part of a control mechanism to limit excessive cell accumulation. What could be the physiological significance of an auto "cell death" signal? Under steady-state conditions, a balance exists between the proportions of cells of the

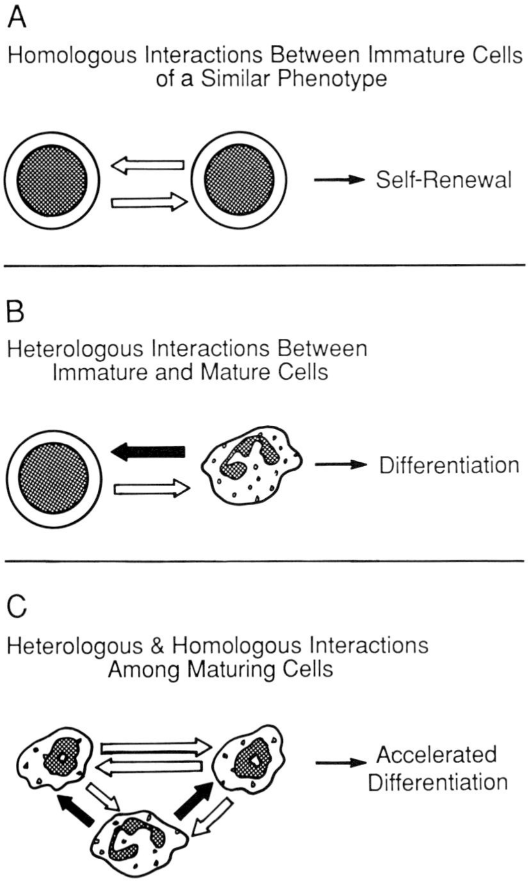

Figure 3 Possible consequences of homologous and heterologous interactions between hemopoietic cells.

various lineages and stages of differentiation. It is conceivable that cells with a high potential for self-renewal may exceed in their number of copies the required total that would permit the maintenance of a steady state. The capacity to generate a death signal beyond a given high concentration provides a means to block the overproduction of immature cells. It is interesting to note that in the B cell lineage the requirement for thiols and the production of autoinhibitors correlate with the differentiation stage. Pre-B and B cell lymphomas are usually thiol-dependent, while plasmacytomas are not. It is thus anticipated that only cells in early stages of hemopoietic differentiation endowed with a self-renewal capacity would be producers of "suicidines." It is also expected that these factors would be cell-lineage- and differentiation-stage-specfic to prevent the accidental kill of bystanders.

III. REGULATION OF HEMOPOIESIS BY STROMAL CELLS

A. Why Do Stem Cells Die in Culture?

Fibroblast cell populations were the first to be cultured for long periods and studied in vitro (reviewed in 81). It took an additional 20 years to find the conditions that allow the in vitro investigation of blood cell formation. Yet some types of hemopoietic cells such as macrophages could be maintained functional for relatively long intervals under simple culture conditions that would not suffice for their progenitors. Hemopoietic stem cells and progenitors are found in the bone marrow at a low incidence, and most studies on the survival of these cells have utilized functional assays. Moreover, specific markers for stem cells have not yet been identified. Consequently, information about survival of stem cells in culture depends upon the use of functional assays.

The in vitro culture of stem cells releases them from constraints that are imposed in vivo. It is found invariably that following short periods of culture stem cells are eliminated. This would occur within a day or, under improved conditions, following a few days of culture. The disappearance of stem cell functions is usually referred to as "stem cell death." Is that indeed the case? Are there any grounds for the assumption that a given hemopoietic cell type is more vulnerable to culture conditions than others?

Many types of cells that would otherwise die and disintegrate in culture can survive when supplied with the appropriate stimulus ("growth factor"). Colony-stimulating factors are capable of inducing proliferation coupled with differentiation of progenitor cells and stem cells (such as Mix-CFC). Consequently, their addition to cultures containing stem cells apparently prevents the death of these cells. Nevertheless, this activity of the stimulating factor actually postpones stem cell "death," which eventually occurs through their differentiation into mature progeny (97). Multi-CSF (IL-3) was found to induce the formation of blastlike colonies in culture (98). In short-term cultures, it can also support the survival of stem cells. It is clear, however, that these activities are transient and eventually terminate in differentiation. Factor-dependent cell lines exhibit dramatic dependence upon IL-3 for their continuous growth (99). Deprivation of inducer causes cell death during overnight incubation. It was found that IL-3 is required for cell survival through the activation of protein kinase C (100). The obvious questions are whether stem cells may be compared to these factor-dependent cell lines and whether it can be inferred that stem cell death in culture is mediated via the absence of IL-3. It appears that IL-3 by itself would not be a sufficient requirement for stem cell survival, let alone self-renewal in vitro. Alternatively, it seems that stem cells put in culture are relieved of restrictions imposed on them in vivo and undergo instantaneous differentiation. Thus, the apparent loss observed when one uses functional assays is a result of progression into a more differentiated nonproliferative cell that requires a specific differentiation factor, rather than cell death. Factor-dependent cell lines may relate to committed stem cells in their requirement for a continuous supply of a specific factor.

B. The Biological Function of CSF: Induction of Terminal Differentiation

I find it necessary to devote an entire section to this point since it is essential for the understanding of the role of stromal cells in the regulation of hemopoiesis. The control of hemopoiesis is often described as a feedback loop in which stimulating factors initiate differentiation. The mature cells that are produced secrete a negative signal that feeds back to the stem cell compartment. Other models that are generally similar suggest a series of signals traveling upstream from the mature cell compartment to the committed cell and finally to the stem cell compartment. These models assume that a single type of molecule, the differentiation inducer, may control the entire differentiation scheme and also account, either directly or indirectly, for stem cell renewal. Nonetheless, this does not seem to be supported by experimental findings. Primarily, no products of mature cells have been identified that satisfy the requirement for a feedback signal. Such a molecule would have to be produced by a mature cell and affect the stem cell in a way that stops the differentiation flow and allows self-renewal to occur. Agents such as prostaglandins (101-103), isoferritins (104), γ-interferon (105), and vitamin D_3 (106) all limit the accumulation of mature cells by accelerating differentiation. Under the influence of these molecules, the progenitor undergoes fewer divisions before it reaches full maturity and concomitant loss of differentiation capacity. The activity of these agents, therefore, assures the supply of highly potent mature cells within a relatively short time interval. Thus, both CSFs (50) and the products of mature cells are engaged primarily in the induction of terminal differentiation and consequent production of additional mature cells (5).

C. Long-Term Maintenance of Stem Cells in Culture Depends on Stromal Cells

Hemopoietic stem cells have been observed in many body sites including circulating blood (107) and the brain (108). These cells are produced, however, primarily in the bone marrow. A pool of spleen colony-forming units (CFU-S) (109) with a high potential for repopulation of peripheral organs is maintained throughout the entire life span (110). It therefore appears that the marrow microenvironment has some specific properties that make it a unique site for stem cell renewal. In Dexter's long-term bone marrow cultures (111), production of CFU-S occurs continuously for many months. These pluripotent stem cells maintain their capacity to repopulate the hemopoietic tissues of recipient mice. The culture system is based upon seeding large inocula of bone marrow cells in preselected horse serum or fetal calf serum supplemented with hydrocortisone, incubation at 33°C, and weekly demidepopulation of the cultures (reviewed in Ref. 112). The precise contribution of each of these ingredients is not completely understood. It is clear though that, in sharp contrast to other culture systems, this allows the formation of multilayers of adherent stromal cells of various types. Hempoietic cells are found engulfed within the adherent layers, attached to the surface of the layer that is exposed to the growth medium, and free in suspension. Stem cells within the adherent layer seem to be vital for long-term hemopoiesis. Transfer of cells from the liquid phase to cultures that do not contain adherent stroma results in loss of stem cells. Media conditioned by the adherent stromal cell layers cannot support stem cell survival or proliferation. Two types of regulator molecules are produced in long-term bone marrow cultures. One is a specific stimulator of DNA synthesis in stem cells, while the other is an inhibitor of cell cycling (113).

D. What Are Stromal Cells?

Trivial as this question may sound, it deserves some attention. "Hemopoietic stromal cells" have already been mentioned here in various contexts. Most authors use this terminology to collectively refer to the mesenchyme-derived connective tissue-like cells that form the tridimensional network that supports hemopoietic cells in situ (1). Others make a distinction between genuine stromal endothelial cells and fibroblasts, although originally Friedenstein regarded the cells that transfer hemopoietic microenvironments as fibroblasts (59). In vitro cultured stromal cells are accepted mostly as those cells that constitute the adherent population growing out of bone marrow inocula, excluding hemopoietic stem cells and their progeny. However, some claims have been made that in humans stromal cells and hemopoietic cells have a common precursor (114). Conversely, in the mouse no evidence for a common origin of hemopoietic cells and stromal cells could be obtained (115). The above definitions of stromal cells are operational and unprecise. It is desirable to obtain specific markers that would distinguish stromal cells from other types of cells. Charbord et al. (116) reported that the monoclonal antibodies CGA-7 and HHF that recognize actin react specifically with stromal cells in actively hemopoietic human long-term cultures. Monoclonal antibodies were also raised against stromal cells from the mouse and appear to react in tissue sections with specific cell types (117).

A step forward in the characterization of stromal cells was made following the derivation of continuous stromal cell lines.

E. Cloned Stromal Cell Lines Represent Distinct Cell Subtypes and Vary in Their Biological Functions

This field of research has been recently reviewed (58). Here the main features of cell lines obtained from hemopoietic tissues and their effects on hemopoiesis will be summarized briefly.

Stromal cell lines have been derived in many laboratories from mouse (94,118-143) and human (144) bone marrow, mouse spleen (145), mouse (146,147) and human (148) thymus, and mouse calvaria (149-151). Their mode of derivation varies considerably from one laboratory to another. A number of laboratories have used similar criteria to identify stromal cells. This allows intercomparisons of the cell lines. Many of the well-characterized cells share some distinct properties such as the capacity to accumulate fat. There is, however, considerable diversity among cells of the latter type in their responses to hormones (120,121,124, 128,149,150) and capacity to support hemopoiesis (94,137,151). Therefore, a whole range of properties were considered when attempting to categorize stromal cell lines into subtypes (58); endothelial-adipose cells are characterized by flattened morphology and long cytoplasmic protrusions in the preadipose stage, fat accumulation and formation of large fat globules, and production of a basal lamina-like extracellular matrix of fibronectin, laminin, and collagen type IV and V. These cells have the most pronounced capacity to support myeloid progenitor cell accumulation and stem cell survival in culture (94,134). A second cell type that is abundant in primary adherent cell layers from hemopoietic organs and has been cloned and propagated as continuous cell lines is a macrophage. The properties of this type of cell do not differ from those of bone marrow macrophages obtained following stimulation with CSF-1 (128). Their relation to resident bone marrow macrophages (RBMM) is unclear. The latter have been isolated from erythroid islands, are negative to Mac-1 antigen, and agglutinate unopsonized erythrocytes (152). Fibroblast cell lines from the bone marrow, also called adventitial reticulum cells, are defined as those making collagen type I and III. This cell is incapable of inducing the in vitro survival of hemopoietic stem cells (94,137). Two other stromal cell types have been identified in our laboratory. The first, an endothelial-like cell, displays spindle-shaped morphology but produces collagen type IV and V. It further exhibits frequent junctional complexes between adjacent cells in culture. A biological function that distinguishes this cell from the rest of the stromal cell lines is the presence of a surface-associated activity that inhibits plasmacytoma cell growth (129). The second is a fibroendothelial cell defined by the composition of the extracellular matrix that it makes, which is a mixture of basal lamina and interstitial collagens. It has not been determined whether cell lines derived from the thymus and other sources and suggested to display tissue-specific function (148) belong to other subtypes of stromal cell. The above five distinct stromal cell types and their corresponding properties are summarized in Table 1.

It is noteworthy that the stromal cell classification was proposed on grounds of our studies with stromal cell lines obtained from normal bone marrow and exhibiting nontumorigenic properties. Experiments performed with normal primary bone marrow cultures substantiate this proposal. Katsuno et al. (153) could distinguish separate colony-forming cells for adipocytes (CFU-A) and fibroblasts (CFU-F). The recovery of only the former following sublethal irradiation correlated

Table 1 Classification of Stromal Cells Based upon Properties of Cloned Cell Lines from Mouse Bone Marrow

Stromal cell subtype	Main collagen types	Fibronectin and laminin	Basic phosphatase	Stem cell support in cultures
Endothelial-adipose	I, IV, V(?)	++	±	+
Fibroblast	I, III	+	++	–
Endothelial-like	IV, V	+	±	–
Fibroendothelial	I, III, IV, V	+	+	–
Macrophage	—	–	–	–

with hemopoietic repopulation (153). Lim et al. (154) identified an additional colony-forming cell, designated reticulofibroblastoid (CFU-RF). The progeny of this precursor made basal lamina and interstitial collagens and resemble therefore the fibroendothelial cell type discussed above.

F. Are Stromal Cells Tissue-Specific?

Long-term proliferation can be initiated by bone marrow cultures and depends, as discussed above, upon marrow stromal cells. It is, however, not certain that this activity is unique to marrow stromal cells since spleen cultures were also found to maintain long-term hemopoiesis (155). An adipocyte cell line derived from mouse calvaria was capable of supporting CFU-S growth in culture (151). It is therefore a matter of further research to define whether the bone marrow contains optimal proportions of stromal cells relevant for induction of stem cell renewal, although similar cells are also present in other tissues. An equally possible alternative is that stromal cells are tissue-specific and the marrow contains unique stromal cell types.

The Whitlock and Witte culture system supports B cell growth rather than myelopoiesis or stem cell renewal (156,157). This could result from the activity of a stromal cell type specific for B cells. However, these types of cultures may be switched to support myelopoiesis and vice versa by changing the culture conditions (158,159).

G. Stromal Cells Produce Cell-Surface-Associated Factors that Restrain Differentiation

Hemopoietic microenvironments were initially conceived as inductive (1). We found evidence, though, for suppressive effects of stromal cells on myeloid differentiation; myeloid progenitors in sparse bone marrow cell suspensions, embedded in semisolid methylcellulose medium, proliferate in response to CSF.

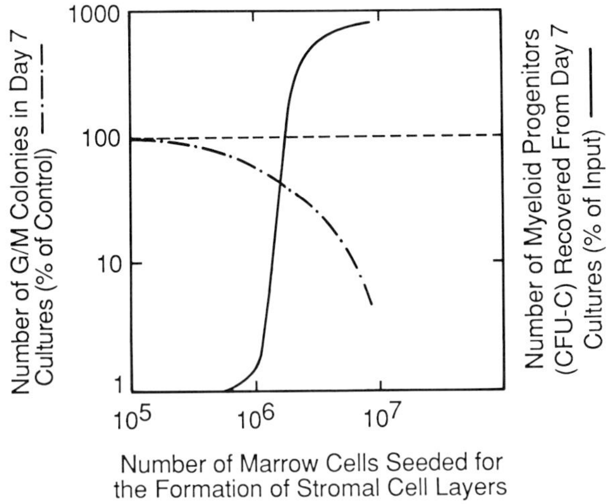

Figure 4 Differentiation-restraining activity of primary stromal cells.

They first divide to form small clusters of relatively immature cells but eventually differentiate and form macroscopic colonies of mature progeny. During this process the progenitors are eliminated from the culture. If such marrow cell suspensions are seeded onto adherent layers of stromal cells from the bone marrow (76), colony formation is inhibited. Concomitantly, myeloid progenitors survive, and their numbers in culture increase beyond the initial input (160,161). These phenomena are mutually dependent, as indicated by the inverse relationship between the degree of inhibition of colony formation and the number of progenitors that accumulate (162) (Fig. 4). Physical separation between the interacting cells relieves the inhibition and prevents the accumulation of progenitors (160-163). This last observation implied that cell-cell interactions may be involved. Indeed, media conditioned by stromal cells were not active. Specific monosaccharides such as β-methylgalactoside partially relieved the inhibition of colony formation caused by stromal cells (161). It is conceivable that surface-associated glycosylated proteins or lipids are involved in this process by serving as "glue" to attach interacting cells or by generating regulatory signals.

H. Stromal Cells May Produce Unique Differentiation Inducers

Media conditioned by primary stromal cell layers or by cells in long-term bone marrow cultures are invariably found to be devoid of significant colony-stimulating activity (161). However, bone marrow cells cocultured with primary stromal cells under conditions that allow direct cell-to-cell contacts develop GM colonies rich in myeloid progenitors (163,164). This occurs without addition of CSF to these cultures, implying that a differentiation-inducing factor is produced by primary stromal cells. This factor may differ from the known species of CSF; it is not found as a secreted form; it overcomes the differentiation-restraining activity that the stroma imposes on M-CSF, GM-CSF, and IL-3; and it is not produced by glucose-starved cells, in contrast to M-CSF, which is secreted in medium containing pyruvate instead of glucose (162-164). Studies with stromal cell lines have led to similar conclusions. An endothelial adipose cell line (14F1.1) was found to support stem cell maintenance and myeloid progenitor accumulation in culture. No other cells, whether from the bone marrow or from other sources, were equally effective (94). The 14F1.1 cell line was examined for its capacity to secrete G, M, GM, and Multi-CSF by use of factor-dependent cell lines. None of these activities could be detected. This could result from the presence of inhibitors of CSFs in the medium or from production of a nonsecreted (membrane-bound?) form of the molecules. These latter possibilities do not appear to be realistic, since a search for GM and Multi-CSF mRNA by sensitive methods such as in situ hybridization and S1 nuclease analysis yielded equally negative results (Zipori and Lee, unpublished observations). It is therefore concluded that stromal cell factors other than the known species of CSF may be involved in the induction of stem cell maintenance and myelopoiesis. The nature of these factors is at the moment unknown.

I. The Spatial Positioning of Stem Cells and Progenitors Relative to Stromal Tissues Determines Their Response to Growth and Differentiation Signals

In the studies of McCulloch and Till it was realized that individual spleen colonies contain cells indistinguishable from the parent CFU-S in their capacity to form clones in secondary hosts. This was taken as an indication for the capacity of CFU-S to self-renew (165). Additional transfers were usually unsuccessful (166). It appears that transfers of bone marrow cells in irradiated mice impose an enormous differentiation pressure on stem cells. This causes an exponential drop in repopulating (self-renewal) ability. Anderson demonstrated that one round of transplantation of bone marrow cells into irradiated recipients causes a reduction in repopulating ability that is more severe than that resulting from the entire life span of the mouse (110). It is therefore inaccurate to deduce the capacity of the CFU-S to self-renew from experiments in which it is placed under strong differentiation stimuli. It is conceivable that under steady-state conditions in the hemopoietic system, stem cells are quiescent. This is controlled by their localization in niches that block their responsiveness to differentiation-inducing signals. Any manipulation that removes stem cells from their niche will result in a cascade of differentiation events. It follows that all in vitro models are based on the use of differentiating cells. Consequently, the knowledge gained by these investigations is primarily relevant to non-steady-state conditions such as during perturbations of hemopoiesis, or to events occurring outside of the stem cell compartment of the bone marrow. A stem cell may not be a stem cell any more when it embarks on a differentiation pathway; that is, at the stem cell level, differentiation and self-renewal are mutually exclusive. Self-renewal would, therefore, be a relative phenomenon in which the progeny of a cell are closely related to it. The production of such cells is encouraged under conditions of low differentiation pressure. With an increase in the latter, the passage of cells along the differentiation pathway is accelerated and fewer cells are self-renewing. Lemischka et al. (167) have used molecular tagging of cells by introducing new genetic markers via retrovirus vectors as a tool to allow for a follow-up of the fate of stem cells in situ. In these studies, only one or two stem cells at the most appeared to be responsible for repopulation of peripheral organs at a given time.

A major role of the stromal tissue in the regulation of hemopoiesis may be to serve as a safeguard for stem cell maintenance (Fig. 5). The existence of a dominant mechanism that interferes with the activity of differentiation-inducing factors within the marrow microenvironment is suggested. In our culture system, myeloid progenitors induced to differentiate by CSF while attached to stromal cells failed to do so. Only small numbers of mature progeny cells were produced. This process was accompanied by accumulation of GM-CFC (160-164). Conversely, when no physical contact between the stromal cells and the target progenitor cells was allowed, terminal differentiation occurred. This model is depicted in Figure 6.

It is interesting to note the resemblance between the above and the events that occur following infection of long-term bone marrow cultures with the recominant virus src (MoMuLV) (reviewed in 168). The balance between mature cells and stem cell production changed, such that the incidence of stem cells became far higher than in control cultures. It appears that the effect of the virus was mediated via changes in the stromal population rather than in the hemopoietic cells.

The differentiation-restraining activity of the stroma is only one part of the mechanism that makes the marrow environment independent of events occurring in the extramedullary space. We have suggested that particular stromal cells produce unique stimulating factors that differ in their biological properties from factors of non-marrow origin (162-164). The stromal "resident CSF" (162) appears to induce large colonies that grow attached to the stromal layer and characteristically contain large numbers of reclonable progenitors (164). It was suggested that these colonies are derived from hemopoietic stem cells. A human analog of this factor may participate in large burst formation induced by the human cell line ST-1 (169). The combined activity of the specific stromal CSF and the differentiation-restraining factor may result in autonomy of the bone marrow with respect to events occurring in the blood stream. For example, an increase in blood CSF titer that may follow an immune reaction would not cause an immediate marrow response due to the antagonistic effect of the restraining factor (Fig. 7).

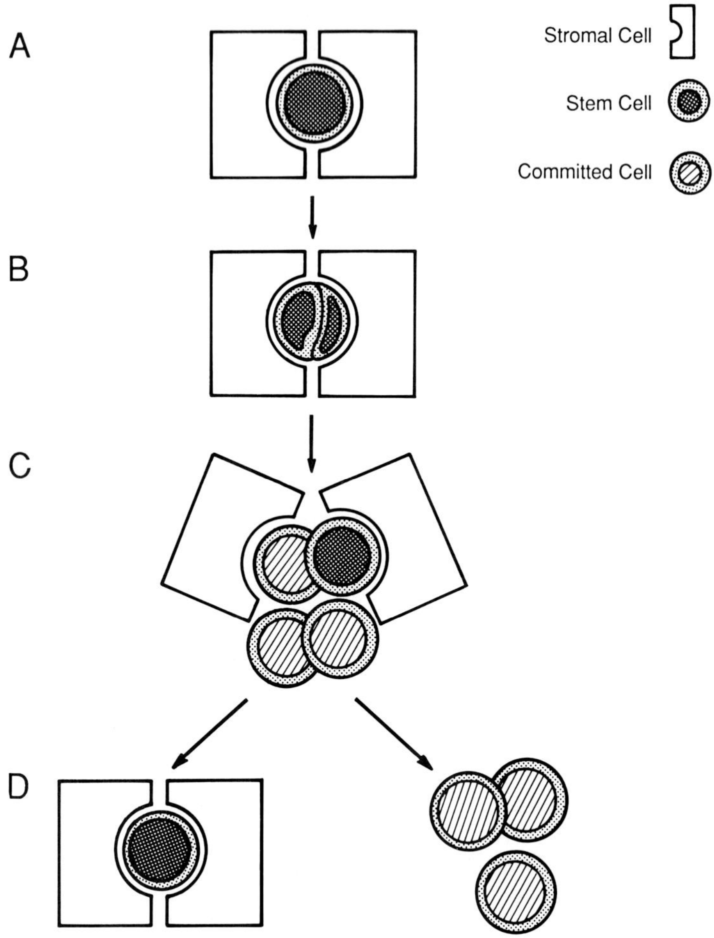

Figure 5 A schematic representation of a putative stem cell "niche," demonstrating the protective role of stromal cells. Stem cell divisions lead to self-renewal due to their isolation from signals from sources other than stromal cells or the stem cells themselves. Self-renewal divisions of stem cells "open" the stromal barrier and release the cells to other compartments. This event may trigger commitment of some stem cells. The reclosing of the niche assures further stem cell production.

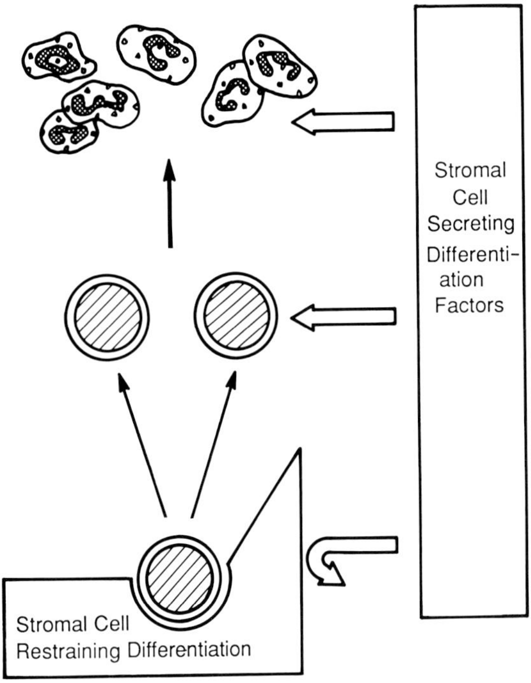

Figure 6 Dual role of stromal cells in the regulation of differentiation: The attachment of a progenitor cell to the stroma prevents it from responding to differentiation signals. On the other hand, when the progenitor is at a distance from the stromal cell, it responds to differentiation inducers secreted by microenvironmental cells.

An additional major contribution to the specific function of the bone marrow is provided by the defined patterns of cell organization within each tissue. Stromal cell activities that may take part in directing cell organization are discussed in the following sections.

J. Stromal Cells Produce Leukemia Cell Inhibitory Activity (LCIA)

The interactions of leukemia cells with cultured stromal cells exemplify the correlations that are found between tumor populations and normal hemopoietic cells. Most primary tumors exhibit poor seeding efficiency in culture, as do proliferative populations of freshly explanted normal hemopoietic cells. Cultured primary stromal cells are not only beneficial for the growth of hemopoietic stem cells but also promote the in vitro growth of a variety of hemopoietic tumors (76,77).

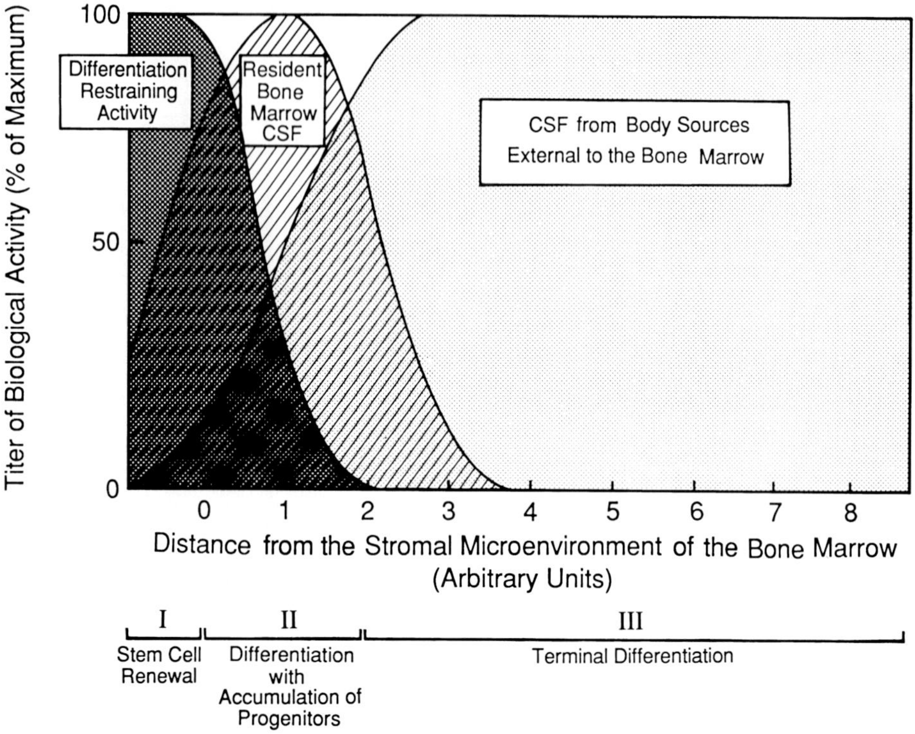

Figure 7 A hypothetical model of stromal cell function: In the proximity of stromal cells two activities are found. One is a differentiation restraining activity. It has a short-range effect and is thus restricted to the bone marrow environment. Its function is to block activity of CSF penetrating the marrow from the blood stream. This assures that the stem cell and progenitor cell pools in the bone marrow will not be subject to constant depletion due to events occurring in extramedullary sites. In addition, stromal cells produce a resident CSF that accounts for local mature cell production. The latter may differ biologically from CSF produced outside of the marrow.

The homogeneity of leukemia cell populations enabled us to monitor quantitatively the fate of various cell types at defined differentiation stages. Whereas pre-B lymphomas that represent an early stage of the B cell differentiation pathway were supported by stromal cells, the growth of plasmacytomas that represent the end stage of this lineage was inhibited (77,170). In contrast, cells of the myeloid lineage were unaffected. These findings correlate well with observations made with normal cell populations. Long-term bone marrow cultures do not support lymphopoiesis (60,61). Furthermore, in a modified long-term culture system, production of pre-B and some B cells could be detected, but mature plasma cells were very scarce (156,157).

The stromal cell type in the heterogeneous primary stroma that mediated the activities could be determined following the cloning of stromal cells and production of cell lines representing distinct cell populations. An endothelial-like cell line (MBA-2.1) was found to have the most pronounced capacity to inhibit plasmacytoma cell growth under coculture conditions (94). This cell line was further found to produce a cell surface associated glycoprotein that exhibited a unique target cell specificity. The factor designated leukemia cell inhibitory activity (LCIA) blocked the growth of plasmacytomas (and hybridomas in which one partner was a plasma cell). Among B and T cell tumors, only some were sensitive to the factor, whereas all pre-B cells were resistant. Myeloid, macrophage, and erythroid tumors were refractory to LCIA (171).

K. Differentiation Stage and Lineage Specific Inhibitors from the Stroma May Direct Pattern Formation in Hemopoietic Tissues

The specificity of LCIA seems to extend beyond the group of tumor cell lines mentioned above. Primarily, hemopoietic stem cells and myeloid progenitors were unaffected by the presence of the factor. LCIA did not affect cell proliferation in a 4-day mitogen stimulation assay of spleen cells but did reduce antibody production in vitro (Zipori and Mozes, unpublished results).

The correlation observed between the effects of LCIA on normal and leukemic populations implies that this molecule is a physiological inhibitor. Its unique specificity makes it a candidate regulator of pattern formation in hemopoietic tissues. The fact that LCIA operates at the cell surface endows it with a capacity to prevent the accumulation of plasma cells in the vicinity of the producer stromal cell. The activity of LCIA and molecules belonging to the same functional family is postulated to be involved in determining which cell types will be found at specific tissue sites.

Is it necessary to assume the existence of such inhibitory molecules? Would the activity of colony-stimulating factors (CSFs) not be sufficient to account for cell organization in the hemopoietic tissue? An unequivocal answer awaits further experimentation. It is, however, quite clear that the production of CSFs is widespread among cells in the organism and that there is a high degree of overlap in target cell specificities of these factors (see Chapter 1). By themselves, therefore, CSFs may not suffice to explain the precise nature of cell organization in hemopoietic tissues.

An important feature in bone marrow organization is the fact that this hemopoietic tissue is intimately associated with bone. The proximity of stem cell proliferation domains to the bone was mentioned above (66,67). In addition, stromal cells may by themselves be involved in induction of bone formation (172). We found that among cloned stromal cell lines, only particular types were capable of inducing bone formation following intraperitoneal implantation in cellulose acetate membranes (Knospe, Huseini, and Zipori, unpublished observations).

L. Modulation of Stromal Cell Functions: Relevance to Hematological Malignancies and Neoplasia

Inoculation of mice with lipopolysaccharide resulted in accumulation of stromal progenitor cells in the spleen (173). This agent was also found to induce in vitro GM-CSF secretion by a mouse bone marrow stromal cell line (Rennick and Lee, unpublished). Cultured human stromal cells respond to platelet-derived growth factor (PDGF) by increasing the incorporation of [^{3}H] thymidine (174). Studies with long-term bone marrow cultures indicated that lithium increases hemopoiesis through an indirect effect on stromal cells (175).

A variety of cytotoxic compounds were found to affect stromal cells. These include benzene (176,177) and agents commonly used in chemotherapy such as cytosine-arabinoside, adriamycin (178), cyclophosphamide derivatives (179), and busulfan (180). Some of the effects persist for prolonged periods of time. Additional studies examined the in vivo sensitivity of stromal cells to ionizing irradiation and heat (181-186). Particular studies showed latent sustained defects in the stroma following irradiation (185). In vitro irradiation of stromal cells was found to modulate CSF production (187,188). It appears premature to determine whether a primary defect in the stromal tissues accounts for particular acquired hemopoietic malfunctions. This is obviously a subject of great clinical importance and is discussed in Chapter 4. It is equally uncertain whether stromal cells are involved in the pathogenesis of aplastic anemia or leukemia, although data implicating this possibility are available (142,189-192).

IV. SUMMARY

The microenvironment in which hemopoietic cells proliferate, differentiate, and execute their biological functions has many components. One of the major variables is the hemopoietic cells themselves, which interact in diverse manners. Schematically, I have classified these interactions into autologous and heterologous. The former relates to interactions wherein cells of a similar phenotype are involved, whereas the latter relates to conditions in which cells of nonidentical phenotypes exchange information. These situations have different consequences and may play a crucial role in the regulation of self-renewal and differentiation. Stromal cells are a major contributor to the formation of the microenvironment. These cells have been characterized and their various functions delineated. Two activities that stromal cells perform may endow the marrow microenvironment with autonomy from events occurring in the extramedullary space and protect the stem cell pool from excess differentiation; stromal cells are capable of antagonizing maturation-inducing factors and produce differentiation-inducing activity associated with the cell surface that may differ from CSFs produced in extramedullary sites. Additional glycoprotein factors isolated from stromal cells exhibit differentiation stage and lineage specificity and may account for the capacity of stromal cells to restrict specifically the accumulation of particular cells, as part of the mechanisms mediating spatial arrangement and pattern formation of cells in hemopoietic tissues.

ACKNOWLEDGMENTS

This chapter was prepared during the author's sabbatical leave at DNAX Research Institute of Molecular and Cellular Biology. It was critically reviewed by Drs. J. Allan Waitz and Pnina Zipori. Mr. Gary Burget performed the word processing, and Mr. Dan Zipori participated in arranging the reference list. The author is an incumbent of the Delta Career Development Chair at the Weizmann Institute of Science.

REFERENCES

1. Trentin, J. J. Influence of hematopoietic organ stroma (hematopoietic inductive microenvironments) on stem cell differentiation. In: *Regulation of hematopoiesis*, Vol. 1. Gordon, A. S. (Ed.). Appleton-Century-Crofts, New York, pp. 161-186 (1970).
2. Bradley, T. R., Metcalf, D. The growth of mouse bone marrow cells in vitro. *Aust. J. Exp. Biol. Med. Sci. 44,* 287-300 (1966).
3. Pluznik, D. H., Sachs, L. The cloning of normal "mast" cells in tissue culture. *J. Cell Comp. Physiol. 66,* 319-324 (1965).
4. Metcalf, D. The granulocyte-macrophage colony-stimulating factors. *Science 229,* 16-22 (1985).
5. Metcalf, D. The molecular biology and functions of the granulocyte-macrophage colony-stimulating factors. *Blood 67,* 257-267 (1986).
6. Metcalf, D. *The hemopoietic colony stimulating factors*, Elsevier, Amsterdam, 1984.
7. Zipori, D., Waitz, J. A. Colony stimulating factors. *Ann. Rep. Med. Chem. 21,* 263-272 (1986).
8. Metcalf, D. The granulocyte-macrophage colony stimulating factors. *Cell 43,* 5-6 (1985).
9. Ihle, J. N., Keller, J., Henderson, L., Klein, F., Palaszynski, E. Procedures for the purification of interleukin-3 to homogeneity. *J. Immunol. 129,* 2431-2436 (1982).
10. Bazil, G. W., Haynes, M., Garland, J., Dexter, T. M. Characterization and partial purification of a hemopoietic cell growth factor in WEHI-3 cell conditioned medium. *Biochem. J. 210,* 747-759 (1983).

11. Yung, Y. P., Eger, R., Tertian, G., Moore, M. A. S. Long-term in vitro culture of murine mast cells. II. Purification of mast cell growth factor and its dissociation from TCGF. *J. Immunol. 127,* 794-799 (1981).
12. Clark-Lewis, I., Kent, S. B. H., Schrader, J. W. Purification to apparent homogeneity of a factor stimulating the growth of multiple lineages of hemopoietic cells. *J. Biol. Chem. 259,* 7488-7494 (1984).
13. Iscove, N. N., Roitsch, C. A., Williams, N., Guilbert, L. J. Molecules stimulating early red cell, granulocyte, macrophage, and megakaryocyte precursors in culture: similarity in size, hydrophobicity and charge. *J. Cell. Physiol. Suppl. 1,* 65-78 (1982).
14. Park, L. S., Friend, D., Gillis, S., Urdal, D. L. Characterization of the cell surface receptor for a multilineage colony-stimulating factor (CSF-2 alpha). *J. Biol. Chem. 261,* 205-210 (1986).
15. Fung, M. C., Hapel, A. J., Ymer, S., Cohen, D. R., Johnson, R. N., Campbell, H. D., Young, I. G. Molecular cloning of cDNA for murine interleukin-3. *Nature 307,* 233-237 (1984).
16. Yokota, T., Lee, F., Rennick, D., Hall, C., Arai, N., Mosmann, T., Nabel, G., Cantor, H., Arai, K. Isolation and characterization of a mouse cDNA clone that expresses mast-cell growth-factor activity in monkey cells. *Proc. Natl. Acad. Sci. USA 81,* 1070-1074 (1984).
17. Lee, F., Yokota, T., Rennick, D., Arai, K. Cloning and expression of murine interleukin-3, a multipotential hematopoietic growth factor. In: *Regulation of the immune system* (UCLA Symp. Mol. Cell. Biol., Vol. 18). Cantor, H., Chess, L., Sercarz, E. (Eds.). Alan R. Liss, New York, pp. 345-353 (1984).
18. Campbell, H. D., Ymer, S., Fung, M. C., Young, I. G. Cloning and nucleotide sequence of the murine interleukin-3 gene. *Eur. J. Biochem. 150,* 297-304 (1985).
19. Miyatake, S., Yokota, T., Lee, F. D., Arai, K. Structure of the mouse interleukin-3 gene that expresses mast cell growth factor activity in L cells. In: *Cellular and molecular biology of lymphokines.* Sorg, C., Schimpl, A., Landy, M. (Eds.). Academic Press, New York, pp. 659-663 (1985).
20. Garland, J. M., Dexter, T. M. Relationship of haemopoietic growth factor to lymphocytes and interleukin-3. *Lymphokine Res. 2,* 13-22 (1983).
21. Palaszynski, E. W., Ihle, J. N. Evidence for specific receptors for interleukin 3 on lymphokine-dependent cell lines established from long-term bone marrow cultures. *J. Immunol. 132,* 1872-1878 (1984).
22. Welte, K., Platzer, E., Lu, L., Gabrilove, J. L., Levi, E., Mertelsmann, R., Moore, M. A. S. Purification and biochemical characterization of human pluripotent hematopoietic colony-stimulating factor. *Proc. Natl. Acad. Sci. USA 82,* 1526-1530 (1985).
23. Gough, N. M., Metcalf, D., Gough, J., Grail, D., Dunn, A. R. Structure and expression of the mRNA for murine granulocyte-macrophage colony stimulating factor. *EMBO J. 4,* 645-653 (1985).
24. Gough, N. M., Gough, J., Metcalf, D., Kelso, A., Grail, D., Nicola, N. A., Burgess, A. W., Dunn, A. R. Molecular cloning of cDNA encoding a murine haematopoietic growth regulator, granulocyte-macrophage colony stimulating factor. *Nature 309,* 763-767 (1984).

25. Sparrow, L. G., Metcalf, D., Hunkapiller, M. W., Hood, L. E., Burgess, A. W. Purification and partial amino acid sequence of asialo murine granulocyte-macrophage colony stimulating factor. *Proc. Natl. Acad. Sci. USA 82,* 292-296 (1985).
26. Miyatake, S., Otsuka, T., Yokota, T., Lee, F., Arai, K. Structure of the chromosomal gene for granulocyte-macrophage colony stimulating factor: comparison of the mouse and human genes. *EMBO J. 4,* 2561-2568 (1985).
27. Wong, G. G., Witek, J. S., Temple, P. A., Wilkens, K. M., Leary, A. C., Luxenberg, D. P., Jones, S. S., Brown, E. L., Kay, R. M., Orr, E. C., Shoemaker, C., Golde, D. W., Kaufman, R. J. Hewick, R. M., Wang, E. A., Clark, S. C. Human GM-CSF: molecular cloning of the complementary DNA and purification of the natural and recombinant proteins. *Science 228,* 810-815 (1985).
28. Cantrell, M. A., Anderson, D., Cerretti, D. P., Price, V., McKereghan, K., Tushinski, R. J., Mochizuki, D. Y., Larsen, A., Grabstein, K., Gillis, S., Cosman, D. Cloning, sequence, and expression of a human granulocyte/macrophage colony-stimulating factor. *Proc. Natl. Acad. Sci. USA 82,* 6250-6254 (1985).
29. DeLamarter, J. F., Mermod, J. J., Liang, C. M., Eliason, J. F., Thatcher, D. R. Recombinant murine GM-CSF from *E. coli* has biological activity and is neutralized by a specific antiserum. *EMBO J. 4,* 2575-2581 (1985).
30. Stanley, E., Metcalf, D., Sobieszczuk, P., Gough, N. M., Dunn, A. R. The structure and expression of the murine gene encoding granulocyte-macrophage colony stimulating factor: evidence for utilization of alternative promoters. *EMBO J. 4,* 2569-2573 (1985).
31. Metcalf, D., Begley, C. G., Johnson, G. R., Nicola, N. A., Vadas, M. A., Lopez, A. F., Williamson, D. J., Wong, G. G., Clark, S. C., Wang, E. A. Biologic properties in vitro of a recombinant human granulocyte-macrophage colony-stimulating factor. *Blood 67,* 37-45 (1986).
32. Tomonaga, M., Golde, D. W., Gasson, J. C. Biosynthetic (recombinant) human granulocyte-macrophage colony-stimulating factor: effect on normal bone marrow and leukemia cell lines. *Blood 67,* 31-36 (1986).
33. Walker, F., Burgess, A. W. Specific binding of radioiodinated granulocyte-macrophage colony-stimulating factor to hemopoietic cells. *EMBO J. 4,* 933-939 (1985).
34. Nicola, N. A., Metcalf, D., Matsumoto, M., Johnson, G. R. Purification of a factor inducing differentiation in murine myelomonocytic leukemia cells. Identification of granulocyte colony-stimulating factor. *J. Biol. Chem. 258,* 9017-9023 (1983).
35. Metcalf, D., Nicola, N. A. Autoinduction of differentiation in WEHI-3B leukemia cells. *Int. J. Cancer 30,* 773-780 (1982).
36. Nicola, N. A., Metcalf, D. Binding of the differentiation-inducer, granulocyte-colony-stimulating factor, to responsive but not unresponsive leukemic cell lines. *Proc. Natl. Acad. Sci. USA 81,* 3765-3769 (1984).
37. Nicola, N. A., Begley, C. G., Metcalf, D. Identification of the human analogue of a regulator that induces differentiation in murine leukaemic cells. *Nature 314,* 625-628 (1985).

38. Nagata, S., Tsuchiya, M., Asano, S., Kaziro, Y., Yamazaki, T., Yamamoto, O., Hirata, Y., Kubota, N., Oheda, M., Nomura, H., Ono, M. Molecular cloning and expression of cDNA for human granulocyte colony-stimulating factor. *Nature 319,* 415-418 (1986).
39. Nagata, S., Tsuchiya, M., Asano, S., Yamamoto, O., Hirata, Y., Kubota, N., Oheda, M., Nomura, H., Yamazaki, T. The chromosomal gene structure and two mRNAs for human granulocyte colony-stimulating factor. *EMBO J. 5,* 575-581 (1985).
40. Stanley, E. R., Heard, P. M. Factors regulating macrophage production and growth. Purification and some properties of the colony stimulating factor from medium conditioned by mouse L cells. *J. Biol. Chem. 252,* 4305-4312 (1977).
41. Stanley, E. R., Guilbert, L. J. Methods for the purification, assay, characterization and target cell binding of a colony stimulating factor (CSF-1). *J. Immunol. Methods 42,* 253-284 (1981).
42. Burgess, A. W., Metcalf, D., Kozka, I. J., Simpson, R. J. Vairo, G., Hamilton, J. A., Nice, E. C. Purification of two forms of colony-stimulating factor from mouse L-cell-conditioned medium. *J. Biol. Chem. 260,* 16004-16011 (1985).
43. Stanley, E. R., Guilbert, L. J., Tushinski, R. J., Bartelmez, S. H. CSF-1: a mononuclear phagocyte lineage-specific hemopoietic growth factor. *J. Cell. Biochem. 21,* 151-159 (1983).
44. Tushinski, R. J., Oliver, I. T., Guilbert, L. J., Tynan, P. W., Warner, J. R., Stanley, E. R. Survival of mononuclear phagocytes depends on a lineage-specific growth factor that the differentiated cells selectively destroy. *Cell 28,* 71-81 (1982).
45. Stanley, E. R. The macrophage colony-stimulating factor, CSF-1. *Methods Enzymol. 116/H,* G. DiSabato, J. J. Langone, H. VanVunakis, Eds., Academic Press, New York, pp. 564-587 (1985).
46. Morgan, C. J., Stanley, E. R. Chemical crosslinking of the mononuclear phagocyte specific growth factor CSF-1 to its receptor at the cell surface. *Biochem. Biophys. Res. Commun. 119,* 35-41 (1984).
47. Guilbert, L. J., Stanley, E. R. Specific interaction of murine colony-stimulating factor with mononuclear phagocytic cells. *J. Cell. Biol. 85,* 153-159 (1980).
48. Sherr, C. J., Rettermier, C. W., Sacca, R., Roussel, M. F., Look, A. T., Stanley, E. R. The c-fms proto-oncogene product is related to the receptor for the mononuclear phagocyte growth factor, CSF-1. *Cell 41,* 665-676 (1985).
49. Kawasaki, E. S., Ladner, M. B., Wang, A. M., Arsdell, J. V., Warren, M. K., Coyne, M. Y., Schweickart, V. L., Lee, M. T., Wilson, K. J., Boosman, A., Stanley, E. R., Ralph, P., Mark, D. F. Molecular cloning of a complementary DNA encoding human macrophage-specific colony-stimulating factor (CSF-1). *Science 230,* 291-296 (1985).
50. Sachs, L., Lotem, J. Haematopoietic growth factors [letter]. *Nature 312,* 407 (1984).

51. Sachs, L. In: *Molecular biology of tumor cells* (Prog. Cancer Res. Therap. Ser., Vol. 32) Wahren, B., Holm, G. (Eds.). Raven Press, New York, pp. 257-280 (1985).
52. Lotem, J., Sachs, L. Control of in vivo differentiation of myeloid leukemic cells. IV. Inhibition of leukemia development by myeloid differentiation-inducing protein. *Int. J. Cancer 33,* 147-154 (1984).
53. Lotem, J., Sachs, L. Mechanisms that uncouple growth and differentiation in myeloid leukemia cells: restoration of requirement for normal growth-inducing protein without restoring induction of differentiation-inducing protein. *Proc. Natl. Acad. Sci. USA 79,* 4347-4351 (1982).
54. Weisinger, G., Sachs, L. DNA-binding protein that induces cell differentiation. *EMBO J. 2,* 2103-2107 (1983).
55. Smith, C. A., Rennick, D. M. Characterization of a murine lymphokine distinct from interleukin 2 and interleukin 3 (IL-3) possessing a T-cell growth factor activity and a mast-cell growth factor activity that synergizes with IL-3. *Proc. Natl. Acad. Sci. USA 8,* 1857-1861 (1986).
56. Lee, F., Yokota, T., Otsuka, T., Meyerson, P., Villaret, D., Coffman, R., Mosmann, T., Rennick, D., Roehm, N., Smith, C., Zlotnik, A., Arai, K. Isolation and characterization of a mouse interleukin cDNA clone that expresses B-cell stimulatory factor 1 activities and T-cell- and mast-cell-stimulating activities. *Proc. Natl. Acad. Sci. USA 83,* 2061-2065 (1985).
57. Noma, Y., Sideras, P., Naito, T., Bergstedt-Lindquist, S., Azuma, C., Severinson, E., Tanabe, T., Kinashi, T., Matsuda, F., Yaoita, Y., Honjo, T. Cloning of cDNA encoding the murine IgG1 induction factor by a novel strategy using SP6 promoter. *Nature 319,* 640-646 (1986).
58. Zipori, D. Cultured stromal cell lines. In: *Regulation of blood cell formation: the role of the hemopoietic microenvironment.* Tavassoli, M. (Ed.). Humana Press, New Jersey, in press (1987).
59. Freidenstein, A. J., Chailakhjan, R. K., Latsink, N. V., Panasyuk, A. F., Keilis-Borok, I. V. Stromal cells responsible for transferring the microenvironment of the hemopoietic tissues. Cloning in vitro and retransplantation in vivo. *Transplantation 17,* 331-340 (1974).
60. Dexter, T. M., Allen, T. D., Lajtha, L. G. Conditions controlling the proliferation of hemopoietic stem cells in vitro. *J. Cell. Physiol. 91,* 335-344 (1977).
61. Allen, T. D., Dexter, T. M. Long term bone marrow cultures: an ultrastructural review. *Scanning Electron Microsc. 4,* 1851-1866 (1983).
62. Alberts, B., Bray, D., Lewis, J., Raff, M., Roberts, K., Watson, J. D. *Molecular biology of the cell,* Garland, New York, p. 873 (1983).
63. Sternberg, P. W., Horvitz, H. R. Pattern formation during vulval development in *C. elegans. Cell 44,* 761-772 (1986).
64. Weiss, L. The histology of the bone marrow. In: *Regulation of hematopoiesis,* Vol. I. Gordon, A. S. (Ed.). Appleton-Century-Crofts, New York, pp. 79-92 (1970).
65. Weiss, L. The hemopoietic microenvironment of bone marrow: an ultrastructural study of the interactions of blood cells, stroma and blood vessels. In: *Blood cell and vessel wall: functional interactions* (Ciba Foundation Series 71). Elsevier, New York, pp. 3-19 (1980).

66. Lambertsen, R. H., Weiss, L. A model of intramedullary hematopoietic microenvironments based on stereologic study of the distribution of endocloned marrow colonies. *Blood 63,* 287-297 (1984).
67. Frassoni, F., Testa, N. G., Lord, B. I. The relative spatial distribution of erythroid progenitor cells (BFUe and CFUe) in the normal mouse femur. *Cell Tissue Kinet. 15,* 447-455 (1982).
68. Kilchherr, F., Baumgartner, S., Bopp, D., Frei, E., Noll, M. Isolation of the paired gene of *Drosophila* and its spatial expression during early embryogenesis. *Nature 321,* 493-499 (1986).
69. Coulter, D., Wieschaus, E. Segmentation genes and the distributions of transcripts. *Nature 321,* 472-474 (1986).
70. Wade, M. H., Trosko, J. E., Schindler, M. A fluorescence photobleaching assay of gap junction-mediated communication between human cells. *Science 232,* 429-522 (1986).
71. Schrader, J. W. Bone marrow differentiation in vitro. *Crit. Rev. Immunol. 4,* 197-277 (1983).
72. Schofield, R. The relationship between the spleen colony-forming cell and the haemopoietic stem cell. *Blood Cells 4,* 7-25 (1978).
73. Grossman, Z. The stem cell concept revisited: self-renewal capacity is a dynamic property of hemopoietic cells. *Leukemia Res. 10,* 937-950 (1986).
74. Grossman, Z. A new approach to the evolution of the blastic crisis from chronic myelocytic leukemia: dynamic interplay of cellular alterations and a changing microenvironment. *EMBO J. 5,* 671-677 (1986).
75. Cooper, M. D., Mulvaney, D., Coutinho, A., Cazenave, P. A. A novel cell surface molecule on early B-lineage cells. *Nature 321,* 616-618 (1986).
76. Zipori, D., Bol, S. The role of fibroblastoid cells and macrophages from mouse bone marrow in the in vitro growth promotion of hematopoietic tumor cells. *Exp. Hematol. 7,* 206-218 (1979).
77. Zipori, D. In vitro proliferation of mouse lymphoblastoid cell lines: growth modulation by various populations of adherent cells. *Cell Tissue Kinet. 13,* 287-298 (1980).
78. Eagle, H., Piez, K. The population-dependent requirement by cultured mammalian cells for metabolites which they can synthesize. *J. Exp. Med. 116,* 29-43 (1962).
79. Burger, M. Requirement of glycine or its polymers in the stimulation of human peripheral lymphocytes by phytohemagglutinin. *FEBS Lett. 73,* 155-158 (1977).
80. Epstein, A. L., Kaplan, H. S. Feeder layer and nutritional requirements for the establishment and cloning of human malignant lymphoma cell lines. *Cancer Res. 39,* 1748-1759 (1979).
81. Tooze, J. *The molecular biology of tumor viruses,* CSH, New York, p. 82 (1973).
82. Ishii, T., Hishinuma, I., Bannai, S., Sugita, Y. Mechanism of growth promotion of mouse lymphoma L1210 cells in vitro by feeder layer or 2-mercaptoethanol. *J. Cell. Physiol. 107,* 283-293 (1981).
83. Click, R. E., Benck, L., Alter, B. J. Enhancement of antibody synthesis in vitro by mercaptoethanol. *Cell. Immunol. 3,* 155-160 (1972).

84. Broome, J. D., Jeng, M. W. Promotion of replication in lymphoid cells by specific thiols and disulfides in vitro. *J. Exp. Med. 138,* 574-591 (1973).
85. Toohey, J. I. Sulfhydryl dependence in primary explant hematopoietic cells. Inhibition of growth in vitro with vitamin B_{12} compounds. *Proc. Natl. Acad. Sci. USA 72,* 73-77 (1975).
86. Hewlett, G., Opitz, H. G., Schlumberger, H. D., Lemke, H. Growth regulation of a murine lymphoma cell line by a 2-mercaptoethanol or macrophage-activated serum factor. *Eur. J. Immunol. 7,* 781-785 (1977).
87. Tanapat, P., Gaetjens, E., Broome, J. D. Growth promoting and inhibitory activities of 3T3 and other cell lines for thiol-dependent lymphoma in vitro. *Proc. Soc. Exp. Biol. Med. 157,* 517-521 (1978).
88. Burger, M. An absolute requirement for 2-mercaptoethanol in the in vitro primary immune response in the absence of serum. *Immunology 37,* 669-671 (1979).
89. Bannai, S., Ishii, T. Transport of cystine and cysteine and cell growth in cultured human diploid fibroblasts: effect of glutamate and homocysteate. *J. Cell. Physiol. 112,* 265-272 (1982).
90. Nara, N., McCulloch, E. A. Membranes replace irradiated blast cells as growth requirement for leukemic blast progenitors in suspention culture. *J. Exp. Med. 162,* 1435-1443 (1985).
91. Tanapat, P., Gaetjens, E., Broome, J. D. Production of autoinhibitory factors by mouse lymphoma cells in vitro and its relationship to thiol dependence. *Proc. Natl. Acad. Sci. USA 75,* 1849-1853 (1978).
92. Horowitz, J. B., Kaye, J., Conrad, P. J., Katz, M. E., Janeway, C. A., Jr. Autocrine growth inhibition of a cloned line of helper T cells. *Proc. Natl. Acad. Sci. USA 83,* 1886-1890 (1986).
93. Lynch, M. P., Nawaz, S., Gerschenson, L. E. Evidence for soluble factors regulating cell death and cell proliferation in primary cultures of rabbit endometrial cells grown on collagen. *Proc. Natl. Acad. Sci. USA 83,* 4784-4788 (1986).
94. Zipori, D., Toledo, J., von der Mark, K. Phenotypic heterogeneity among stromal cell lines from mouse bone marrow disclosed in their extracellular matrix composition and interactions with normal and leukemic cells. *Blood 66,* 447-455 (1985).
95. Resnitzky, D., Yarden, A., Zipori, D., Kimchi, A. Autocrine β-related interferon controls c-myc suppression and growth arrest during hematopoietic cell differentiation. *Cell 46,* 31-40 (1986).
96. Marx, J. L. The yin and yang of cell growth control. *Science 232,* 1093-1095 (1986).
97. Suda, J., Suda, T., Kubota, K., Ihle, J. N., Saito, M., Miura, Y. Purified interleukin-3 and erythropoietin support the terminal differentiation of hemopoietic progenitors in serum-free culture. *Blood 67,* 1002-1006 (1986).
98. Suda, T., Suda, J., Ogawa, M., Ihle, J. N. Permissive role of interleukin 3 (IL-3) in proliferation and differentiation of multipotential hemopoietic progenitors in culture. *J. Cell. Physiol. 124,* 182-190 (1985).
99. Dexter, T. M., Garland, J., Scott, D., Scolnick, E., Metcalf, D. Growth of factor-dependent hemopoietic cell lines. *J. Exp. Med. 152,* 1036-1047 (1980).

100. Farrar, W. L., Thomas, T. P., Anderson, W. B. Altered cytosol/membrane enzyme redistribution on interleukin 3 activation of protein kinase C. *Nature 315,* 235-237 (1985).
101. Kurland, J. I., Moore, M. A. S. Modulation of hemopoiesis by prostaglandins. *Exp. Hematol. 5,* 357-373 (1977).
102. Kurland, J. I., Bockman, R. S., Broxmeyer, H. E., Moore, M. A. S. Limitation of excessive myelopoiesis by the intrinsic modulation of macrophage derived prostaglandin E. *Science 199,* 552-555 (1978).
103. Kurland, J. I., Pelus, L. M., Ralph, P., Bockman, R. S., Moore, M. A. S. Induction of prostaglandin E synthesis in normal and neoplastic macrophages: role of colony stimulating factor(s) distinct from effects on myeloid progenitor cell differentiation. *Proc. Natl. Acad. Sci. USA 76,* 2326-2330 (1979).
104. Broxmeyer, H. E., Piacibello, W., Juliano, L., Platzer, E., Berman, E. Gamma interferon induces colony forming cells of the human monoblast cell line U937 to respond to inhibition by lactoferrin, transferrin and acidic isoferritins. *Exp. Hematol. 14,* 35-43 (1986).
105. Piachibello, W., Rubin, B., Broxmeyer, H. E. Prostaglandin E counteracts the gamma interferon induction of major histocompatibility complex class-II antigens on U937 cells and induction of responsiveness of U937 colony forming cells to suppression by lactoferrin, transferrin, acidic isoferritins and prostaglandin E. *Exp. Hematol. 14,* 44-50 (1986).
106. Ishikura, H., Okazaki, T., Mochizuki, T., Izumi, Y., Tashima, M., Sawada, H., Uchino, H. Effect of antimetabolites and thymidine blockage on the induction of differentiation of HL-60 cells by retinoic acid or 1α-25-dihydroxyvitamin D_3. *Exp. Hematol. 13,* 981-988 (1985).
107. Baptiste, L. C., Reid, C. D. L. Effect of T cells and monocytes on globin chain synthesis in erythroid bursts cultured from human peripheral blood burst forming units (BFU-e). *Exp. Hematol. 13,* 507-511 (1985).
108. Bartlett, P. F. Pluripotential hemopoietic stem cells in adult mouse brain. *Proc. Natl. Acad. Sci. USA 79,* 2722-2725 (1982).
109. McCulloch, E. A., Till, J. E. Proliferation of hemopoietic colony forming cells transplanted into irradiated mice. *Rad. Res. 22,* 383-397 (1966).
110. Harrison, D. E., Astle, C. M. Loss of stem cell repopulating ability upon transplantation: effect of donor age, cell number and transplantation procedure. *J. Exp. Med. 156,* 1767-1778 (1982).
111. Dexter, T. M., Moore, M. A. S., Sheridan, A. P. C. Maintenance of hemopoietic stem cells and production of differentiated progeny in allogeneic and semiallogeneic bone marrow chimeras. *J. Exp. Med. 145,* 1612-1616 (1977).
112. Dexter, T. M., Spooncer, E., Simmons, P., Allen, T. D. Long term marrow culture: an overview of techniques and experience. In: *Long-term bone marrow culture*, Alan R. Liss, New York, KROC Foundation Ser. (USA), pp. 57-96 (1984).
113. Toksoz, D., Dexter, T. M., Lord, B. I., Wright, E. G., Lajtha, L. G. The regulation of hemopoiesis in long-term bone marrow cultures II. Stimulation and inhibition of stem cell proliferation. *Blood 55,* 931-936 (1980).

114. Islam, A. Haemopoietic stem cell: a new concept. *Leukemia Res. 9,* 1415-1432 (1985).
115. Chertkov, J. L., Drize, N. J., Gurevitch, O. A., Samoylova, R. S. Origin of hemopoietic stromal progenitor cells in chimeras. *Exp. Hematol. 13,* 1217-1222 (1985).
116. Charbord, P., Gown, A. M., Keating, A., Singer, J. W. CGA-7 and HFF, two monoclonal antibodies that recognize muscle actin and react with adherent cells in human long-term bone marrow culture. *Blood 66,* 1138-1142 (1985).
117. Piersma, A. J., Ploemacher, R. E., Brockbank, K. G. M., Ottenheim, C. P. E. Monoclonal antibodies identify specific determinants on reticular cells in murine embryonic and adult hemopoietic stroma. In: *Experimental hematology today–1985.* Baum, S. J., Pluznik, D. H., Rozenszajn, L. A. (Eds.). Springer Verlag, New York, pp. 50-54 (1986).
118. Haas, M., Meshorer, A. Reticulum cell neoplasms induced in C57BL/6 mice by cultured virus grown in stromal hematopoietic cell lines. *J. Natl. Cancer Inst. 63,* 427-436 (1979).
119. Haas, M., Reshef, T. Non-thymic malignant lymphomas induced in C57BL/6 mice by cloned dualtropic viruses isolated from hematopoietic stromal cell lines. *Eur. J. Cancer 16,* 909-917 (1980).
120. Anderson, R. W., Mann, S. L., Crouse, D. A., Sharp, J. G. Modulation of one of three murine bone marrow stromal cell lines to adipose cells by serum and insulin. *J. Supramol. Struct. Cell. Biochem. 16,* 377-384 (1981).
121. Harigaya, K., Cronkite, E. P., Miller, M. E., Shadduck, R. K. Murine bone marrow cell line producing colony-stimulating factor. *Proc. Natl. Acad. Sci. USA 78,* 6963-6966 (1981).
122. Cronkite, E. P., Harigaya, K., Garnett, H., Miller, M. E., Honikel, L., Shadduck, R. K. Production of colony-stimulating factor by murine bone marrow cell line derived from the Dexter adherent layer and other properties of this cell line. In: *Experimental hematology today–1982.* Baum, S. J., Ledney, G. D., Thierfelder, S. (Eds.). S. Karger, Basel, pp. 11-18 (1982).
123. Lanotte, M., Allen, T. D., Dexter, T. M. Histological and ultrastructural characteristics of a cell line from human bone marrow stroma. *J. Cell. Sci. 50,* 281-297 (1981).
124. Lanotte, M., Scott, D., Dexter, T. M., Allen, T. D. Clonal preadipocyte cell lines with different phenotypes derived from murine marrow stroma: factors influencing growth and adipogenesis in vitro. *J. Cell. Physiol. 111,* 177-186 (1982).
125. Hines, D. Lipid accumulation and production of colony-stimulating activity by the 266AD cell line derived from mouse bone marrow. *Blood 61,* 397-402 (1983).
126. Godard, C. M., Augery, Y. L., Ginsbourg, M., Jasmin, C. Established cell lines of mouse marrow adherent cells producing differentiation factor(s) for the granulocyte-macrophage lineage. *In Vitro 19,* 897-902 (1983).
127. Fujita, J., Yoshida, O., Miyanomae, T., Mori, K. J. A colony-stimulating-factor producing cell line derived from mouse bone marrow cells transfected with adenovirus DNA. *Gann 74,* 334-337 (1983).

128. Zipori, D., Friedman, A., Tamir, M., Silverberg, D., Malik, Z. Cultured mouse marrow cell lines: interactions between fibroblastoid cells and monocytes. *J. Cell. Physiol. 118,* 143-152 (1984).
129. Zipori, D., Duksin, D., Tamir, M., Argaman, A., Toledo, J., Malik, Z. Cultured mouse marrow stromal cell lines. II. Distinct subtypes differing in morphology, collagen types, myelopoietic factors and leukemic cell growth modulating activities. *J. Cell. Physiol. 122,* 81-90 (1985).
130. Greenberger, J. S., Sakakeeny, M. A., Davis, L. M., Moloney, W. C., Reid, D. Biologic properties of factor-independent nonadherent hematopoietic and adherent preadipocyte cell lines derived from continuous bone marrow culture. *Leukemia Res. 8,* 363-375 (1984).
131. Li, C. L., Johnson, G. R. Stimulation of multipotential, erythroid and other murine haematopoietic progenitor cells by adherent cell lines in the absence of detectable multi-CSF (IL-3). *Nature 316,* 633-636 (1985).
132. Song, Z. X., Shadduck, R. K., Innes, D. J., Jr., Waheed, A., Quesenberry, P. J. Hematopoietic factor production by a cell line (TC-1) derived from adherent murine marrow cells. *Blood 66,* 273-281 (1985).
133. Katsuno, M., Motomura, S., Kaneko, S., Sakai, H., Ibayashi, H. A preadipocyte cell line derived from murine bone marrow stroma: characterization of morphological, enzymatic and functional nature of the cells. *Int. J. Cell Cloning 3,* 81-90 (1985).
134. Zipori, D. Stromal cell lines from mouse bone marrow: a model system for the study of the hemopoietic microenvironment. In: *Experimental hematology today–1985.* Baum, S. J., Pluznik, D. H., Rozenszajn, A. (Eds.). Springer-Verlag, New York, pp. 55-63 (1986).
135. Naparstek, E., Donnelly, T., Shadduck, R. K., Waheed, A., Wagner, K., Kase, K. R., Greenberger, J. S. Persistent production of colony-stimulating factor (CSF-1) by cloned bone marrow stromal cell line D2XRII after x-irradiation. *J. Cell. Physiol. 126,* 407-413 (1986).
136. Garnett, H. M., Harigaya, K., Cronkite, E. P. Characterization of a murine cell-line derived from cultured bone marrow stromal cells. *Stem Cells 2,* 11-23 (1982).
137. Garnett, H. M., Harigaya, K., Cronkite, E. P. Influence of a fibroblastoid cell line derived from murine bone marrow (H-1 cells) on stem cell proliferation. *Proc. Soc. Exp. Biol. Med. 175,* 70-73 (1984).
138. Lanotte, M., Metcalf, D., Dexter, T. M. Production of monocyte/macrophage colony stimulating factor by preadipocyte cell lines derived from murine marrow stroma. *J. Cell. Physiol. 112,* 123-127 (1982).
139. Garnett, H. M., Cronkite, E. P., Harigaya, K. Regulation of the colony-stimulating activity produced by a murine marrow-derived cell line (H-1). *Proc. Natl. Acad. Sci. USA 79,* 1545-1548 (1982).
140. Cronkite, E. P., Miller, M. E., Garnett, H., Harigaya, K. Regulation of hemopoiesis: inhibitors and stimulators produced by a murine bone marrow stromal cell line (H-1). In: *Haemopoietic stem cells.* Alfred Benzon Symposium 18. Killmann, S. A., Cronkite, E. P., Muller-Berat, C. N. (Eds.). Munksgaard, Copenhagen, pp. 266-284 (1983).

141. Shah, G., Dexter, T. M., Lanotte, M. Interferon production by human marrow stromal cells. *Brit. J. Haematol. 54,* 365-372 (1983).
142. Umiel, T., Friedman, S., Zaizov, R., Cohen, I. J., Gozes, Y., Epstein, N., Kobiler, D., Zipori, D. Long term culture of infant leukemia cells: dependence upon stromal cells from the bone marrow and bilineage differentiation. *Leukemia Res. 10,* 1007-1013 (1986).
143. Fujita, K., Shimomura, Y., Fujita, J., Mori, K. J. Granulocytosis induced in vivo by a mouse marrow stromal cell line BMA1 which produces colony stimulating factor. *Experientia 41,* 504-505 (1985).
144. Harigaya, K., Handa, H. Generation of functional clonal cell lines from human bone marrow stroma. *Proc. Natl. Acad. Sci. USA 82,* 3477-3480 (1985).
145. Piersma, A. H., Brockbank, K. G. M., Ploemacher, R. E. Regulation of in vitro myelopoiesis by a hematopoietic stromal fibroblastic cell line. *Exp. Hematol. 12,* 617-623 (1984).
146. Itoh, T., Kasahara, S., Mori, T. A thymic epithelial cell line IT-45R1 induces the differentiation of prethymic progenitor cells into postthymic cells through direct contact. *Thymus 4,* 69-75 (1982).
147. Itoh, T. Establishment of an epithelial cell line from rat thymus. *Am. J. Anat. 156,* 99-104 (1979).
148. Hays, E. F., Beardsley, T. R. Immunologic effects of human thymic stromal grafts and cell lines. *Clin. Immunol. Immunopathol. 33,* 381-390 (1984).
149. Kodama, H., Amagai, Y., Koyama, H., Kasai, S. A new preadipose cell line derived from newborn mouse calvaria can promote the proliferation of pluripotent hemopoietic stem cells in vitro. *J. Cell. Physiol. 112,* 89-95 (1982).
150. Kodama, H., Amagai, Y., Koyama, H., Kasai, S. Hormonal responsiveness of a preadipose cell line derived from newborn mouse calvaria. *J. Cell. Physiol. 112,* 83-88 (1982).
151. Kodama, H., Sudo, H., Koyama, H., Kasai, S., Yamamoto, S. In vitro hemopoiesis within a microenvironment created by MC3T3-G2/PA6 preadipocytes. *J. Cell. Physiol. 118,* 233-240 (1984).
152. Crocker, P. R., Gordon, S. Isolation and chracterization of resident stromal macrophages and hematopoietic cell clusters from mouse bone marrow. *J. Exp. Med. 162,* 993-1014 (1985).
153. Katsuno, M., Motomura, S., Kaneko, S., Hirata, J., Ibayashi, H. Quantitative study of marrow stromal precursor cells in sublethal x-irradiated mice. *Acta Hematol. Jap. 48,* 924-938 (1985).
154. Lim, B., Izaguirre, C. A., Aye, M. T., Huebsch, L., Drouin, J., Richardson, C., Minden, M. D., Messner, H. A. Characterization of reticulofibroblastoid colonies (CFU-RF) derived from bone marrow and long-term marrow culture monolayers. *J. Cell. Physiol. 127,* 45-54 (1986).
155. Arnold, E. A., Katsnelson, I., Hoffman, G. J. Proliferation and differentiation of hematopoietic stem cells in long-term cultures of adult hamster spleens. *J. Exp. Med. 155,* 1370-1384 (1982).

156. Whitlock, C. A., Witte, O. N. Long-term culture of B lymphocytes and their precursors from murine bone marrow. *Proc. Natl. Acad. Sci. USA 79,* 3608-3612 (1982).
157. Whitlock, C. A., Robertson, D., Witte, O. N. Murine B cell lymphopoiesis in long-term culture. *J. Immunol. Methods 67,* 353-369 (1984).
158. Dorshkind, K. In vitro differentiation of B lymphocytes from primitive hemopoietic precursors present in long-term bone marrow cultures. *J. Immunol. 136,* 422 (1986).
159. Johnson, A., Dorshkind, K. Stromal cells in myeloid and lymphoid long-term bone marrow cultures can support multiple hemopoietic lineages and modulate their production of hemopoietic growth factors. *Blood 68,* 1348-1354 (1986).
160. Zipori, D., Sasson, T. Adherent cells from mouse bone marrow inhibit the formation of colony-stimulating factor (CSF) induced myeloid colonies. *Exp. Hematol. 8,* 816-817 (1980).
161. Zipori, D., Sasson, T., Frenkel, A. Myelopoiesis in the presence of stromal cells from mouse bone marrow. I. Monosaccharides regulate colony formation. *Exp. Hematol. 9,* 656-662 (1981).
162. Zipori, D. Cell interactions in the bone marrow microenvironment: role of endogenous colony-stimulating activity. *J. Supramol. Struct. Cell. Biochem. 17,* 347-357 (1981).
163. Zipori, D., Sasson, T. Myelopoiesis in the presence of stromal cells from mouse bone marrow. II. Mechanism of glucose dependent colony formation. *Exp. Hematol. 9,* 663-673 (1981).
164. Zipori, D., Sasson, T., Friedman, S. Bone marrow resident colony stimulating factor activity (CSA) produced by stromal cells. In: *Experimental hematology today–1982.* Baum, S. J., Ledney, G. D., Thierfelder, S. (Eds.). S. Karger, Basel, pp. 19-26 (1982).
165. Siminovitch, L., McCulloch, E. A., Till, J. E. The distribution of colony-forming cells among spleen colonies. *J. Cell Comp. Physiol. 62,* 327-336 (1963).
166. Siminovitch, L., Till, J. E., McCulloch, E. A. Decline in colony-forming ability of marrow cells subjected to serial transplantation into irradiated mice. *J. Cell Comp. Physiol. 64,* 23-32 (1964).
167. Leminschka, I. R., Raulet, D. H., Mulligan, R. C. Developmental potential and dynamic behavior of hematopoietic stem cells. *Cell 45,* 917-927 (1986).
168. Dexter, T. M., Whetton, A. D., Spooncer, E., Heyworth, C., Simmons, P. The role of stromal cells and growth factors in hemopoiesis and modulation of their effects by the src oncogene. *J. Cell Sci. Suppl. 3,* 83-95 (1985).
169. Tsai, S., Sieff, C. A., Nathan, D. G. Stromal cell-associated erythropoiesis. *Blood 67,* 1418-1426 (1986).
170. Zipori, D. Conditions required for the inhibition of in vitro growth of a mouse myeloma cell line by adherent bone marrow cells. *Cell Tissue Kinet. 14,* 479-488 (1981).
171. Zipori, D., Tamir, M., Toledo, J., Oren, T. Differentiation stage and lineage specific inhibitor from mouse stroma that restricts lymphoma cell growth. *Proc. Natl. Acad. Sci. USA 83,* 4547-4551 (1986).

172. Ashton, B. A., Allan, T. D., Howlett, C. R., Eaglesom, C. C. Hattori, A., Owen, M. Formation of bone and cartilage by marrow stromal cells in diffusion chambers in vivo. *Clin. Orthopaed. Related Res. 151,* 294-307 (1980).
173. Brockbank, K. G., Ploemacher, R. E., van Peer, C. M. Splenic accumulation of stromal progenitor cells in response to bacterial lipopolysaccharides. *Exp. Hematol. 11,* 358-363 (1983).
174. Rosenfeld, M., Keating, A., Bowen-Pope, D. F., Singer, J. W. Ross, R. Responsiveness of the in vitro hematopoietic microenvironment to platelet-derived growth factor. *Leukemia Res. 9,* 427-434 (1985).
175. Quesenberry, P. J., Coppola, M. A., Gualtieri, R. J., Wade, P. M., Song, Z., Doukes, M. A., Shideler, C. E., Baker, D. G., McGrath, E. H. Lithium stimulation of murine hematopoiesis in liquid culture: an effect mediated by marrow stromal cells. *Blood 63,* 121-127 (1984).
176. Gaido, K., Wierda, D. In vitro effects of benzene metabolites on mouse bone marrow. *Toxicol. Appl. Pharmacol. 76,* 45-55 (1984).
177. Garnett, H. M., Cronkite, E. P., Drew, R. T. Effect of in vivo exposure to benzene on the characteristics of bone marrow adherent cells. *Leukemia Res. 7,* 803-810 (1983).
178. Ben-Ishay, Z., Prindull, G., Sharon, S., Borenstein, A. Effects of chemotherapy on bone marrow stroma in mice with acute myelogenous leukemia. Correlation with CFU-C and CFU-D. *Leukemia Res. 9,* 1059-1067 (1985).
179. de Jong, J. P., Nikkels, P. G., Brockbank, K. G., Ploemacher, R. E. Voerman, J. S. Comparative in vitro effects of cyclophosphamide derivatives on murine bone marrow-derived stromal and hemopoietic progenitor cell classes. *Cancer Res. 45,* 4001-4005 (1985).
180. McManus, P. M., Weiss, L. Busulfan-induced chronic bone marrow failure: changes in cortical bone, marrow stromal cells, and adherent cell colonies. *Blood 64,* 1036-1041 (1984).
181. Gallicchio, V. S., Chen, M. G., Watts, T. D. Regeneration of murine megakaryocytopoiesis and the hematopoietic inductive microenvironment after sublethal whole body irradiation by treatment with an anabolic steroid. *Acta Haematol. 73,* 80-85 (1985).
182. Piersma, A. H., Brockbank, K. G., Ploemacher, R. E., Ottenheim, C. P. Recovery of hemopoietic stroma progenitor cells after lethal total-body irradiation and bone marrow transplantation. *Transplantation 40,* 198-201 (1985).
183. Laver, J., Ebell, W., Castro-Malaspina, H. Radiobiological properties of the human hematopoietic microenvironment: contrasting sensitivities of proliferative capacity and hematopoietic function to in vitro irradiation. *Blood 67,* 1090-1097 (1986).
184. Hendry, J. H. The cellular basis of long-term marrow injury after irradiation. *Radiother. Oncol. 3,* 331-338 (1985).
185. Ploemacher, R. E., Brockbank, K. G. M., Brons, R. H. C., de Ruiter, H. Latent sustained injury of murine hemopoietic organ stroma induced by ionizing irradiation. *Haematologica 68,* 454-468 (1983).

186. Wang, S. B., Hendry, J. H., Testa, N. G. Thermal sensitivity of haemopoietic and stromal progenitor cells in different proliferative states. *Brit. J. Cancer 52,* 51-54 (1985).
187. Gualtieri, R. J., Shadduck, R. K., Baker, D. G., Quesenberry, P. J. Hematopoietic regulatory factors produced in long-term murine bone marrow cultures and the effect of in vitro irradiation. *Blood 64,* 516-525 (1984).
188. Naparstek, E., Donnelly, T., Kase, K., Greenberger, J. S. Biologic effects of in vitro x-irradiation of murine long-term bone marrow culture on the production of granulocyte-macrophage colony-stimulating factor. *Exp. Hematol. 13,* 701-708 (1985).
189. Zipori, D., Reichman, N., Arcavi, L., Shtalrid, M., Berrebi, A., Resnitzky, P. In vitro functions of stromal cells from human and mouse bone marrow. *Exp. Hematol. 13,* 603-609 (1985).
190. Juneja, H. S., Gardner, F. H. Functionally abnormal marrow stromal cells in aplastic anemia. *Exp. Hematol. 13,* 194-199 (1985).
191. Ben-Ishay, Z., Prindull, G., Borenstein, A., Sharon, S. Bone marrow stromal deficiency in acute myeloid leukemia in mice. *Leukemia Res. 8,* 1057-1064 (1984).
192. Zipori, D., van Bekkum, D. W. Changes in the fibroblastoid colony-forming unit population from mouse bone marrow in early stages of Soule virus induced murine leukemia. *Exp. Hematol. 7,* 137-144 (1979).

3

Myelosuppressive Effects of Antineoplastic Chemotherapy

ROBERT PETER GALE
University of California–Los Angeles School of Medicine, Los Angeles, California

I. INTRODUCTION

Substantial advances have been made in the development and use of antineoplastic drugs in humans. Several cancers can now be cured by chemotherapy. Much of this progress relates to the design of combination chemotherapy regimens utilizing active drugs in optimal dose and schedule.

The efficacy of most antineoplastic drugs is dose-dependent; higher doses result in increased response rates and a higher proportion of cures (1,2). The major dose-limiting toxicity of many anticancer drugs is myelosuppression. Table 1 summarizes the relative degree of myelosuppression associated with several commonly used drugs at conventional doses. These drugs can be separated into three groups: some drugs are rarely associated with bone marrow toxicity; a second group typically cause mild to moderate myelosuppression; the third is associated with predictable and potentially severe dose-limiting hemopoietic toxicity.

The rate at which myelosuppression is produced by drugs is also variable. Hemopoietic toxicity occurs rapidly with some drugs, usually within 2-3 days. For example, hydroxyurea produces a rapid decrease in granulocytes. Anthracyclines and antimetabolites typically reduce granulocytes after 1-3 weeks. Nitrosoureas and mitomycin C in standard doses result in more delayed myelosuppression with granulocyte nadirs at 6-8 weeks. At higher doses these drugs produce more rapid suppression of bone marrow function. The myelosuppressive effects of anticancer drugs are also schedule- and route-dependent. Factors thought to be important in determining the degree of bone marrow suppression with antineoplastic drugs are summarized in Table 2. As indicated, the antitumor activity for many anticancer drugs is also dose-dependent. A similar relationship frequently exists

Table 1 Levels of Severity in Myelosuppressive Effects of Antineoplastic Drugs by Group

Absent to mild	
Vincristine	Hormones
Bleomycin	Tamoxifen
L-Asparaginase	
Moderate	
Vinblastine/vindesine	Methotrexate
Actinomycin D	Purine analogs
Epipodophyllotoxins	Hexamethylmelanine
Cisplatin	Procarbazine
Severe	
Alkylating agents	Anthraquinones
Anthracyclines	Mitomycin C
Nitrosoureas	Pyramidine analogs
Methotrexate	Hydroxyurea

Table 2 Factors Affecting the Time Course of Myelosuppression

Nature of drug
Mechanism of action
Dose (total dose as well as dose per treatment)
Schedule of administration
Route of administration
Combined chemotherapy with other drugs
Prior chemotherapy
Prior radiation therapy

for the myelosuppressive effects of these agents. Consequently there is often only a minimal or no therapeutic margin of these drugs for tumor cells versus normal bone marrow cells.

II. MECHANISMS OF MYELOSUPPRESSION

Mechanisms by which antineoplastic cells produce bone marrow suppression are summarized in Table 3. Drug-related myelosuppression can be divided into two major groups: direct and indirect. Direct refers to the interaction of a drug or its

Table 3 Mechanisms of Myelosuppression

Direct	
	Myeloid cell
	Hemopoietic stem cells
	Lethality vs. proliferative defects
	Imbalances in self-renewal, differentiation, maturation
Indirect	
	Microenvironment
	Hemopoietic growth factors
	Immune system
	Blood vessels
	Hemolytic-uremic syndrome
	Activation of coagulation
	Azotemia

Table 4 Immune Mechanisms of Drug-Induced Myelosuppression

Imbalances in T cells or macrophages
Effects on lymphokines
Antibody synthesis
Immune suppression leading to infection

metabolites with myeloid cells or their progenitors. The precise nature of these interactions has not been studied extensively in most instances. Possible mechanisms include a direct toxic effect, induction of a proliferative defect, or an imbalance between self-renewal and cell differentiation or maturation. Conceptually the result is either to decrease the size of the myeloid compartment or to change the distribution of stem cells and their progeny within the compartment; likely both occur (3-10). These concepts are reviewed by Lohrmann and Schreml in Chapter 14, this volume.

Antineoplastic drugs can also affect hemopoietic cells indirectly by interactions with the bone marrow microenvironment or by affecting hemopoietic growth or regulatory factors. An example is busulfan, which is toxic to bone marrow stromal cells as well as to hemopoietic stem cells. Hemopoietic suppression can also occur via immune-mediated mechanisms such as by causing imbalances in regulatory cells or factors or by inducing an antibody response to hemopoietic cells after binding of the drug or its metabolite to the cell membrane. Finally, administration of immunosuppressive drugs predisposes the patient to infections that secondarily inhibit hemopoiesis. Examples include disseminated cytomegalovirus infections in bone marrow transplant recipients (11,12) and non-A, non-B hepatitis (13,14). Possible immune interactions are summarized in Table 4.

Several other indirect interactions also occur between antineoplastic drugs and hemopoietic cells. For example, mitomycin C affects endothelial cells that line blood vessels and can result in microangiopathic hemolytic anemia (15). In rare instances this can eventuate in bone marrow failure. The use of antileukemia drugs in patients with acute progranulocytic leukemia can result in disseminated intravascular coagulation (DIC) (16,17). Actinomycin D is also associated with a DIC-like syndrome. Coagulation factors are also affected by drugs that inhibit protein synthesis, such as L-asparaginase (18,19). Factors II (prothrombin), V, VII, and VIII are typically affected. Finally, several antineoplastic drugs are nephrotoxic and can cause uremia; examples are cisplatin and mitomycin C. These agents indirectly affect hemopoiesis, since uremia is a well-documented cause of anemia and leukopenia; the precise mechanism of this effect is complex.

III. KINETICS OF MYELOSUPPRESSION

As indicated, the time course of myelosuppression that follows treatment with antineoplastic drugs is variable and depends on several factors including the nature of the drug, the mechanism of bone marrow suppression, dose, schedule, route, interactions with other drugs, the extent of prior chemotherapy and/or radiation, and other factors. Antineoplastic drugs can be divided into four groups based on whether they cause immediate, early, delayed, or latent bone marrow suppression (Table 5). Drugs such as hydroxyurea or prednisone cause a rapid reduction in blood cells detectable within 12-48 hr. With prednisone, this may result from a redistribution of cells rather than from their destruction. An immediate response is, however, unusual; most antineoplastic agents produce an early predictable reduction in blood counts occurring 1-3 weeks after administration. Usually this results from the effect of these agents on immature hemopoietic cells that becomes evident as more mature cells die and require replacement. Granulo-

Table 5 Types of Myelosuppression Following Antineoplastic Drugs

	Time	Examples
Immediate	0-48 hr	Hydroxyurea, radiation[a]
Early	1-3 weeks	Alkylators, anthracyclines
Delayed	6-8 weeks	Nitrosoureas, mitomycin C
Latent	–	Busulfan

[a]High-dose radiation.

cytes have the shortest life span (24-48 hr); as a consequence, a reduction in granulocytes is often the first detectable effect of antineoplastic drugs. Platelets (life span 10 days) are usually the next affected cell type followed by red blood cells (life span 120 days). Rarely, drugs such as the nitrosoureas and mitomycin C cause a delayed form of myelosuppression 4-8 weeks after drug administration. This delayed type of myelosuppression is thought to result from a relatively selective effect on immature hemopoietic stem cells. This effect requires several weeks to become evident. Recent data indicate that the time of occurrence of this delayed effect on hemopoiesis is dose-dependent; two- to threefold escalation of drug doses results in suppression of hemopoiesis within 1 week.

A fourth type of drug-induced myelosuppression is referred to as latent. This effect has been studied primarily in animal models (20-23). Under appropriate experimental conditions busulfan-treated mice maintain normal levels of circulating blood cells but have markedly decreased myeloid stem cells (GM-CFC) in their bone marrow. This defect may be evident only when the animals are stressed (24). The pathophysiologic basis of this abnormality is complex and is likely related to busulfan-induced damage to stem cells, to the bone marrow microenvironment, and possibly to lymphoid cells.

The precise mechanisms by which antineoplastic drugs inhibit hemopoiesis are largely undefined and do not necessarily reflect the mode by which the drugs affect neoplastic cells. For example, bone marrow target cells of several alkylating agents are dissimilar (Fig. 1). Cyclophosphamide, a potent alkylating agent, is thought to have a greater effect on mature than on immature hemopoietic stem cells (4). In contrast, busulfan seems to affect predominantly immature stem cells. The action of melphelan (L-phenylalanine mustard) is intermediate. Vinca alkaloids, which act primarily by inhibition of tubulin, also have diverse effects on hemopoiesis (Fig. 2). Vincristine is relatively devoid of myelosuppressive activity; in contrast, this is the dose-limiting toxicity of vinblastine. Vindesine is similar to vincristine but is more often associated with bone marrow toxicity. Epipodophyllotoxins, such as etoposide and teniposide, are myelosuppressive, but this is rarely their dose-limiting toxicity.

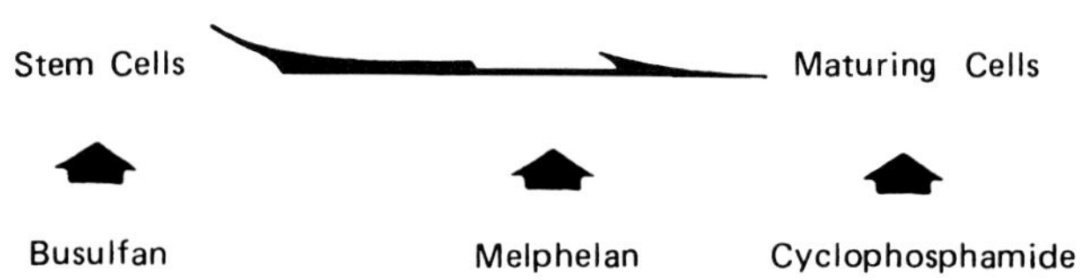

Figure 1 Differential myelosuppression of alkylating agents, showing the different points at which different drugs may act in the sequence of hematopoietic cell differentiation and maturation.

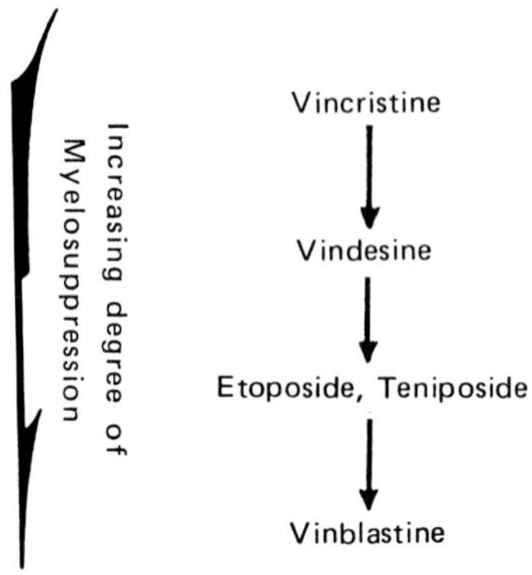

Figure 2 Myelosuppressive effects of tubulin-binding drugs, showing the variations in myelosuppressive activity of the vinca alkyloids.

IV. EVALUATION OF MYELOSUPPRESSION

Myelosuppression is a frequent and clinically important consequence of antineoplastic drugs. One important problem concerns how best to analyze these myelosuppressive effects. Potential approaches are indicated in Table 6. Some tests, such as blood counts and bone marrow cellularity, are relatively easily performed. Unfortunately, these tests may not detect subtle damage to hemopoietic cells. Detailed analyses of hemopoietic stem cells are now possible. Some are described elsewhere in this volume (Chapters 1, 4, 17, 18). Considerable data in animals and humans indicate that there can be disparities between blood counts, bone marrow cellularity, and assays of hemopoietic stem cells. Therefore, the precise

Table 6 Assessment of Myelosuppression

Techniques applicable to both humans and animals

1. Peripheral blood cell counts, WBC granulocytes, platelets, RBC
2. Bone marrow cellularity measurements
3. Bone marrow and marginal pool reserve estimates
4. Assays of committed hemopoietic stem cells. Includes quantitation and proliferation of GM-CFC, BFU-E, CFU-E, CFU-DG, Mix-CFC, and CFU-F in conventional and long-term cultures

Techniques applicable only in animals

1. CFU-S (pluripotent hemopoietic stem cell) assay
2. Serial transplantation of bone marrow cells through several sets of irradiated recipients

clinical interpretation and biological relevance of the stem cell assays is not certain. For example, we and others studied recovery of GM-CFCs in recipients of bone marrow transplants (25-29). We found that these patients had markedly reduced or absent GM-CFCs despite the presence of normal blood counts and bone marrow cellularity. This abnormality could be corrected by depletion of T lymphocytes in some, but not all, instances. These data suggest that some patients have intrinsic abnormalities in GM-CFCs, whereas others may have immune-mediated suppression of hemopoiesis (25). Several investigators have reported similar GM-CFC defects in transplant recipients and in patients receiving chemotherapy for leukemia (30-32). These data are reviewed by Emerson and myself, by Testa and co-workers, and by Miller and Weiner in this volume. Recently, long-term culture systems of bone marrow cells have been developed. Although these cultures are difficult to perform and evaluate, they may prove useful in assessing drug-induced damage to the bone marrow microenvironment (33).

In animals, serial transplantation studies and in vivo assays of pluripotent hemopoietic stem cells (CFU-S) are the most sensitive and biologically relevant means of detecting toxicity to hemopoietic stem cells. This technique is not applicable to humans, and it is therefore necessary to use the less direct and less sensitive approaches such as in vitro assays of stem cells in semisolid matrices or long-term cultures. Recently new stem cell assays such as the blast cell assay or Mix-CFC-macro have also been reported that may more closely correlate with in vivo bone marrow repopulating capacity.

V. FUTURE DIRECTIONS

Increasingly sophisticated studies of the myelosuppressive effects of antineoplastic drugs are in progress. Several recent studies are summarized in this volume. Potential directions of this research and implications for cancer therapy are indicated in Table 7. Hopefully these studies will more precisely define mechanisms responsible for

Table 7 Future Directions

1. Achieve a more precise definition of mechanism of myelosuppression.
2. Distinguish antitumor from myelosuppressive mechanisms.
3. Develop means to circumvent myelosuppression.
4. Design new drugs.
5. Develop less myelotoxic combination chemotherapy.
6. Investigate autologous bone marrow transplants.
7. Develop antibody targeting of tumor cells.
8. Develop liposome-delivery mechanisms for chemotherapy.
9. Investigate the applicability of regional chemotherapy.

the myelosuppressive effects of antineoplastic drugs. If this can be accomplished, it may be possible to distinguish those features of drugs responsible for antitumor effects from those responsible for bone marrow toxicity. These two activities need not be identical. Alternatively, it may be possible to develop dose, schedule, or route modifications that increase therapeutic index. Data generated from these studies may also facilitate development of new drugs or congeners that decrease myelosuppression.

Several techniques have been developed to circumvent or decrease the myelosuppressive effects of antineoplastic drugs. These include bone marrow autotransplantation or "rescue," liposome-entrapped drugs, antibody-directed drugs, radionuclides or immunotoxins, regional chemotherapy, and others.

Bone marrow autotransplantation is already reasonably advanced. It is well established that otherwise irreversible myelosuppression can be circumvented by rescue with autologous cryopreserved bone marrow cells (for reviews see Refs. 34-37). Several interesting conclusions are suggested by these data. First, it is possible to achieve long-term disease-free survival in a small proportion of patients whose cancer is resistant to conventional doses of drugs and radiation. Second, the degree of dose escalation achievable with this approach is limited to one- to threefold rather than the several log-orders typical of tumor resistance in experimental systems. This implies that if bone marrow autotransplants are to succeed they should be performed earlier in the course of the disease. Several controlled trials comparing bone marrow autotransplants with intensive consolidation chemotherapy are in progress. Recent reports suggest favorable results in selected tumors including Hodgkin and non-Hodgkin lymphoma, neuroblastoma, testicular cancer, breast cancer, myeloma, ovarian cancer, melanoma, and others (38). Autotransplants are also being used to treat leukemia with favorable results (39); controlled trials, however, have not been reported.

The observation that the dose of antineoplastic drugs that could be administered in most instances can be increased by only one- to threefold even in the context of bone marrow autotransplantation suggests that it will be necessary to contend with the myelosuppressive effects of antineoplastic drugs in the immediate future. Hopefully, studies of the type proposed will lead to increased understanding and optimal use of antineoplastic drugs.

Another important area of investigation relates to the use of adjuvant chemotherapy or radiation (40). Substantial numbers of individuals with cancer are now treated with adjuvant chemotherapy; many will become long-term survivors. Hemopoiesis in these individuals is now being studied (4,41,42). Clearly these data will be important in determining the risk-benefit ratio of this approach. These data are reviewed by Lohrman and Schreml in this volume.

VI. SUMMARY

Antineoplastic drugs have diverse effects on hemopoiesis. Some drugs directly affect myeloid stem cells or their progenitors; others affect hemopoiesis indirectly.

Drugs with a direct effect usually decrease blood cells and bone marrow cellularity; at high doses they cause bone marrow aplasia. This type of toxicity is usually reversible. Antineoplastic drugs can also alter normal hemopoiesis by affecting the bone marrow microenvironment or by interactions with cells or factors that regulate hemopoiesis. The most common means of directly assessing the myelosuppressive effects of antineoplastic drugs involves measurements of blood cells or of bone marrow cellularity. More detailed analyses include assessment of hemopoietic stem cells or of bone marrow reserve. Bone marrow microenvironmental abnormalities are difficult to evaluate critically in humans, as are effects on the immune system. The recent development of assays of hemopoietic growth regulatory factors (erythropoietin, colony-stimulating factors, interleukins) may permit a more precise basis for the assessment of drug effects on bone marrow function. It is likely that an increased understanding of the mechanisms of myelosuppression induced by antineoplastic drugs will lead to the development of drugs with increased therapeutic ratios or to the more effective use of current drugs. Alternatively, the use of molecular cloned hemopoietic growth factors, such as GM-CSF or Interleukin-3, either pre- or postchemotherapy, may permit the use of higher doses of myelotoxic drugs.

REFERENCES

1. Frei, E., III, Canellos, G. P. Dose: a critical factor in cancer chemotherapy. *Am. J. Med. 69,* 585 (1980).
2. Hryniuk, W., Bush, H. The importance of dose intensity in chemotherapy of metastatic breast cancer. *J. Clin. Oncol. 2,* 1281-1288 (1984).
3. Lohrmann, H.-P., Schreml, W. Cytotoxic drugs and the granulopoietic system. *Rec. Res. Cancer Res. 81,* (1982).
4. Schreml, W., Lohrmann, H.-P., Anger, B. Stem cell defects after cytoreductive therapy in man. *Exp. Hematol. 13* (*Suppl. 16*), 31-42 (1985).
5. Schofield, R. The relationship between the spleen colony-forming cell and the haemopoietic stem cell. A hypothesis. *Blood Cells 4,* 7-25 (1978).
6. Botnick, L. E., Hannon, E. C., Hellman, S. Limited proliferation of stem cells surviving alkylating agents. *Nature 162,* 68-70 (1976).
7. Botnick, L. E., Hannon, E. C., Hellman, S. Multisystem stem cell failure after apparent recovery from alkylating agents. *Cancer Res. 38,* 1942-1947 (1978).
8. Hellman, S., Botnick, L. E., Hannon, E. C., Vigneulle, R. M. Proliferative capacity of murine hematopoietic stem cells. *Proc. Natl. Acad. Sci. USA 75,* 490-494 (1978).
9. Fried, W., Barone, J. Residual marrow damage following therapy with cyclophosphamide. *Exp. Hematol. 8,* 610-614 (1980).
10. Hellman, S., Botnick, L. E. Stem cell depletion: an explanation of the late effects of cytotoxins. *Int. J. Radiat. Oncol. Biol. Phys. 2,* 181-184 (1977).
11. Winston, D. J., Ho, W. G., Gale, R. P., Champlin, R. E. Treatment and prevention of interstitital pneumonia after bone marrow transplant. In: *Progress in bone marrow transplantation.* Gale, R. P., Champlin, R. E. (eds.). Alan R. Liss, New York, pp. 525-544 (1987).

12. Meyers, J. D., Shepp, D. H., Bowden, R. A., Reed, R. C. Viral infections in marrow transplant recipients. In: *Progress in bone marrow transplantation.* Gale, R. P., Champlin, R. E. (eds.). Alan R. Liss, New York, pp. 454-562 (1987).
13. Zeldis, J. B., Dienstag, J. L., Gale, R. P. Aplastic anemia and non-A, non-B hepatitis. *Am. J. Med. 74,* 64-68 (1983).
14. Hagler, L., Pastore, R. A., Bergin, J. J. Aplastic anemia following viral hepatitis: report of two fatal cases and literature review. *Medicine* (*Baltimore*) *54,* 139-164 (1975).
15. Carter, S. K., Crooke, S. T. (eds.). *Mitomycin C: current status and new developments.* Academic Press, New York (1979).
16. Gralnick, H. R., Abrell, E. Studies of the procoagulant and fibrinolytic activity of promyelocytes in acute promyelocytic leukemia. *Brit. J. Haematol. 24,* 89-99 (1973).
17. Collins, A. J., Bloomfield, C. D., Peterson, B. A., McKenna, R. W., Edison, J. R. Acute progranulocytic leukemia. Management of the coagulopathy during daunorubicin-prednisone induction. *Arch. Intern. Med. 138,* 1677-1680 (1978).
18. Haskell, C. M., Canellos, G. P., Leventhal, B. G., et al. L-Asparaginase: therapeutic and toxic effects in patients with neoplastic disease. *New Engl. J. Med. 281,* 1028-1034 (1969).
19. Sills, R. H., Nelson, D. A., Stockman, J. A., III. L-Asparaginase induced coagulopathy during therapy of acute lymphocytic leukemia. *Med. Pediatr. Oncol. 4,* 311 (1978).
20. Morley, A., Blake, J. An animal model of chronic aplastic marrow failure. I. Late marrow failure after busulfan. *Blood 44,* 49-56 (1974).
21. Morley, A., Blake, J. Haemopoietic precursor cells in experimental hypoplastic marrow failure. *Aust. J. Exp. Biol. Med. Sci. 52,* 909-914 (1974).
22. Morley, A., Trainor, K., Blake, J. A primary stem cell lesion in experimental chronic hypoplastic marrow failure. *Blood 45,* 681-688 (1975).
23. Morley, A. A., Trainor, K. J., Seshadri, R. S. Chronic hypoplastic marrow failure and residual injury. *Blood Cells 4,* 253-266 (1978).
24. Fitchen, J. H., Cline, M. J. The effect of granulopoietic stress in mice with 'latent' bone marrow failure. *Exp. Hematol. 8,* 788-794 (1980).
25. Li, S., Champlin, R. E., Fitchen, J. H., Gale, R. P. Abnormalities of myeloid progenitor cells following "successful" bone marrow transplantation. *J. Clin. Invest. 75,* 234-241 (1985).
26. Arnold, R., Schmeiser, T., Heit, W., Frickhofen, N., Pabst, G., Heimpel, H., Kubanek, B. Hematopoietic reconstitution after bone marrow transplantation. *Exp. Hematol. 14,* 271-277 (1986).
27. Raghavachan, A., Frickhofen, N., Arnold, R., Schmeiser, T., Prozsolt, F., Heimpel, H. Hematopoietic colony formation after allogeneic bone marrow transplantation: enhancement by cyclosporin A and anti-γ-(immune) interferon antiserum *in vitro. Exp. Hematol. 14,* 621-625 (1986).
28. Arnold, R., Heit, W., Heimpel, H., Frickhofen, N., Schneiser, T., Kubanek, B. The reconstitution of haemopoietic precursors after bone marrow transplantation. *Exp. Hematol. 10* (*Suppl. 10*), 79-82 (1982).
29. Gale, R. P., Emerson, S. G. Hematopoietic engraftment and differentiation following bone marrow transplantation. This volume, Chapter 15.

30. Haworth, C., Morris-Jones, P. H., Testa, N. G. Long-term bone marrow damage in children treated for ALL: evidence from *in vitro* colony assays (GM-CFC and CFU-F). *Brit. J. Cancer 46,* 918-923 (1982).
31. Paschel, C., Kowalinka, G., Geissler, D., Braunsteiner, H. In vitro growth of erythropoietic progenitor cells in long-term remission of acute leukemia. *Int. J. Cell Cloning 4,* 186-191 (1986).
32. Ganser, A., Hoelzer, D. Effect of intensified chemotherapy on the pluripotent haematopoietic progenitor cells CFU-GEMM in adult acute lymphoblastic leukaemia. *Brit. J. Haematol. 64,* 169-178 (1986).
33. Hays, E. F., Hale, L., Villarreal, B., Fitchen, J. H. Stromal and haemopoietic stem cell abnormalities in long term cultures of marrow from busulphan treated mice. *Exp. Hematol. 10,* 383-392 (1982).
34. Goldstone, A. H. (ed.). *Autologous bone marrow transplantation. Clinics in hematology,* Vol. 15. W.B. Saunders, Philadelphia (1986).
35. Dicke, K. A., Spitzer, G., Zander, A. Autologous bone marrow transplantation. M.D. Anderson Hospital Proceedings, Houston, 1985.
36. International Autologous Bone Marrow Transplant Registry. Bone marrow autotransplantation in man: report of an international cooperative study. *Lancet ii,* 960-962 (1986).
37. Phillips, G. L. Current clinical trials with intensive therapy and autologous bone marrow transplantation (ABMT) for lymphomas and solid tumors. In: *Recent advances in bone marrow transplantation.* Gale, R. P. (ed.). Alan R. Liss, New York, pp. 567-598 (1983).
38. Antman, K. A., Gale, R. P. Bone marrow autotransplants in breast cancer. *Ann. Intern. Med.,* in press (1988).
39. Linch, D. C., Goldstone, A. H. Autologous bone marrow transplantation in acute leukemia. *Bone Marrow Transplant. 2,* 291-225 (1987).
40. Jones, S. E., Salmon, S. E. (eds.). *Adjuvant therapy of cancer,* Vol. II. Grune and Stratton, New York, 1979.
41. Lohrmann, H.-P., Schreml, W., Lang, M., Betzler, M., Fliedner, T. M., Heimpel, H. Changes of granulopoiesis during and after adjuvant chemotherapy of breast cancer. *Brit. J. Haematol. 40,* 369-381 (1978).
42. Schreml, W., Lohrmann, H.-P. Hematotoxicity of adjuvant therapy. In: *Adjuvant therapy of cancer,* Vol. II. Jones, S. E., Salmon, S. E. (eds.). Grune and Stratton, New York, pp. 63-70 (1979).

4

Long-Term Bone Marrow Damage After Cytotoxic Treatment

Stem Cells and Microenvironment

NYDIA G. TESTA, JOLYON H. HENDRY, and GRAHAM MOLINEUX
Paterson Institute for Cancer Research, Christie Hospital and Holt Radium Institute, Manchester, England

I. INTRODUCTION

The production of mature cells by hemopoietic tissue is the final result of a finely regulated and complex series of proliferation and differentiation events that start at the level of the multipotential stem cells. The number of mature blood cells that a normal human adult replaces daily is of the order of 2×10^{11} red blood cells and similar numbers of granulocytes, in addition to lymphoid cells and marrow megakaryocytes. The hemopoietic tissue also has the capacity to respond swiftly and effectively to an increased need for mature functional cells (for example, after blood loss or infection) and is able to maintain an adequate response to hemopoietic stress for long periods of time.

It is known that the stem cell population is not impaired by exhaustion either in normal old age (1,2) or after severe proliferation pressure induced by cell depletion in situ (3,4). However, there is a considerable amount of experimental evidence that some cytotoxic treatments may induce long-term hemopoietic damage expressed at the level of stem and progenitor cell populations, which is sometimes translated into hemopoietic failure. This chapter analyzes the relative contribution of damage to these hemopoietic cell populations and to the regulatory microenvironment within which hemopoiesis takes place, to the long-term function of the tissue. In order to do this, we have taken as main examples two drugs: busulfan, which induces stem cell damage, and cyclophosphamide, which spares selectively the most immature stem cells.

II. STEM CELL DAMAGE

A. Quantitative Damage

The classic studies of Morley and colleagues (5,6) established that after repeated doses of busulfan totaling 70 mg per kilogram of body weight, mice developed long-term injury manifested by low numbers of multipotential spleen colony-forming cells (CFU-S) in the bone marrow and at later times by low leukocyte counts and a hypoplastic syndrome. The observation that the effect was largely corrected by a transplant of normal bone marrow led to the conclusion that stem cell damage was responsible for the hypoplastic syndrome. This concept was also supported by the converse experiment: bone marrow from busulfan-treated mice had a poorer repopulation capacity than normal marrow when transplanted into irradiated mice. This effect was even more noticeable after serial transplantation (7). However, the former experiments also indicated the existence of an (undefined) environmental defect in busulfan-treated mice transplanted with normal bone marrow.

The comparison between the acute kill of CFU-S which represent the stem cell population and that of a population of progenitors of stromal fibroblastoid-reticular cells (CFU-F) after treatment with busulfan is seen in Figure 1*a*. Their levels in the long term after treatment are seen in Figure 1*b*. These low values persist for at least half the life span of mice and may therefore be considered permanent. It is of interest that although the acute kill of CFU-S is dose-dependent, in the long term the number of CFU-S does not show dose dependency within a wide range of doses. This indicates that the long-term damage is not related to the degree of the acute CFU-S kill induced by busulfan and might imply, as will be discussed below, that a constraint is applied to the CFU-S by damaged regulatory cells, which may be the limiting feature in the expression of the damage.

B. Qualitative Damage

One of the classic parameters that measure the quality of stem cells is their self-reproduction capacity, usually determined by measuring the mean numbers of new CFU-S generated by the test CFU-S in the spleen colony assay (see Chapter 1). After treatment with busulfan, the self-reproduction capacity of the CFU-S is not diminished significantly after doses of up to 30 mg/kg (a dose at which the maximum long-term reduction in CFU-S numbers is already observed; see Fig. 1), although at higher doses self-reproduction is markedly and persistently subnormal (Table 1). Even moderate doses of busulfan that cause little reduction in the self-renewal capacity of CFU-S in the short term can cause a long-term reduction in the number of CFU-S per colony. The degree of this long-term damage is similar to that caused by much higher doses of busulfan, which have a greater acute effect on the self-renewal capacity of the CFU-S (Table 1). Extensive studies in mice have shown that busulfan reduces considerably the ability of the

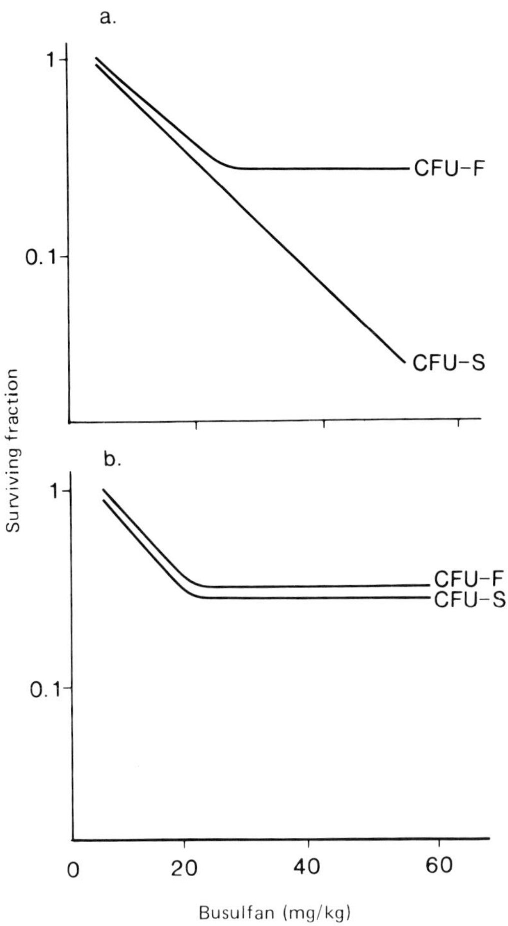

Figure 1 Long-term levels of spleen colony-forming units (CFU-S) in the bone marrow of mice treated with busulfan. (a) Initial kill of CFU-S is entirely dose-dependent, kill of CFU-F only partially so. (b) Long-term levels of CFU-S and CFU-F correlate closely. Data taken from Ref. 17.

bone marrow to regenerate the hemopoietic system after serial transplantation in mice (7). This effect was also seen after BCNU, but not after L-phenylalanine mustard (L-PAM), 5-fluorouracil (5-FU), or cyclophosphamide (Cy). Although these data were interpreted at the time in terms of stem cell failure, there are alternative considerations. Damaged regulatory cells, either transferred with the transplanted marrow or remaining in the ablated host, may have abnormal functions. Cell-cell interactions may be interfered with, as might the ability to produce

Table 1 Self-Reproduction Capacity of Spleen Colony Forming Cells (CFU-S) After Treatment with Busulfan or Cyclophosphamide

		Self-Reproduction Capacity of CFU-S (% of control)		
Treatment	Dose (mg/kg)	Acute Effect[a]	Steady State, Postregeneration	Ref.
Busulfan	10	95 (2 days)	100 (125-600+ days)	16
	20	85	60	36
	30	77	61	
	40	13	72	
	50	15	48[b]	
	60	ND	62	
Cyclophosphamide	200	687 (1 day)	56 (15 days)	Unpublished
			85 (60-450 days)	
			52 (15 days)	Unpublished
	4 X 200[c]	874 (1 day after last dose)	62 (50-570 days after last dose)	

ND = Not done.
[a]Time after treatment shown in parentheses.
[b]Similar results were obtained with a single or fractionated dose (20-20-10 mg/kg at 14-day intervals).
[c]Four doses separated by 2-week intervals.

or release regulatory growth factors. These possibilities are now being studied actively in the context of experimental and clinical bone marrow transplantation (see Chapters 15 and 17). In this situation the effects of the conditioning regime (in the case of mice, whole body irradiation) on the regulatory cells of the host may have to be considered.

Treatment with Cy was not found to cause a long-term reduction in the numbers of CFU-S in mice (8) or an altered capacity for repopulation upon serial transplantation (7). However, we found a moderate decrease in CFU-S numbers after Cy (Table 1, Fig. 2). Also, about 8% of the mice treated with a repeated administration schedule to the maximum tolerated dose (5 doses of 200 mg/kg) showed hemopoietic dysfunction expressed as anemia or granulocytopenia, sometimes with signs of myelodysplasia (9).

Cyclophosphamide is known to spare selectively the most immature cells in the CFU-S population, and presumably even earlier cells (10,11), as can be shown by the high self-reproduction capacity of the surviving CFU-S shortly after treatment (Table 1). This effect of Cy is remarkably similar to that of 5-FU, which also spares selectively the most immature CFU-S (12). It may therefore be speculated

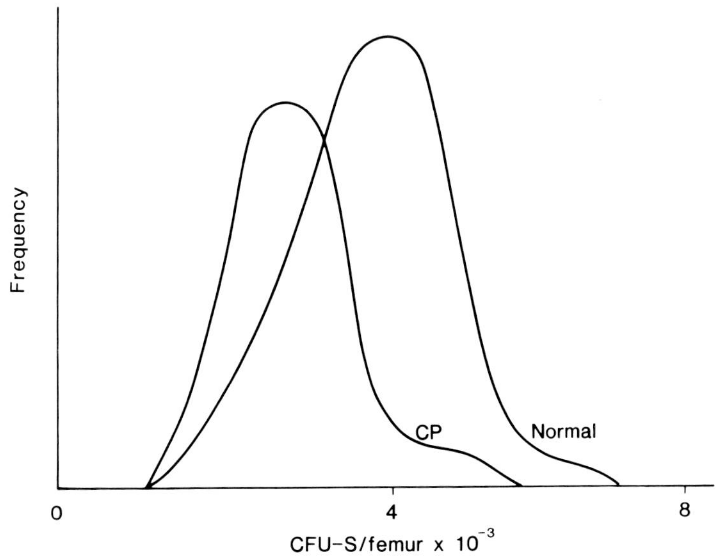

Figure 2 The distribution of numbers of spleen colony-forming units (CFU-S) in the femora of mice assessed individually after no treatment or after cyclophosphamide (CP; 200 mg × 5 at 14-day intervals) at least 100 days previously. Data taken from Ref. 9.

Table 2 Proliferation Stress by Transplantation Accentuates Long-Term Damage After Cytotoxic Treatment

			In Situ (Bone Marrow)[b]			Transplanted (Spleen Colonies)[b]		
Group	Dose[a]	Time of Assays	CFU-S	GM-CFC	Cellularity	CFU-S	GM-CFC	Cellularity
BCNU	4 × 20, 25, or 30 mg/kg	Up to 250 days	62	71	111	24	31	54
Cyclophosphamide	4 × 150, 175, or 200 mg/kg	Up to 150 days	89	89	104	64	66	68

[a]Doses were repeated 4 times at 3-week intervals.
[b]Results expressed as percent of the adequate control: In situ = normal bone marrow; transplanted = spleen colonies derived from normal bone marrow. As no dose effect was observed in these experiments, the results from all groups treated with different doses were pooled. Data taken from Ref. 22.

that the high quality surviving stem cells may reconstitute the CFU-S population, since it is known that induced proliferative stress per se does not result in any exhaustion of the system. The reconstitution was demonstrated by measuring the numbers of CFU-S after intense and repeated proliferation stress induced by treatment with hydroxyurea (HU) or triethylenemelamine (TEM): After up to 10 doses of TEM, each producing a depopulation of the order of 99% in the CFU-S compartment, the recovery patterns were similar with regard to the rate of regeneration and the final (normal) level reached (4). Similarly, after repeated treatment with HU, it was shown that the considerable proliferation stress induced by the drug did not alter the self-reproduction capacity of the CFU-S for the rest of the life span of the mice (3). However, in spite of the remarkable sparing of CFU-S with high self-reproduction capacity after Cy (Table 1), a late, long-lasting, presumably permanent, defect both in numbers and in self-reproduction capacity of CFU-S is seen (Tables 1 and 2). Although the mean numbers of CFU-S per femur show only a moderate difference from controls, measurements performed in individual mice indicate that a proportion of the treated mice have very low numbers of CFU-S (Fig. 2).

III. ENVIRONMENTAL DAMAGE

Several assays have been used to measure the capacity of the hemopoietic environment to support hemopoiesis. One classic method measures the number of progenitors of fibroblastoid-reticular cells (CFU-F) by their capacity to generate colonies in vitro (13). As described above, the numbers of CFU-F in mice are persistently subnormal after treatment with busulfan (Fig. 1*b*) and follow a pattern strikingly similar to that shown by CFU-S.

After repeated treatment with Cy, the mean level of the femoral CFU-F is 70% of the controls, a level similar to that reached by the CFU-S (Table 2; Ref. 9). However, examination of individual mice shows that again, as in the CFU-S population, a proportion had markedly subnormal numbers of CFU-F. These low values were observed up to at least 15 months after treatment and may therefore be considered permanent.

Another assay consists of implanting a femoral bone subcutaneously in mice and then measuring the capacity of its stroma to support hemopoiesis (14). The bones from mice treated with busulfan (at a dose of 40-48 mg/kg) have an environment able to support lower numbers of CFU-S lodged in it than femora of control mice. In contrast, the environment in the femur of Cy-treated mice (15) normalized between 13 and 24 weeks. However, it is possible that the implanted femur assay reflects in part the capacity for regeneration of a competent endothelial capillary system; because of the length of the femoral shaft, an extensive blood supply system may have to be established before hemopoiesis can develop fully in the shaft.

Table 3 Long-Term Effects on the Hemopoietic System of Mice After Treatment with Busulfan or Cyclophosphamide[a]

	Marrow Hemopoietic Cells			Circulating Cells		
Stroma[b]	CFU-S	GM-CFC	Total Cells	Erythrocytes	Leukocytes	Ref.
Busulfan						
	++	++	++++	++++	++++	38
+	+++	+	++++			19
++++	++++					39
	++					40, 7, 26
	++		++++			41, 42
+++	++		++++→+			5, 6
++	++					43, 18, 44
Cyclophosphamide						
++	++++					44
+++	++	++	+++			45
	++++		++++		++++	46
+++	+++		++++	++++→+		9

[a]++++, normal; +++, slight, but detectable, damage; ++, significant damage; +, severe, possibly life-threatening damage; →, progression with time.

[b]Tests used to measure stromal damage include: growth of transplanted normal bone marrow in drug-treated recipient mice, CFU-F assays, long-term bone marrow cultures, and ectopic marrow implants.

A further assay involves the implantation of bone marrow tissue under the kidney capsule in mice (16). A donor-derived microenvironment develops that is adequate for the support of host-derived hemopoiesis. The environment provided by the implanted marrow (from busulfan-treated mice, 50 mg/kg single dose) assayed up to 170 days after treatment is able to support only subnormal hemopoiesis, at a level of about 50-60% of the control implant of normal marrow (17).

In long-term bone marrow cultures, where active hemopoiesis depends on the functional integrity of an adherent layer of stromal cells (18), adherent layers established from normal donor mice were able to support roughly comparable levels of hemopoiesis (75-80% of the adequate control) when inoculated with bone marrow cells from either normal or busulfan-treated mice (19). In contrast, the converse experiment (adherent layers derived from busulfan-treated bone marrow inoculated with either normal or treated cells) showed that the stroma from busulfan-treated marrow was able to support only about 20% of the level of hemopoiesis seen in cultures of normal stroma inoculated with normal cells (19). It has also been found that nonadherent cells from normal bone marrow cultures can compensate for the defect if added in sufficient numbers, probably because they are able to provide normal stromal progenitors (20).

The data on the behavior of bone marrow from Cy-treated mice in long-term cultures is limited, but results to date suggest that the variability seen in individual mice is reflected in cultures. If cultures from single donors are performed, the production of mature hemopoietic cells and the numbers of progenitor cells and CFU-S may be close to control levels in some mice, though markedly deficient in others (Molineux, Dexter, and Testa, unpublished).

The data reviewed above indicate that both busulfan and Cy induce considerable environmental damage, probably to more than one component of the hemopoietic stroma; such damage is persistent and shows little tendency to repair with time. Both drugs may induce long-term hemopoietic failure, more noticeable for busulfan than for cyclophosphamide (Table 3).

IV. EVALUATION OF LONG-TERM DAMAGE

A. Dose Dependency

In contrast to acute myelotoxicity, the increase in dosage may not result in measurably greater damage to the CFU-S or progenitor cell levels (17,20; Fig. 1; Table 1). This unexpected phenomenon is observed after treatment with busulfan, cyclophosphamide, and BCNU [but not after radiation (21-23)]. The damage coexists with normal levels of hemopoietic cells in the bone marrow and in the peripheral blood and may not become apparent if only a normal demand for mature cells is imposed on the system. It may be logical to expect, however, that the latent damage may be expressed in a dose-dependent manner if further injury is applied to the tissue. No experimental data are yet available to clarify this point. However, it is known that in Cy-treated mice there is a slower recovery of the CFU-S population after subsequent exposure to sublethal irradiation (15). It would be of interest to investigate whether the rate of recovery after subsequent acute injury shows dependency on the dose of previously administered agents that induce long-term bone marrow damage.

In interpreting experimental results, it has to be considered that the doses are in general larger than those used for treatment in accepted clinical protocols. However, there is a tendency to use more intense chemotherapy. This tendency is likely to continue, not least because the use of hemopoietic growth factors (CSFs) in clinical trials is now being considered as a means to overcome acute toxicity to the hemopoietic system (see Chapters 1 and 16). Furthermore, it is difficult to extrapolate the *degree* of damage (in contrast to the type of damage) from experimental animals to humans. In this context it is relevant that experimental protocols are often based on maximum tolerated doses, which may provide a good basis for interspecies comparisons. Finally, some of the doses used in the clinic are within the range used for experiments reviewed here (24).

B. Stem Cell Damage Versus Environmental Damage

The known damage to stem cells and other hemopoietic cells induced by several myelotoxic drugs exemplified here by busulfan may not, as already suggested above, be the limiting factor in the expression of late damage. The normal stem cells have a considerable reserve capacity to respond to intense proliferative stress (3,4), which has been calculated as being sufficient to support hemopoiesis for at least five normal life spans in mice (25). It is possible, therefore, that even a considerably damaged stem cell population may be able to comply with the normal demands for mature cell production. However, further proliferative stress, for example when cytotoxic treatment is needed for a secondary malignancy, may precipitate hemopoietic failure. In this context, it is well known that little tolerance to treatment is shown by patients of secondary acute nonlymphocytic leukemia, which develops after treatment for lymphoma or other malignancies. Further proliferative stress may be of particular importance in children treated for malignancies, since their hemopoietic system may still be expanding and also because of their longer life expectancy.

One important factor to be considered when assessing damage induced by cytotoxic drugs is that the status of the stem cell population can vary from full recovery, both quantitative and qualitative, seen after treatment with hydroxyurea (3), TEM (4), or 5-FU (12) to permanent and marked depression in numbers together with loss of quality after, for example, treatment with busulfan (17), BCNU (8,22), or TCNU (26). A more comprehensive list of agents is given in Table 4. There are several factors to be considered:

1. Different agents have selective effects on some subpopulations of the stem cell hierarchy, some (busulfan, BCNU) injuring preferentially CFU-S with high

Table 4 Differing Effects of Selected Chemicals on the Spleen Colony-Forming Cells (CFU-S) of Mouse Bone Marrow

Drug	Self-Reproduction Capacity Immediately after Treatment (% control)	Long-Term CFU-S Numbers (% control)	Ref.
Hydroxyurea (HU)	–	100	3
Triethylenemelamine (TEM)	–	100	4
Isopropylmethane sulfonate (IMS)	–	100	27
5-Fluorouracil (5-FU)	75	100	8,37
Methotrexate (MTX)	100	100	8
6-Mercaptopurine (6-MP)	95	100	8
Cyclophosphamide (Cy)	776	96	9
Vinblastine (VBL)	100	85	8
Dimethylsulfonoxy octane (ODMS, $n = 8$)[a]	182	100	38
Dimethylsulfonoxy propane (Pr-DMA, $n = 3$)	100	90	38
Dimethylsulfonoxy ethane (EDMS, $n = 2$)	73	85	38
Dimethylsulfonoxy pentane (PeDMs, $n = 5$)	100	85	38
	55	90	38
1,2-Dimethylsulfonoxy cyclopentane (1,2c-PDMS)			
Dimethylsulfonoxy heptane (HpDMS, $n = 7$)	236	100	38
1,3-Dimethylsulfonoxy cyclopentane (1,3c-PDMS)			
Dimethylsulfonoxy nonane (NDMS, $n = 9$)	182	75	38
(±)-Dimethyl myleran (DMM)	90	85	38
L-Phenylalanine mustard (L-PAM)		65	38
Dimethylsulfonoxy methane (MDMS, $n = 1$)	36	60	38
meso-Dimethyl myleran (*meso*-DMM)	60	53	38
Tauryl chloroethyl nitrosourea (TCNU)	100	50	25
Busulfan (BUS, BDMS, $n = 4$)	11	30	8
	38	60	16
Bischloroethylnitrosourea (BCNU)	24	60	21
	25	30	8

[a] n value for dimethylsulfonoxy alkanes refers to molecular chain length (for example, busulfan, $n = 4$). Initial depletion of CFU-S was greater than 90% in all cases except for dimethyl sulfonoxy propane, where the initial depletion was 50%, and the dimethyl mylerans (± and *meso*), where the initial depletion was 80%.

self-reproduction capacity, while others such as isopropyl methane sulfonate (IMS), cyclophosphamide, and 5-FU kill preferentially the more mature stem cells (9,27,28). A damaged stem cell population composed mainly of cells with low self-reproduction capacity will be more sensitive to further hemopoietic stress.

2. Compounds having identical functional groups may have different effects on stem cells. For example, different members of the series of straight-chain dialkane sulfonates (to which busulfan belongs) have qualitatively different effects on CFU-S both in the short and long term after administration, even when administered at doses that induce similar levels of acute kill (Kelly and Schofield, personal communication; Table 4). An extreme example of this occurs with the dimethyl derivative of busulfan (dimethyl myleran, DMM). The ends of this molecule are structurally similar, and it is optically active. It has been shown that the racemic mixture [i.e., the (+) form mixed with the (−) form, (±)-DMM] has quite different consequences upon the blood-forming tissues than the much more obviously damaging *meso*-DMM, where one end of the molecule is (+) and the other end (−). *meso*-DMM causes a profound degree of long-term damage (CFU-S levels are at 60% of the level in age-matched control mice), whereas (±)-DMM results in a fall of only 15% in CFU-S numbers. These levels were attained after equivalent (80%) initial reductions in the CFU-S population size (Table 4).

3. The capacity of stromal cells to respond to cytotoxic injury is likely to be considerably less than that shown by stem cells. Stromal cells have a slow turnover (29) and probably have a long life span, although there may be considerable variation among the different cell types that are part of the bone marrow microenvironment. Injury to them, therefore, may be expected to take a long time to be expressed because after cytotoxic treatment they may continue to function normally and may be eliminated only if they attempt cell division. In this context, it is of interest to note that a transient normalization in stem and progenitor cells may be achieved after cytotoxic treatment; for example, normal values of CFU-S are observed around 100 days after busulfan treatment, but, as described above, they are not maintained (17). This agrees with the concept of damaged stromal cells remaining functional for a long time after cytotoxic treatment. It is also likely that the proliferation capacity of at least some populations of stromal cells is much more limited than that of the hemopoietic stem cells. Therefore, marked and repeated depopulation may result in exhaustion of certain stromal cell types.

Another feature of the system that may make the regulatory microenvironment a critical target of cytotoxic treatment is that not only may the integrity of several cell populations be required for the normal function of regulatory networks, but also the correct cell-cell associations may have to take place (see Chapters 1 and 2) and the correct ratios of different cell types maintained (see Chapters 15 and 16).

There are several problems in the experimental study of the hemopoietic microenvironment (reviewed in Ref. 30). One is the variety of available assays, which measure very different end points: The CFU-F assay relies on the proliferation capacity of a precursor of fibroblastic-reticular cells but does not provide a functional assay of the regulatory role of that cell type. Long-term bone marrow cultures, on the other hand, allow the assessment of a functional end point (production of hemopoietic cells), but the cultures require a complex cellular network composed of different cell types to support hemopoiesis. The analysis of the role of each individual component has proved difficult (see Chapter 2), not least because the behavior of each cell type in isolation may not (or not wholly) reflect its role in an intact microenvironment (Chapter 1).

Ectopic hemopoiesis in femora implanted subcutaneously, or in ossicles formed following implantation of bone marrow under the kidney capsule in mice, also provides a functional end point: The microenvironment provided by the graft is able to support the growth and differentiation of hemopoietic cells provided by the host. However, the host may influence in yet unknown ways the development of the microenvironment (31,32). Furthermore, each assay is likely to measure different limiting cell types in the formation of a functional microenvironment: because of its shape and size, a femoral shaft may be more dependent on the development of a vascular system than a kidney capsule implant as a prerequisite for hemopoiesis. Experimental evidence has already established that after low-dose-rate irradiation the recovery of the CFU-F reaches 70% of control while the hemopoietic microenvironment, as measured by bone marrow implanted under the kidney capsule, reaches only 20% of control (33,34) in spite of the similar sensitivity to acute irradiation. This suggests that there are other populations besides CFU-F that are needed for ossicle formation and that those populations either require longer times for recovery or are unable to recover to the same level.

In summary, although the performance of the stem cells determines the level of production of hemopoietic cells, their ability to self-renew and to differentiate depends upon the survival and function of the regulatory microenvironment. Although less is known about the latter, partly due to the difficulties inherent in its study, data on long-term hemopoietic damage after treatments that apparently do not damage stem cells (for example after Cy) can be attributed to microenvironmental alterations.

C. Evolution

The defects found in hemopoietic and stromal cell populations in mice appear to be stable, with no tendency to recover once the acute phase of regeneration has been completed. Although these defects are not always manifested as a clinical syndrome, in some cases there may be delayed hemopoietic failure (5,9) as shown also after repeated irradiation by a long-term decline in blood counts (35).

V. SUMMARY

Long-term damage to the hemopoietic system induced by cytotoxic treatment is more noticeable at the level of the more immature cells and may coexist with normal numbers of mature cells in the bone marrow and in the peripheral blood. The coexistence is maintained by increased cycling and increased amplification of the precursor cells (30). However, hypoplastic or myelodysplastic syndromes may be seen at later times.

Hemopoietic stress, such as may be induced by (1) further cytotoxic treatment, (2) the need for hemopoietic expansion after bone marrow transplantation into syngeneic irradiated mice (a situation comparable to autologous transplants in humans), or (3) the transplant procedure itself, may cause damage, previously not expressed by a lower production of mature cells, to become apparent. An example is seen in Table 2: After repeated treatment of groups of mice with a range of BCNU or cyclophosphamide doses, which induced damage at the level of stem and progenitor cells (CFU-S and GM-CFC) but not mature cells, the numbers of CFU-S and GM-CFC harvested from spleen colonies derived from bone marrow of those treated mice transplanted to syngeneic irradiated recipients are much lower than those in spleen colonies derived from normal marrow. Furthermore, a lower level of production of mature cells is apparent.

In contrast to the clear dose response in the long-term hemopoietic effects seen after irradiation, no significant dose reponse has been observed within a wide range of doses of busulfan, Cy, or BCNU. It is not yet clear how general this phenomenon is, because comparable studies using other drugs are not available. At least in experimental mice, the long-term damage appears to be stable and shows no tendency to recover with time.

In spite of the well-defined stem cell damage induced by some agents, it appears likely that even damaged stem cells may be able to produce adequate numbers of mature cells in the absence of further increased proliferative stress. They may, however, be more sensitive (as a population) to alterations in regulatory cell networks induced by further cytotoxic treatment. The latter type of damage may in some cases be the limiting factor in the expression of hemopoietic injury.

ACKNOWLEDGMENTS

The authors thank the Cancer Research Campaign (UK) for supporting this research.

REFERENCES

1. Botnick, L. E., Hannon, E. C., Obaggy, J., Hellman, S. The variation of hematopoietic stem cell self-renewal capacity as a function of age: further evidence for heterogeneity of the stem cell compartment. *Blood 60,* 268-271 (1982).

2. Schofield, R., Dexter, T. M., Lord, B. I., Testa, N. G. Comparison of haemopoiesis in young and old mice. *Mech. Ageing Develop. 34,* 1-12 (1986).
3. Ross, E. A. M., Anderson, N., Micklem, H. S. Serial depletion and regeneration of the murine hematopoietic system. *J. Exp. Med. 155,* 432-444 (1982).
4. Valeriote, F., Tolen, S. Extensive proliferative capacity of haemopoietic stem cells. *Cell Tissue Kinet. 16,* 1-6 (1983).
5. Morley, A., Blake, J. An animal model of chronic aplastic marrow failure. I. Late marrow failure after busulphan. *Blood 44,* 49-56 (1974).
6. Morley, A., Trainor, K., Blake, J. A primary stem cell lesion in experimental chronic hypoplastic marrow failure. *Blood 45,* 681-688 (1975).
7. Botnick, L. E., Hannon, E. C., Hellman, S. Multisystem stem cell failure after apparent recovery from alkylating agents. *Cancer Res. 38,* 1942-1947 (1978).
8. Trainor, K. J., Morley, A. A. Screening of cytotoxic drugs for residual bone marrow damage. *J. Natl. Cancer Inst. 57,* 1237-1239 (1976).
9. Molineux, G., Xu, C. X., Hendry, J. H., Testa, N. G. A cellular analysis of long-term haematopoietic damage in mice after repeated treatment with cyclophosphamide. *Cancer Chemother. Pharmacol. 18,* 11-16 (1986).
10. Porcellini, A., Manna, A., Talevi, N., Sparaventi, G., Marchetti-Rossi, M.-T., Baronciani, D., De Biagi, M. Effect of two cyclophosphamide derivatives on haemopoietic progenitor cells and pluripotential stem cells. *Exp. Hematol. 12,* 863-866 (1984).
11. De Jong, J. P., Nikkels, P. G., Brockbank, K. G. M., Ploemacher, R. C., Voerman, J. S. A. Comparative in vitro effects of cyclophosphamide derivatives on murine bone marrow derived stromal and hemopoietic progenitor cell classes. *Cancer Res. 48,* 4001-4005 (1985).
12. Hodgson, G. S., Bradley, T. R. Properties of stem cells surviving 5-fluorouracil treatment: evidence for a pre-CFU-S cell? *Nature 281,* 381-382 (1979).
13. Friedenstein, A. J., Gorskala, U. F., Kulagina, N. N. Fibroblast precursors in normal and irradiated mouse haemopoietic organs. *Exp. Hematol. 4,* 267-274 (1976).
14. Fried, N., Musseini, S., Knospe, W. H., Trobaugh, F. E. Studies on the source of haematopoietic tissue in the marrow of subcutaneously implanted femurs. *Exp. Hematol. 1,* 29-35 (1973).
15. Fried, W., Adler, S. Late effects of chemotherapy on hematopoietic progenitor cells. *Exp. Hematol.* (*Suppl. 16*) *13,* 49-56 (1985).
16. Friedenstein, A. J., Chailakhjan, R. K., Latsinik, N. V., Panasynk, A. F., Keiliss-Borok, I. V. Stromal cells responsible for transferring the microenvironment of hemopoietic tissues. *Transplantation 17,* 331-340 (1974).
17. Molineux, G., Testa, N. G., Massa, G., Schofield, R. An analysis of haemopoietic and microenvironmental populations of mouse bone marrow after treatment with busulphan. *Biomedicine 40,* 215-220 (1986).
18. Allen, T. D., Dexter, T. M. Cellular interrelationships during in vitro granulopoiesis. *Differentiation 6,* 191-194 (1976).
19. Anderson, R. W., Matthews, K. I., Crouse, D. A., Sharp, J. G. In vitro evaluation of haematopoiesis in mice treated with busulphan or nitrogen mustard. *Biomedicine 36,* 149-152 (1982).

20. Hays, E. F., Hale, L., Villarreal, B., Fitchen, J. H. Stromal and haemopoietic stem cell abnormalities in long term cultures of marrow from busulphan treated mice. *Exp. Hematol. 10,* 383-392 (1982).
21. Hendry, J. H., Wang, S. B., Testa, N. G. Greater sparing of stromal progenitor cells than of haemopoietic stem cells in γ-irradiated mouse marrow using low dose-rates. *Biomedicine 38,* 356-358 (1984).
22. Xu, C. X., Molineux, G., Testa, N. G., Hendry, J. H. Long-term damage to haemopoietic cell subpopulations in mice after repeated treatment with BCNU or cyclophosphamide. *Brit. J. Cancer 53, Suppl. VIII,* 174-176 (1986).
23. Xu, C. X., Hendry, J. H., Testa, N. G. The response of stromal progenitor cells in mouse marrow to graded repeated doses of x-rays or neutrons. *Radiat. Res. 96,* 82-89 (1983).
24. Blazar, B. R., Ramsay, N. K. C., Kersey, J. H., Krivit, W., Arthur, D. C., Filiporich, A. H. Pretransplant conditioning with busulphan (myleran) and cyclophosphamide for nonmalignant disease. *Transplantation 39,* 597-603 (1985).
25. Harrison, D. E., Astle, C. M. Loss of stem cell repopulating ability on transplantation. Effects of donor age, cell number and transplantation procedure. *J. Exp. Med. 156,* 1767-1779 (1982).
26. Molineux, G., Schofield, G., Testa, N. G. The haemopoietic effects of TCNU in mice. *Cancer Treatment Rep. 71,* 837-841 (1987).
27. Botnick, L. E., Hannon, E. C., Hellman, S. A long-lasting proliferative defect in the haematopoietic stem cell compartment following cytotoxic agents. *Int. J. Radiat. Oncol. Biol. Phys. 5,* 1621-1625 (1979).
28. Schofield, R., Lajtha, L. G. Effects of isopropyl methane sulphonate (IMS) on haemopoietic colony forming cells. *Brit. J. Haematol. 25,* 195-202 (1973).
29. Castro-Malaspina, H., Gay, R. E., Jhanwar, S. C., Hamilton, J. A., Chiarieri, D. R. Meyers, P. A., Gay, S., Moore, M. A. S. Characteristics of bone marrow fibroblasts colony-forming cells (CFU-F) and their progeny in patients with myeloproliferative disorders. *Blood 59,* 1046-1054 (1982).
30. Testa, N. G., Hendry, J. H., Molineux, G. Long-term bone marrow damage in experimental systems and in patients after radiation or chemotherapy. *Anti-Cancer Res. 5,* 101 (1985).
31. Schofield, R. Standardisation of procedures for ectopic marrow grafting. I. Influence of sex of recipient. *Exp. Hematol. 14,* 66-71 (1986).
32. Molineux, G., Schofield, R., Hendry, J. H., Testa, N. G. Standardisation of procedures for ectopic marrow grafting. II. Influence on recipients of radiation dose and field size. *Exp. Hematol. 15,* 676-678 (1987).
33. Wang, S. B., Hendry, J. H., Testa, N. G. Sensitivity and recovery of stromal progenitor cells (CFU-F) in mouse bone marrow given γ-irradiation at 0.65 Gy per day. *Biomedicine 41,* 48-50 (1987).
34. Molineux, G., Testa, N. G., Hendry, J. H., Schofield, R. The radiation sensitivity of the haemopoietic microenvironment—effect of dose rate on ectopic ossicle formation. *Radiother. Oncol.* (in press).

35. Hendry, J. H., Xu, C. X., Testa, N. G. A cellular analysis of residual haemopoietic deficiencies in mice after 4 repeated doses of 4.5 gray x-rays. *Int. J. Radiat. Oncol. Biol. Phys. 9,* 1641-1646 (1983).
36. Molineux, G., Schofield, R., Testa, N. G. Development of spleen CFU-S colonies from day 8 to day 11: relationship to self-renewal capacity. *Exp. Hematol. 14,* 710-713 (1986).
37. Van Zant, G. Studies of haematopoietic stem cells spared by 5-fluorouracil. *J. Exp. Med. 159,* 679-690 (1984).
38. Kelly, M. D. Personal communication.
39. Fitchen, J. H., Cline, M. J. The effect of granulopoietic stress in mice with "latent" bone marrow failure. *Exp. Hematol. 8,* 788-794 (1980).
40. Delmonte, L. Effect of myleran on murine hemopoiesis. I. Granulocytic cell line specificity of action on progenitor cells. *Cell Tissue Kinet. 11,* 347-358 (1978).
41. Udupa, K. B., Okamura, H., Reissmann, K. R. Granulopoiesis during myleran-induced suppression of transplantable hematopoietic stem cells. *Blood 39,* 317-325 (1972).
42. Blackett, N. M., Millard, R. E. Different recovery patterns of mouse haemopoietic stem cells in response to cytotoxic agents. *J. Cell Physiol. 89,* 473-480 (1976).
43. Boggs, D. R., Boggs, S. S., Chervenick, P. A., Patrene, K. D. Murine recovery from busulphan induced haematopoietic toxicity as assessed by three assays for colony forming cells. *Amer. J. Hematol. 8,* 43-54 (1980).
44. Wathen, L. M., DeGowin, R. L., Gibson, D. P., Knapp, S. A. Residual injury to the hemopoietic microenvironment following sequential radiation and busulphan. *Int. J. Radiat. Oncol. Biol. Phys. 8,* 1315-1322 (1982).
45. Fried, W., Kedo, A., Barone, J. Effects of cyclophosphamide and of busulphan on spleen colony forming units and on haemopoietic stroma. *Cancer Res. 37,* 1205-1209 (1977).
46. Wathen, L. M., Knapp, S. A., DeGowin, R. L. Suppression of marrow stromal cells and microenvironmental damage following sequential radiation and cyclophosphamide. *Int. J. Radiat. Oncol. Biol. Phys. 7,* 935-941 (1981).

5

Long-Term Bone Marrow Damage After Irradiation

WILLIAM H. KNOSPE
Rush-Presbyterian-St. Luke's Medical Center and Rush Medical College, Chicago, Illinois

Delayed effects of irradiation on bone marrow depend to a major extent on injury to the hemopoietic microenvironment or stroma. The hemopoietic stroma remains a poorly defined entity composed of cellular constituents, including sinusoidal endothelial cells, fibroblasts, fat cells and macrophages, noncellular matrix components, and the biochemical products of stromal cells that modulate hemopoietic stem cells and their differentiated lineages. Delayed effects of irradiation affect, to a lesser extent, hemopoietic stem cells or their progeny, through injury to the proliferative capacity of the cell. At least in vivo the hemopoietic stroma appears relatively radioresistant, and little damage has been detected from exposures below 10 Gy. Thus, the study of the effect of doses greater than 15 Gy on the stroma restricts such observations to localized rather than whole body exposures.

This chapter reviews what is known about delayed effects on the marrow in laboratory animals and in humans, comparing localized to whole body exposures. In humans these effects have occurred in patients receiving radiation therapy or in accidentally exposed subjects involved in the atomic bombings in Japan or in reactor accidents.

I. EXPERIMENTAL DELAYED EFFECTS OF RADIATION ON BONE MARROW IN ANIMALS

My own interest in radiation effects on the marrow was stimulated by the work of George W. Casarett at the University of Rochester. He proposed that a significant portion of late radiation injury of parenchymal elements had its origin in primary injury to fine vasculature. A reduction in fine vasculature resulted in reduced perfusion, hypoxia, and loss of parenchyma. An important part of this concept was that injury to fine vasculature was in part acute and in part delayed, with reduction of fine vasculature occurring progressively over months after initial radiation exposure (1). Several early investigators studying the delayed or long-term effects of irradiation on the marrow reported that doses of 20 Gy or more resulted in permanent marrow aplasia, but their observations were limited to periods less than 4 months after irradiation (2-6).

A. Localized Effects of Irradiation on In Situ Marrow

In 1962 long-term effects of irradiation on bone marrow were begun in collaboration with Blom and Crosby. Our goal was to develop an experimental model that would illuminate several obscure aspects of bone marrow structure and function. Crosby had observed patients with fatal aplastic anemia and severe pancytopenia, with scattered foci of hemopoiesis containing all three myeloid lineages. Active hemopoiesis in these foci appeared to be supported by pluripotent hemopoietic stem cells (HSCs). Why did these HSCs not migrate into the surrounding aplastic sites and mediate marrow regeneration? Crosby suspected that damage to the marrow stroma was present. He had observed a fascinating patient at Walter Reed Army Hospital who had been injured by a land mine in World War II. This patient had fragments of hand bones from a fellow soldier impacted into his buttocks area, and the bony fragments contained active marrow. This suggested that marrow stroma could be transplanted, regenerate, and support hemopoiesis (7).

We developed a simple model of radiation-induced aplasia in rat limbs. Single exposures of 20-100 Gy of 250 kVp x-rays were delivered to the distal half of the femur and the entire tibia. Rats were killed after intervals of up to 12 months, and irradiated and nonirradiated marrow was examined histologically. The first point was at 14 days, and we were surprised to find a remarkable degree of cellularity at all radiation doses given, even 100 Gy. Examination at shorter times after radiation exposure demonstrated aplasia after 4 days followed by an influx of hemopoietic elements and normal hemopoietic regeneration at 14 days after exposure. Extensive injury to marrow sinusoids was observed between 24 and 48 hr followed by repair of sinusoids at 4 days with a reconstituted, intact pattern of functioning sinusoids (Figs. 1-3).

A secondary wave of marrow aplasia was observed 1-3 months after irradiation. Concurrently, there was a loss of sinusoids associated with extensive extravasation of erythrocytes and increasing amounts of fibrosis along endosteal surfaces (Fig. 4).

After 20 Gy, sinusoidal regeneration occurred after 6-12 months and diffuse hemopoietic regeneration was also evident (Figs. 5-7). Regeneration of hemopoiesis did not occur after 40-100 Gy (Fig. 8). Some regenerated sinusoid-like vessels were surrounded by dense eosinophilic material. Fibrosis progressively increased after 60-100 Gy (Fig. 9).

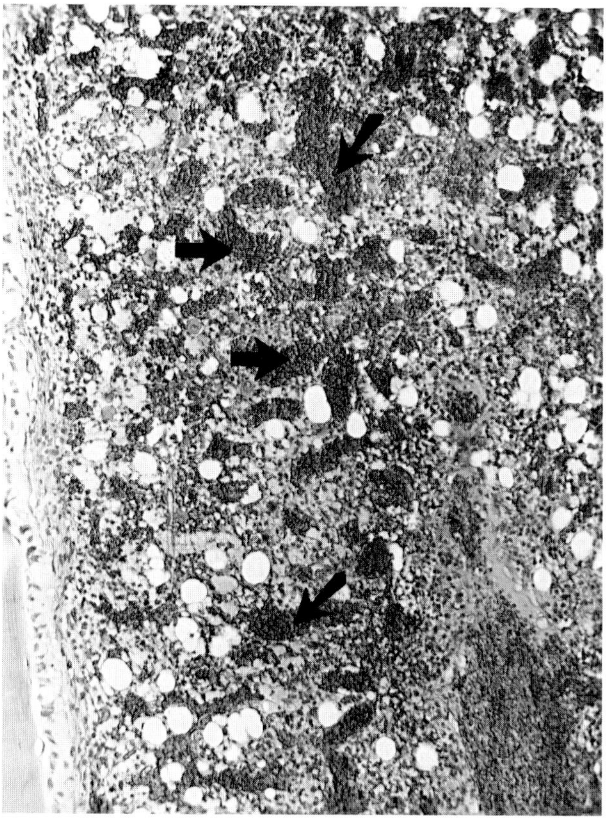

Figure 1 20 Gy, 4 days, femur (140X). Fat is increased and hemopoiesis is severely depressed. Sinusoids (arrows) are dilated and often disrupted with extravasation of erythrocytes into parenchymal areas. From Ref. 8.

We concluded that functional marrow depended on an intact sinusoidal microcirculation. Cells that morphologically appeared transitional between reticulum cells, fat cells, and sinusoidal elements were observed. We speculated that all of these lines originated in a stromal stem cell. We also concluded that regeneration of a relatively radioresistant sinusoidal cell [or precursor stromal cell(s)] with a very slow turnover time mediated marrow regeneration after 20 Gy. After 40 Gy this cell was destroyed and no marrow regeneration occurred (8). Earlier work by Bloom had noted that reticulum cells (or histiocytes) were phagocytically active up to doses of 30 Gy, indicating an equivalent radiation sensitivity of phagocytic cells to sinusoidal or endothelial cells (9).

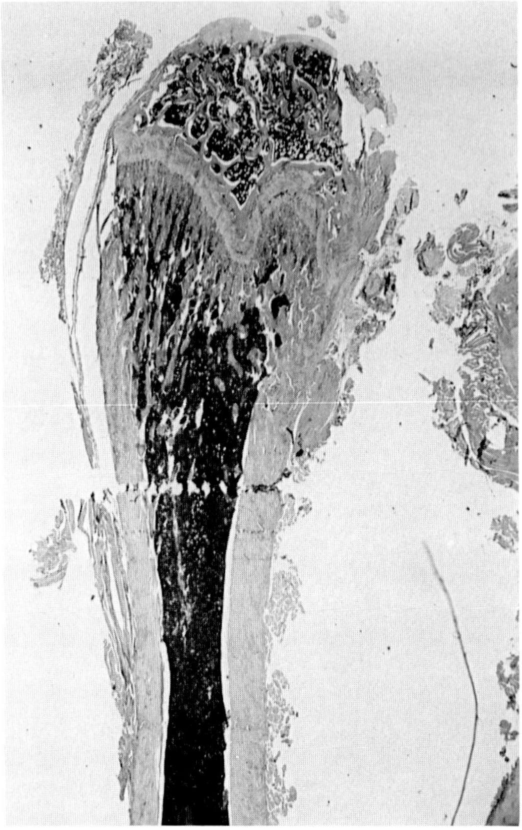

Figure 2 20 Gy, 14 days, femur (13X). Cellularity appears almost normal. From Ref. 8.

An extension of this work in the rat used a model of permanently induced aplasia after 40 Gy to evaluate several types of experimental maneuvers intended to induce regeneration of the marrow. Three months after 40 Gy of local limb irradiation, rats were treated with (1) intravenous syngeneic bone marrow, (2) intramedullary curettage to remove injured stroma and stimulate endosteal regeneration, and (3) combination of intramedullary curettage followed by local infusion of syngeneic marrow into the curetted, aplastic cavity. Neither IV infusion of syngeneic marrow nor local curettage alone was effective in inducing regeneration of hemopoiesis in the limbs exposed to 40 Gy. However, the combination of intramedullary curettage followed by local infusion of syngeneic marrow resulted in regeneration of marrow including stromal sinusoidal regeneration and

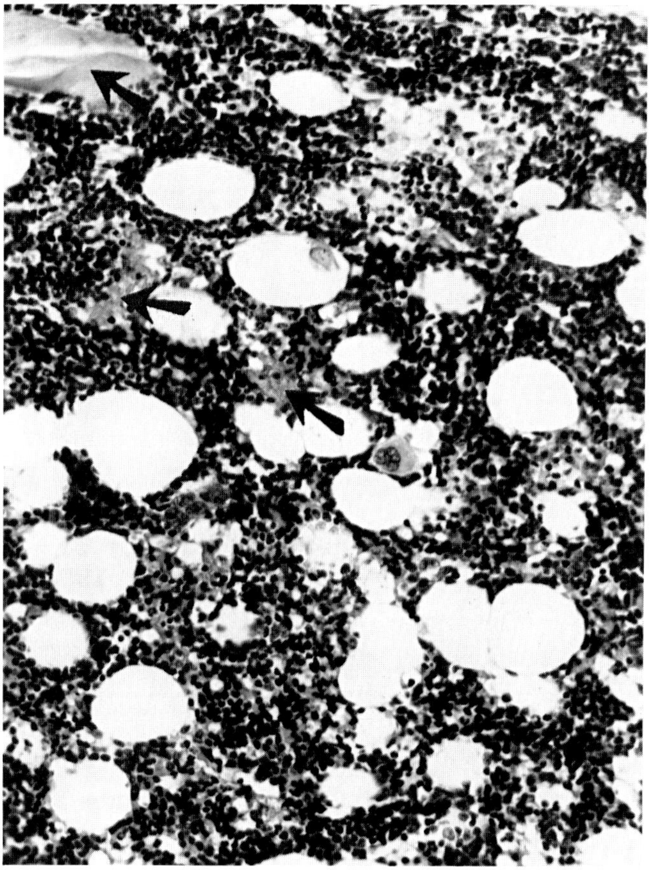

Figure 3 20 Gy, 14 days, tibia (340X). Diffuse hemopoietic activity is present with regeneration of sinusoidal elements (arrows). From Ref. 8.

parenchymal hemopoietic regeneration. We concluded that 40 Gy permanently injured the sinusoidal structures of marrow, rendering the marrow permanently aplastic. The IV infusion of marrow failed to provide stromal cells capable of circulating and migrating into the aplastic irradiated marrow and mediating regeneration (10). Earlier studies by Steinberg and Martin and Steinberg and Hufford of marrow curettage in rabbits suggested that complete stromal regeneration followed from the endosteal layer, which possessed the capability of developing a complete stroma including vascular structures, fat cells, and reticular elements (11,12). That sinusoidal, stromal, and hemopoietic regeneration occurred after

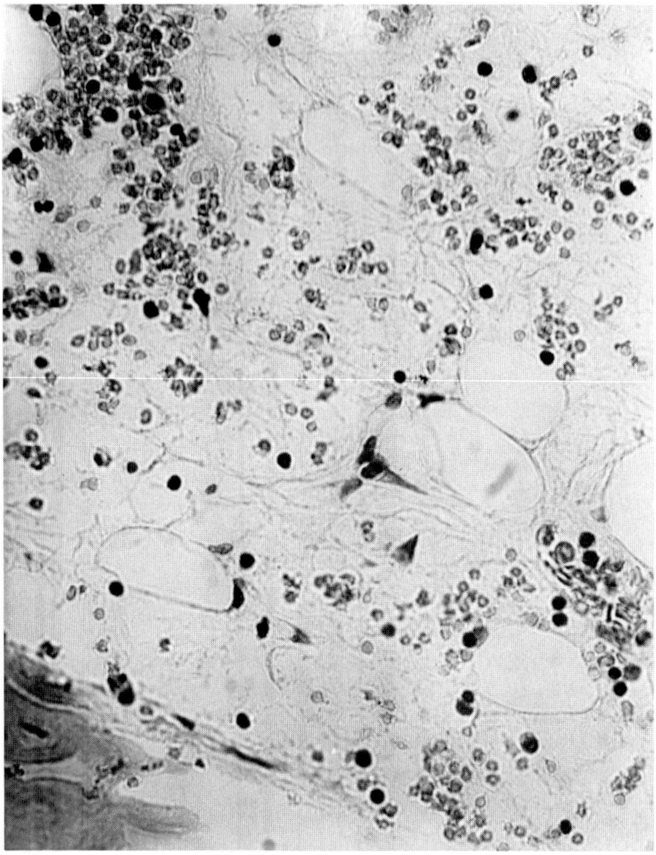

Figure 4 20 Gy, 3 months, femur (520X). Hemopoiesis is absent, and erythrocytes are scattered through areas of fat. Sinusoids have disappeared. From Ref. 8.

medullary curettage followed by local infusion of marrow (with stromal cells) indicated that noncirculating, nonmigrating stromal elements implanted locally were required to regenerate the permanently aplastic irradiated cavities (10).

Nelp et al. studied the effects of 250 keV x-rays on the marrow of the hind legs of rabbits. They monitored the uptake of ^{59}Fe and carbon particles into the irradiated legs. Five rabbits were given 20 Gy to the leg and studied up to 15 months later. Forty-eight hours after irradiation there was obliteration of hemopoietic elements with prominence of reticuloendothelial (RE) cells containing carbon. After 2 months there was irregularity of sinusoidal structure and marked reduction of hemopoietic elements. At 15 months, marrow architecture was entirely

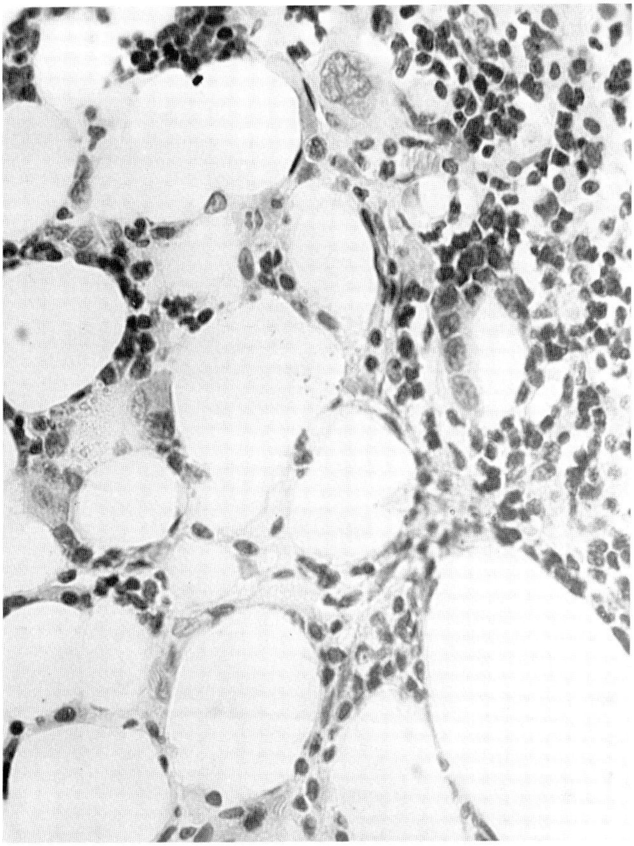

Figure 5 20 Gy, 6 months, tibia (520X). Diffuse activity of all hemopoietic elements is present, but fat remains increased and the marrow remains hypocellular. From Ref. 8.

disorganized, with an irregular and indistinct sinusoidal pattern. Most of the central marrow space was replaced by a homogeneous eosinophilic staining material. RE cells were difficult to identify, and hemopoietic elements were markedly reduced, located peripherally in the marrow spaces, and reduced to 50% of controls. This represented a secondary recovery from aplasia and was similar to the secondary wave of recovery observed by Knospe et al. (8,13).

Rubin studied the effects of dose fractionation on marrow injury and regeneration in rabbits. Localized doses of 20-50 Gy were given at rates varying from 2 Gy/day to 10 Gy/week. Marrow function was monitored using uptake of ^{99m}Tc-sulfur colloid and ^{59}Fe to measure RE and erythroid activity. At 20 and 30 Gy,

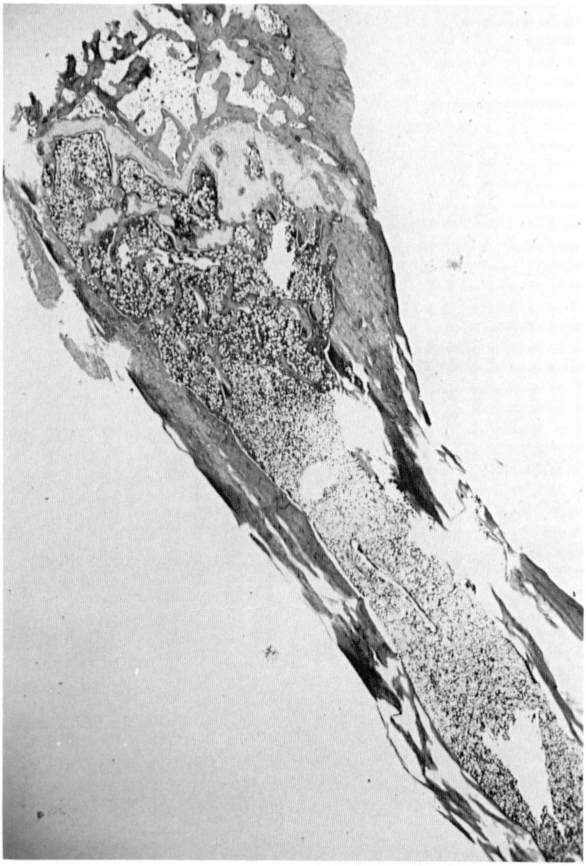

Figure 6 20 Gy, 1 year, femur (13X). Scattered hemopoietic activity is present throughout most of the marrow, although cellularity has not returned to normal. Several areas in the diaphysis and epiphysis remain severely hypoplastic. There is marked disorganization and replication of the epiphyseal plate. From Ref. 8.

marrow of irradiated limbs regenerated to 80-90% of contralateral control limbs after 6 months. At 40-50 Gy, marrow regeneration was 75-85% of control limbs. Marrow tolerance (resistance) was clearly greater with fractionated radiation than for single-exposure radiation (14).

Maloney et al. studied HSC domains in locally irradiated mice given 10-30 Gy four to five months previously. Compared to unirradiated contralateral marrow, fewer spleen colony-forming cells (CFU-S) either reached previously irradiated marrow or were seeded into sites that could support growth. The initial exponen-

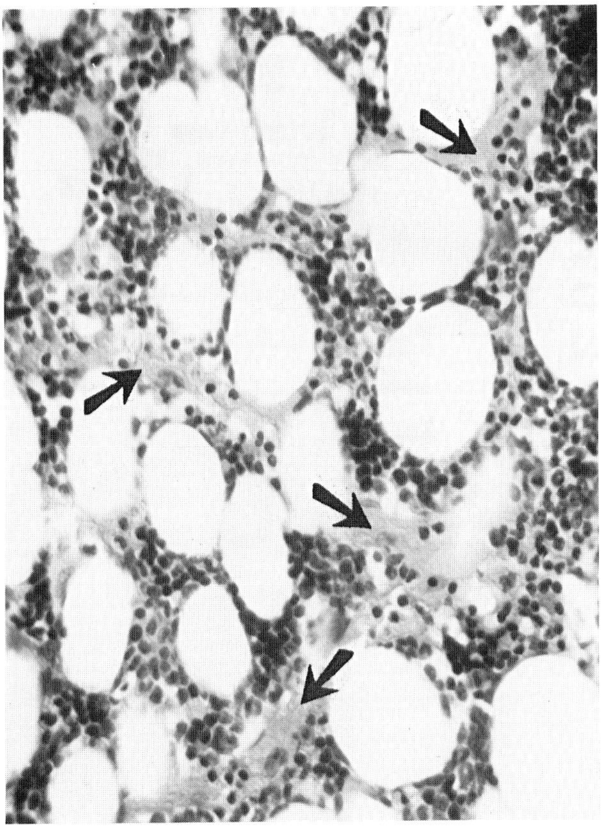

Figure 7 20 Gy, 1 year, tibia (520X). Diffuse hemopoietic activity is present. Many sinusoids filled with erythrocytes are seen (arrows). From Ref. 8.

tial growth of effectively seeded CFU-S was unchanged, but growth deceleration (inflection point) occurred at a lower level of CFU-S in the previously irradiated marrow. The decrease in effective stem cell domains was calculated to be 35% and reflected delayed radiation damage to the marrow microenvironment (15).

B. Delayed Effects of Whole Body Irradiation (Assayed by Transplantation of Irradiated Stroma into Normal Animals)

Several years later Fried and I adapted the technique of transplantation of marrow reported by Tavassoli and Crosby to assess marrow stromal function after irradiation and freezing injury to the marrow. Our technique took femora from normal +/+ and coisogeneic Sl/Sl^d mice were given whole body irradiation at doses

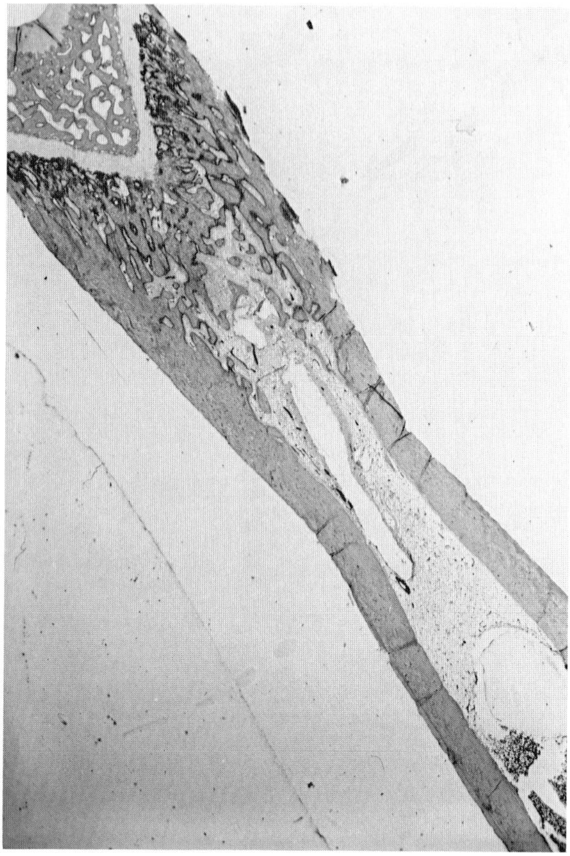

Figure 8 40 Gy, 1 year, femur (13X). Severe hypoplasia is present without evidence of hemopoietic or sinusoidal regeneration. Several large cystic areas are seen within the medullary cavity. From Ref. 8.

of 9.5 and 25 Gy one day before or in vitro freezing injury to extirpated femora following which the femora were transplanted to a subcutaneous site. Femora from normal mice that received no irradiation or in vitro freezing regenerated stroma after 8 weeks. Hemopoietic regeneration occurred, and the femora had a near-normal content of CFU-S. In vivo whole body irradiation or in vitro irradiation injured the hemopoietic stroma and reduced the capacity of the transplanted femora to support hemopoiesis. CFU-S were markedly reduced following 9.5 Gy whole body irradiation to the donors of the femora and completely inhibited after 25 Gy whole body x-irradiation. Chromosome sex markers of regenerated cells in the implants indicated that 100% of the cells were of host type after 9.5 Gy whole body x-irradiation. These data argued that the relatively radioresistant stromal cells of

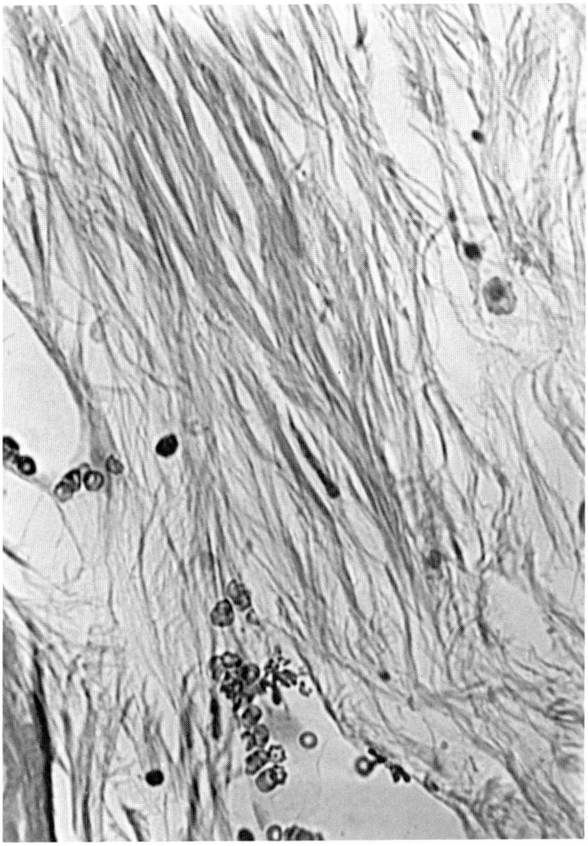

Figure 9 100 Gy, 1 year, femur (520X). The medullary cavity is almost obliterated by a dense deposit of collagen. No hemopoietic activity is present. Several large vessels are seen. From Ref. 8.

the donor were capable of mediating hemopoietic stromal cell regeneration. Pluripotent HSC derived from the donor did not survive the process of subcutaneous transplantation. The CFU-S in the implants derived from circulating cells of the host and migrated into the transplanted regenerated stroma of donor origin (16).

Similar studies were done on normal CBA mice irradiated 24 hr previous to sacrifice with 7.5 or 9.5 Gy whole body x-rays. Assay of CFU-S in these femora transplanted to subcutaneous sites of unirradiated normal CBA hosts indicated a reduction of CFU-S content to 20% and 1%, respectively, of normal unirradiated control donors assayed similarly. The use of a T_6/T_6 marker chromosome indicated that 100% of the CFU-S in the regenerated marrow transplants from mice irradiated with 7.5 or 9.5 Gy whole body x-rays were of host type, indicating that the stromal cells mediating hemopoietic regeneration were more radioresistant than the sensitive CFU-S (17).

Maniatis et al. reported studies in the rat indicating that stromal cells were more radioresistant than HSC (18). They assayed stromal function after irradiation by transplanting marrow to subcutaneous sites and analyzing histologically the regeneration of bone and hemopoiesis. They observed that doses of 10 Gy markedly impaired stromal and hemopoietic regeneration and 20 Gy ablated both stroma and hemopoiesis. Their data suggested that in vivo irradiation was less damaging than in vitro irradiation (18).

Chamberlin et al. compared the rates of recovery of CFU-S and of hemopoietic stroma. Mice were exposed to 9.5 Gy whole body x-rays, after which they received 10^6 marrow cells from nonirradiated donors. After intervals of 1-6 weeks, mice were sacrificed, the number of CFU-S was determined in the right femur, and the left femur was assayed for stromal function by transplanting it into an unirradiated host. Six weeks later, CFU-S in the implants were assayed. In a second group of experiments the same studies were done 1, 6, and 9 weeks after irradiation. CFU-S in the right femur returned to preirradiation levels in 6 weeks, but the hemopoietic stroma assayed in the left femur did not recover significantly in 9 weeks. Although the numbers of CFU-S in bone marrow or spleen were not significantly different 6 weeks after exposure to 9.5 Gy, hemopoietic stromal function as assayed by transplantation of these organs to subcutaneous sites was severely depressed 6 weeks after irradiation. The number of CFU-S per implant was less than 10% of nonirradiated control femora and spleens. After 18 weeks, CFU-S content of femur implants rose to 80% of control implants whereas spleen implants from irradiated mice showed an insignificant recovery. Chamberlin et al. also investigated factors influencing regeneration in irradiated versus nonirradiated hosts. The number of CFU-S was assayed in femur implants from unirradiated donors transplanted into donors given 9.5 Gy + 10^6 marrow cells. Femora transplanted into irradiated hosts contained more CFU-S than femora transplanted into control unirradiated hosts 2 and 4 weeks after implantation. Six weeks after implantation the numbers of CFU-S in the two groups were comparable. These results indicated that radiation damage to the stroma of marrow was repaired slowly and had not yet returned to normal (80%) after 18 weeks. Proliferation of CFU-S in the implants was affected by factors extraneous to the implants and stimulated, presumably by humoral factors, in the irradiated hosts (19).

Fried et al. further studied the effects of radiation on the hemopoietic stroma by exposing mice to whole body x-irradiation doses of 3-10 Gy. Mice exposed to 8 Gy or more were rescued with 10^6 normal marrow cells. Two days and six weeks after irradiation exposure mice were killed; CFU-S content of the right femur was assayed, and stromal function was assayed by implanting the left femur to a subcutaneous site in an unirradiated host. They also studied the effects of radiation doses with minimal effects on the hemopoietic stroma. One group of mice was exposed to 5 Gy and three control groups received 0, 5, or 10 Gy followed by 10^6 syngeneic marrow cells. Mice from the experimental group (5 Gy) received a second dose of 5 Gy 1, 6, or 27 days later. One day after the second radiation exposure, or 2, 7, and 28 days after the initial exposure, mice were killed and stromal function assayed by transplantation of their femora to subcutaneous sites of normal host mice. Exposure to less than 5 Gy caused no detectable injury to the stroma. CFU-S levels declined to undetectable levels (less than 1% of CFU-S in marrow from unirradiated controls). Exposure to 5 Gy resulted in a small decrease in stromal function measured by the ability to support CFU-S proliferation in some but not all experiments. Stromal injury was increasingly evident after exposures of 6-10 Gy. CFU-S numbers recovered to control levels within 6 weeks at all radiation levels. However, stromal function showed no detectable recovery at 6 weeks at exposure levels of 7 Gy or greater (20). Exposure to 10 Gy as a single dose decreased stromal function to less than one-third of control levels, and no significant recovery occurred within 4 weeks. While a single exposure to 5 Gy resulted in no significant injury to stroma after any of the intervals studied, two doses of 5 Gy resulted in significant stromal damage, and the amount of injury was similar when the doses were separated by intervals of 1-28 days. Exposures to 10 Gy as a single dose caused greater damage to marrow stromal function than did exposure to two doses of 5 Gy (20).

A variety of stromal cells have been identified apart from vascular endothelial cells including fat cells, phagocytic and nonphagocytic reticular cells, and fibroblasts. The previously cited studies by Bloom and Rubin indicate that phagocytic cells of the RE system are functionally active up to doses of 50 Gy in vivo (9, 14). Little information relating to radiation effects on specific stromal cell types is available other than for fibroblasts. Wilson et al. have studied radiation response of clonogenic fibroblastic cells in vitro (CFU-F), comparing them to GM-CFC. Relative to GM-CFC, CFU-F exhibited increased radioresistance. Whole body x-irradiation doses of 0-600 R were given. D_0 (D_{37}) of 200-300 R was obtained which showed substantially more radioresistance than GM-CFC (21). Similar results were reported by Xu et al. following repeated, graded doses of x-rays or neutrons (22).

These studies clearly showed that the hemopoietic stroma was more radioresistant than CFU-S as evidenced by the observation that doses of 5 Gy or less do not consistently affect the hemopoietic stroma whereas they destroy more than 99% of CFU-S. Whereas CFU-S rapidly recover to normal at 6 weeks, radiation-induced stromal injury recovered very slowly and only to 80% of controls after 18 weeks (21).

C. Delayed Effects of Irradiation In Vitro on Marrow Stroma

Tavassoli studied the effects of varying doses of ^{137}Cs gamma irradiation upon murine bone marrow stroma using long-term bone marrow cultures (23). Mice were irradiated in vivo with total body irradiation before establishing stromal layers in vitro. In vitro irradiation of stroma was done by establishing stromal layers and irradiating in vitro immediately after placing the stroma in the flask or 3 weeks after. Doses of irradiation ranged from 2.5 to 40 Gy, and cultures were studied up to 8 weeks after establishment. Doses of irradiation as small as 5 Gy either in vitro or in vivo interfered with the attachment of the stromal layer. Stromal cells did not adhere to or spread over the surface, and there was no formation of cellular stromal islands. No established stromal layer could be detected up to 2 weeks after the initiation of cultures. Once established, after three weeks of in vitro culture similar doses of irradiation interfered with its potential to support the proliferation and maintenance of the hemopoietic stem cell. Doses of 2.5 Gy permitted the development of a stromal layer, but GM-CFCs were assayed at a lower concentration than in control, nonirradiated cultures (24).

Zuckerman et al. have studied the effects of 0-500 Gy on murine marrow stromal cell layers in long-term bone marrow cultures. They reported that established stromal cell layers showed no morphologic changes up to 100 Gy. Hemopoiesis stopped immediately after 9 Gy and did not resume over 10 weeks of observation. RNA and protein synthesis recovered within 3 weeks of irradiation up to 100 Gy. Adherent stroma irradiated with 9-500 Gy supported long-term hemopoiesis by Sl/Sl^d marrow cells and showed no substantial death of cells in the stromal layer over 6 weeks. Once established in vitro, stromal cell layers can tolerate large doses of irradiation up to 200 Gy. Although incapable of proliferating, they can support significant GM-CFC proliferation (25).

Naparstek et al. performed similar studies of in vitro irradiation of stromal layers using doses up to 100 Gy. They observed that production of a colony-stimulating factor (CSF_1) by the stromal layers persisted up to 7 weeks after 100 Gy and that the layers were able to support overlying GM-CFC colonies (26,27). In other experiments they showed that these stromal cells produced increased levels of cell-contact-mediated hemopoietins including factor(s) that stimulate production of certain other GM-CSF/IL-3 dependent hemopoietic progenitor cell lines as well as factor-dependent malignant variant cell lines. Transformation of factor-dependent to factor-independent cells has been associated with malignant change attributed to transforming growth factors or to action of retroviral gene products and activation of protooncogenes. The authors presented these changes in the heavily irradiated stromal cell layers as a possible model system for interactions involved between normal and leukemogenic hemopoietic microenvironments (28).

We used a technique of regenerating hemopoietic stromal cells by applying murine stromal cells from bone marrow, bone, regenerating endosteal mesenchyme, or spleen to cellulose ester membranes (CEMs) subsequently folded into open-ended tubes and implanted intraperitoneally into syngeneic murine recipients. After 6 months the transplanted stromal cells regenerate to form bone cells, sinusoidal endothelium, fat cells, reticular elements, fibroblasts, and macrophages.

We assumed that hemopoietic stromal cell regeneration derived from living stromal cells from the donor hemopoietic tissue. To prove this hypothesis, CEMs coated with stromal cells from bone or bone marrow were irradiated in vitro immediately after placement upon CEM using doses of ^{137}Cs gamma irradiation of 10, 20, or 40 Gy. Doses of 10-40 Gy completely inhibited stromal cell regeneration from marrow. Stromal cells from bone were significantly more radioresistant. CEM coated with stromal cells from bone irradiated with 10 Gy in vitro had no impairment of stromal or hemopoietic regeneration. CEM coated with stromal cells from bone irradiated with 20 Gy had about 50% impairment of hemopoietic regeneration, and 40 Gy completely inhibited stromal and hemopoietic regeneration. It is unclear why stromal cells from bone were more radioresistant than those from marrow. It is also unclear why stromal cells irradiated in vivo appear more radioresistant than stromal cells irradiated in vitro (29).

Hemopoietic stromal cell sensitivity to radiation has been variable. Knospe et al. reported that stromal cells irradiated in vivo and in situ were quite radioresistant to localized x-irradiation. Regeneration occurred 6 months after 20 Gy but only after a nadir of injury to sinusoidal endothelium at 3 months (8). Although the experiments utilized different assay techniques, Fried's results suggested very severe injury at exposures of 10 Gy (20).

Friedenstein et al. transplanted marrow to subcapsular sites of the kidney. They studied stromal cell regeneration and the formation of a hemopoietic microenvironment, which they attributed to a fibroblastic cell. Dispersal of stromal cells in this model prevented stromal regeneration (30,31). Chertkov et al. studied regeneration of marrow-derived stromal cells and noted the effects on the regenerative process of stromal cell dispersion versus compaction of stromal cells by centrifugation. Dispersion prevented regeneration (32). These several studies support the concept that regeneration of marrow stroma and radiation repair is enhanced by structural orderliness or spatial organization with stromal cells remaining in close proximity to each other. Stromal cells remaining in situ may possess greater radioresistance than stromal cells that are disrupted or separated from an intact circulation. The capacity of stromal cells to repair radiation injury may be much greater in an intact marrow, with sinusoidal cells, fat cells, macrophages, and fibroblasts interrelating in an organized way. Ultrastructural analysis of the marrow has shown that certain reticular cells extend cytoplasmic processes for long distances through the marrow and that these processes surround and sustain hemopoietic cells. Such spatial and intercellular relationships of the stromal cells may be essential for optimal repair. In the CEM experiments, irradiated stromal cells from bone were encased in small particles (up to 800 or 1000 μm in diameter) of bone, which may have made them more resistant to radiation injury by preserving spatial intercellular relations (29).

Reincke et al. studied residual injury in murine marrow cells using long-term marrow cultures. Cultures were established, and 21 days after inoculation irradiated in vitro with 0.5, 3, or 5.5 Gy from a ^{137}Cs gamma source. Very substantial suppression of granulopoietic cellular proliferation was observed at 3 and 5 Gy exposure without recovery at 24 weeks after exposure, and this was attributed to injury to surviving hemopoietic stem cells. The authors suggested that this injury resulted from inherent limits on cellular regeneration following radiation-induced reduction in the stem cell pool (33).

D. Delayed Effects of Whole Body Irradiation on Hemopoiesis in Animals

Baum and Wyant studied hemopoietic recovery in beagles given 1.5 Gy as a single exposure of x-rays or mixed neutron-gamma irradiation. Ninety days later the dogs were irradiated a second time, and 90 days later a third irradiation dose of 1.5 Gy was given. X-rays appeared to be more injurious and resulted in greater lethality than gamma-neutron irradiation. Dogs given two doses of 1.5 Gy x-rays had a 15% mortality compared to 3% in the twice-irradiated gamma-neutron group. The reasons for this mortality were not clear, as there were only slightly lower leukocyte levels in the dogs given x-rays. Hematocrits after 200 days were slightly below preirradiation control levels (50%), with levels slightly more depressed in the group given 1.5 Gy X 3 (hematocrits of 30-40% versus 40-50%). The poorer response of previously irradiated dogs was attributed to residual injury in previously irradiated HSCs (34). Gong et al. exposed rats to 170 R (200 kVp) x-irradiation; at intervals of 3-60 weeks postirradiation the rats were bled one-third or two-thirds their calculated blood volume and the overall marrow content of nucleated red blood cells was determined by ^{59}Fe uptake in the marrow 24-48 or 48-66 hr, respectively, after bleeding. The increase in numbers of erythroid precursors in bled irradiated rats was less at each interval studied than in the control rats. Erythroid response increased with time from 16% to 80% of controls after 3-60 weeks. The half-recovery time of this component of residual injury was 29.2 weeks. In nonbled irradiated rats this component of residual injury was not detected (35). Baum presented evidence that in the nonstressed state the erythropoietic system of rats exposed to 300 R would return to normal between 2 and 13 weeks postexposure. These several investigations were consistent with the concept of a diminished pluripotent stem cell pool, in part reparable, which progressively returned toward normal (36). Valentine et al. reported the effects of four whole body exposures of 200 R to cats over 18 months. Hemoglobin regeneration was slightly slower after the fourth and last irradiation. Leukocytes did not appear to be affected (37). Testa et al. studied long-term marrow injury following irradiation exposure in mice exposed to 4-5-Gy x-rays separated by 3-week intervals. The exponential regeneration of CFU-S and GM-CFC was decreased with a population doubling time of 48 hr instead of 28 hr in mice exposed to a single dose. CFU-S in repeatedly irradiated mice were less competent in repopulating ablated hemopoietic tissue. Single exposure to 5 Gy also resulted in reduced CFU-S regeneration to about 50% of normal (38). The defect was also expressed as an inability to maintain normal numbers of CFU-S in long-term bone marrow cultures (39). Similar changes were seen in GM-CFCs of mice in a similar model of fractionated exposures (40,41). Hendry et al. showed that repeatedly irradiated mice are less competent in repopulating ablated hemopoietic tissue when transplanted (40). Residual damage was observed after single sublethal doses of 5 Gy and was comparable to that seen after an equivalent fractionated dose. CFU-S recovered to only 50% of normal. This suggested that there was no sparing effect of fractionated versus single doses of long-term effects on hemopoiesis (42,43). Schofield and Dexter reported that an irradiated (15 Gy gamma irradiation) adherent layer of long-term marrow cultures was able to support hemopoiesis at normal levels of CFU-S and GM-CFC compared to unirradiated controls (44).

These delayed effects of whole body irradiation were probably the result of injury to hemopoietic stem cells through a mechanism of injury to DNA and the proliferative machinery of the cell.

Calvo et al. studied bone marrow histology in dogs given 12 Gy x-irradiation as a single-exposure total body dose. The animals were then rescued with cryopreserved autologous leukocytes collected by leukophoresis. Following recovery from the acute radiation syndrome, the dogs were observed for 260 days or 700-898 days. Hemopoiesis appeared normal with marrow differential counts showing M:E ratios close to normal with lymphocytes 40% of normal in the dogs observed for the longer period. Blood counts were similar to preirradiation levels except for one dog with slight anemia. A dense endosteal fibrosis was observed along trabecular surfaces of bone, and at these areas osteoblasts were absent. These changes were observed in 6 of 7 dogs and were progressive (45).

E. Chronic, Continuous Low-Dose Irradiation Effects in Experimental Animals

Seed et al. have performed long-term, continuous-exposure studies of beagles irradiated continuously (22 hr/day) with ^{60}Co gamma rays at rates varying from 35 to 0.4 cGy/day. Two distinct patterns of response were noted. At the higher dose levels of 35 and 17 cGy/day, aplastic anemia and death predominated, with a mean survival time of 53 days and 156 days, respectively. At 10 and 5 cGy/day exposures, mean survival times were 256 and 1834 days, respectively. These survival times represented reductions of observed life spans of 7.1 and 50.8% (extended median survival time of 3613 days for the nonirradiated colony controls). LD_{50} was estimated to be: 35 cGy/day, 14.42 Gy; 17 cGy/day, 21.24 Gy; 10 cGy/day, 20.39 Gy; and 5 cGy/day, 71.61 Gy. An interesting feature of the survival curves at the higher daily dose rates was a narrow shoulder, whereas the longer surviving lower daily exposures developed a broader shoulder, suggesting the development of radioresistance (46,47).

The clinical hemopathologic syndromes changed at the lower daily dose of 5 cGy/day with a dramatic reduction of aplastic anemias and an increasing incidence of nonlymphocytic acute leukemia (6.3%) and acute endosteal myelofibrosis with myeloid metaplasia of the spleen (4%). The incidence of nonlymphoblastic acute leukemia in the control, nonirradiated population of dogs was 0%, and that of acute lymphoblastic leukemia, 1% (48).

The radiosensitive subgroup prone to aplastic anemia had a marked decrease in blood counts, marrow cellularity, and an irreversible depletion of GM-CFCs, whereas the leukemia-prone group exposed to lower doses of 5 cGy/day showed initial depletion of GM-CFCs and a drop in blood counts followed by a partial restoration and later accommodative, cyclic maintenance of this compartment's size and function. Depletion of the GM-CFCs was accompanied by an aberrant, intense granulomonocytic proliferation of marrow, with a clonal outgrowth of preleukemic progenitors with radically altered clonogenic properties and a restriction of proliferative capacity of early progeny of these clonogenically hyperactive cells. The authors speculated that the cellular mechanisms involved included (1) acquired radioresistance as a primary mechanism of recovery and accommodation. Although (2) enhanced stem cell-cell cycling with shortened cycle times, (3) broadened proliferative zones, and (4) altered cell transit patterns may play a minor role, these mechanisms could not be invoked for prolonged periods at the relatively high rates of exposure received by the leukemia-prone group without eventually depleting stem cell compartments below the threshold levels necessary to maintain a minimum level of hemopoiesis. They demonstrated that GM-CFCs from the marrow of leukemia-prone dogs (5 cGy/day) were markedly more radioresistant than the more sensitive cells isolated from the aplasia-prone animals or from nonirradiated controls. This radioresistance was acquired at the time of hemopoietic recovery, and not gradually. They interpreted these results to mean that the mode of acquisition of radioresistance was not "simple selection" but more likely a process of gene modification, perhaps gene amplification. Several patterns of development of radioresistance were observed, with elevated D_0 values (suppressed dose-dependent lethality rates) followed by increased D_Q values (increased sublethal damage capacity) and a final pattern of greatest radioresistance in which cells showed both elevated D_0 and D_Q values (48,49).

Others have shown that chronic irradiation is associated with the emergence of radioresistant stem cells having altered buoyant light density. These were observed in human patients with polycythemia vera and myelofibrosis (50,51). This pattern of altered lighter stem cells is also seen in fetal hemopoietic GM-CFCs (52). The authors speculated that the leukemia-inducing 5 cGy/day exposures in some way trigger the reemergence of a radioresistant type of hemopoiesis, perhaps by an induction of the fetal type of hemopoiesis (49).

Brecher et al. studied rats exposed to 70 cGy/day. Aplasia of marrow was followed by extramedullary hemopoiesis in the spleen and recovery of blood counts after 90 days of exposure (53). Knospe et al. investigated hemopoiesis in mice exposed to doses of 70, 45, and 25 cGy/day of ^{60}Co gamma irradiation. Mice exposed to 45 and 70 cGy/day progressed rapidly to marrow aplasia, severe cytopenias, and death between 60 and 90 days. Mice exposed to 25 cGy/day rapidly developed leukopenia, anemia, and marrow aplasia with nadirs around 6 months. Between 8 and 10 months, splenomegaly and splenic hemopoiesis were followed by recovery of leukocytes and red cells. Platelet levels were relatively preserved with only slight to moderate reductions, and megakaryocytic hyperplasia was observed in both marrow and spleen. At the time of red cell and leukocyte recovery, CFU-S and GM-CFC levels were markedly depressed. These results were consistent with a subpopulation of rapidly cycling radioresistant stem cells as mediators of hemopoietic recovery. The aplastic marrow showed extensive evidence of sinusoidal hemorrhage and reductions of sinusoidal number. These changes suggested damage to the hemopoietic microenvironment of marrow similar to previously reported single-exposure localized irradiation at a comparable total dosage (8). The results in chronic, continuously irradiated mice suggested a greater sensitivity to chronic irradiation injury of the marrow stroma compared to the spleen (54).

The low-level continuous radiation studies of Seed et al. and Knospe et al. both resulted in syndromes of acute leukemia or myeloproliferative disease. Both of these models resulted in very large total body exposures of radiation approaching 75 Gy total doses. Such injury may induce changes in the stroma that mediate cell transformation to malignancy, perhaps by mechanisms inducing stromal cell factor-derived independence for proliferating cell lines as suggested by Naparstek et al. (26-28).

II. DELAYED EFFECTS OF RADIATION ON THE BONE MARROW IN HUMANS

The majority of effects of irradiation studied in human subjects have been in patients given local radiation therapy for cancer or rheumatoid spondylitis. Another population studied has comprised the victims of atomic bomb irradiation in Japan and scattered other patients exposed to fallout or reactor accidents. More recently, patients subjected to bone marrow transplantation represent a growing pool of subjects given whole body doses of irradiation in the lethal range (10 Gy whole body).

A. Local Irradiation for Cancer

Hutaff and Belding studied 12 patients with cancer of the cervix treated with fractionated localized x-ray doses of 2400 R (in air). Some of these patients received radium implants locally into the cervix. Four patients had marrow examined 67-104 days after therapy was completed. They reported significant regeneration of marrow elements (55).

Sykes et al. studied changes in the marrow after localized irradiation for cancer of the breast, kidneys, lung, and cervix. Fractionated doses of 30-65 Gy of x-rays were given over 3-7 weeks. Calculated doses to bone marrow were less and ranged from 19 to 65 Gy. Autopsy studies of the marrow within irradiated fields in 7 patients showed it to be markedly depressed in 5 of the 7. Cellularity varied, being aplastic in 2 patients, hypocellular in 3 patients, and apparently regenerated in 2 patients. The bone marrow dose in the 2 patients with regenerated marrow was 56 and 19 Gy. Two patients were noted to have regenerated marrow 2 months after irradiation but 2 months later reverted to a permanently hypoplastic marrow. Eighteen patients had marrow examined prior to death and at intervals of 2-18 months after irradiation. Only one showed marrow regeneration. In the other 17 patients failure to recover was attributed to permanent damage to HSCs or physiological alteration of blood vessels or supporting syncytium (56).

Goswitz et al. studied 6 patients with cancer of the bladder and 2 patients with cancer of the lung who received fractionated ^{60}Co tumor doses of 29-60 Gy. Bone marrow doses were 12.5-45 Gy. Marrow cellularity in irradiated sites fell to 10% of normal. However, some regeneration was reported after 3-4 months even at 50 Gy marrow doses, and all three myeloid lineages were observed to be present (57).

DeGowin et al. investigated the ablation and regeneration of erythropoiesis in locally irradiated fields of 5 patients with malignant lymphoma using marrow scanning with ^{59}Fe. Radiation doses varied from 12 to 40 Gy. Regeneration was inhibited and delayed for at least 1-3 years (58).

Stewart and Dische studied the effects of x-ray therapy on the marrow of patients with ankylosing spondylitis. Marrow doses varied from 1020 to 1640 R. In 12 of 28 patients, total marrow cell counts outside the irradiated fields were above the upper limit of normal, with a generalized hyperplasia of erythroid, myeloid, megakaryocytic, and lymphoid lineages. This suggested a stimulation of hemopoiesis outside the irradiated fields. In 4 of 5 patients whose irradiated marrow was examined 73-189 days posttreatment, the marrow cellularity remained markedly depressed. Ten patients were studied who had been irradiated 15-142 months earlier. In 2 cases the marrow was still aplastic more than 9 years after treatment. In 5 patients regeneration was inadequate and the marrow remained hypoplastic. In only 3 patients was the marrow normal. These marrow changes were associated with neutrophil leukopenia and lymphopenia in the blood (59).

Knospe et al. studied the regeneration and extension of marrow in 25 patients with malignant lymphoma given marrow ablative doses of irradiation. Most of these patients received so-called total nodal irradiation (mantle + inverted Y fields). ^{52}Fe whole body marrow scanning was used to determine the degree of suppression and recovery of erythropoietic marrow after doses of ^{60}Co that varied from 12 to 48 Gy, although most patients received 40-48 Gy. The interval between completion of irradiation and time of scanning varied from immediately posttreatment to 73 months. Only one patient was scanned before and after treatment. Patients were selected to include representative time intervals between radiation and erythropoietic bone marrow imaging. The intervals selected for analysis were 0-12, 12-24, and greater than 24 months. Three questions were posed: (1) What level of total radiation dose results in permanent marrow aplasia? (2) What interval is required for marrow regeneration to occur? (3) Does significant expansion of the active marrow organ occur into the inactive peripheral skeleton normally containing yellow marrow?

Significant inhibition of erythropoiesis was observed in all patients at intervals less than 1 year after completion of radiation therapy, and the magnitude of suppression was maximal in patients scanned less than 6 months after irradiation (Fig. 10). Less suppression was observed at intervals of 6-12 months. Between 12 and 24 months, moderate recovery occurred in one or more radiation fields in 7 of 8 patients (Fig. 11). However, in 6 of 8 patients, one or more fields showed marked residual suppression at intervals greater than 24 months after completion of irradiation. All patients treated with multiple fields showed excellent recovery of erythropoietic function in the first field treated, but 4 of 9 patients showed poor recovery in the last field treated. Pelvic fields more frequently showed impaired recovery or residual inhibition than marrow in mantle fields, and the pelvic fields were usually the last irradiated.

Four of ten patients showed expansion of erythropoietic marrow into the peripheral skeleton or long bones in the intervals less than 12 months after irradiation. Between 12 and 24 months after irradiation only 1 of 8 patients showed evidence of marked expansion and 6 of 8 patients showed evidence of minimum long bone activation of erythropoiesis. The patients graded as 2+ expansion were also those patients with initial marked suppression of erythropoiesis. After intervals longer than 24 months, 7 of 9 patients showed either no expansion or minimal expansion (0 to 2+), and only one showed 3+ expansion.

There was no correlation between total radiation dose and the degree of marrow suppression. Regeneration regularly occurred at doses of 40-44 Gy and was seen 1 year after doses of 45 and 46 Gy in 2 patients. It appeared that the fractionated dose causing permanent aplasia was well over 44 Gy.

Cytopenias were frequent during the first year after irradiation, with 8 of 10 patients anemic, 6 of 10 leukopenic, and 5 of 10 thrombocytopenic. Between 12 and 24 months, cytopenias were less frequent: 2 of 8 patients were anemic, none were leukopenic, and 2 of 8 were thrombocytopenic. After 24 months, 9 patients were studied and none was anemic or thrombocytopenic; 1 patient was leukopenic. In the treatment intervals after 12 months, 3 of the cytopenic patients also received chemotherapy and 1 was hypersplenic.

Autopsy material was available on 1 patient who received 35-46 Gy 35-38 months prior to death. The marrow was variably cellular with areas of focal regeneration alternating with aplasia. The ^{52}Fe scans showed patchy or irregular regeneration of erythropoiesis (60).

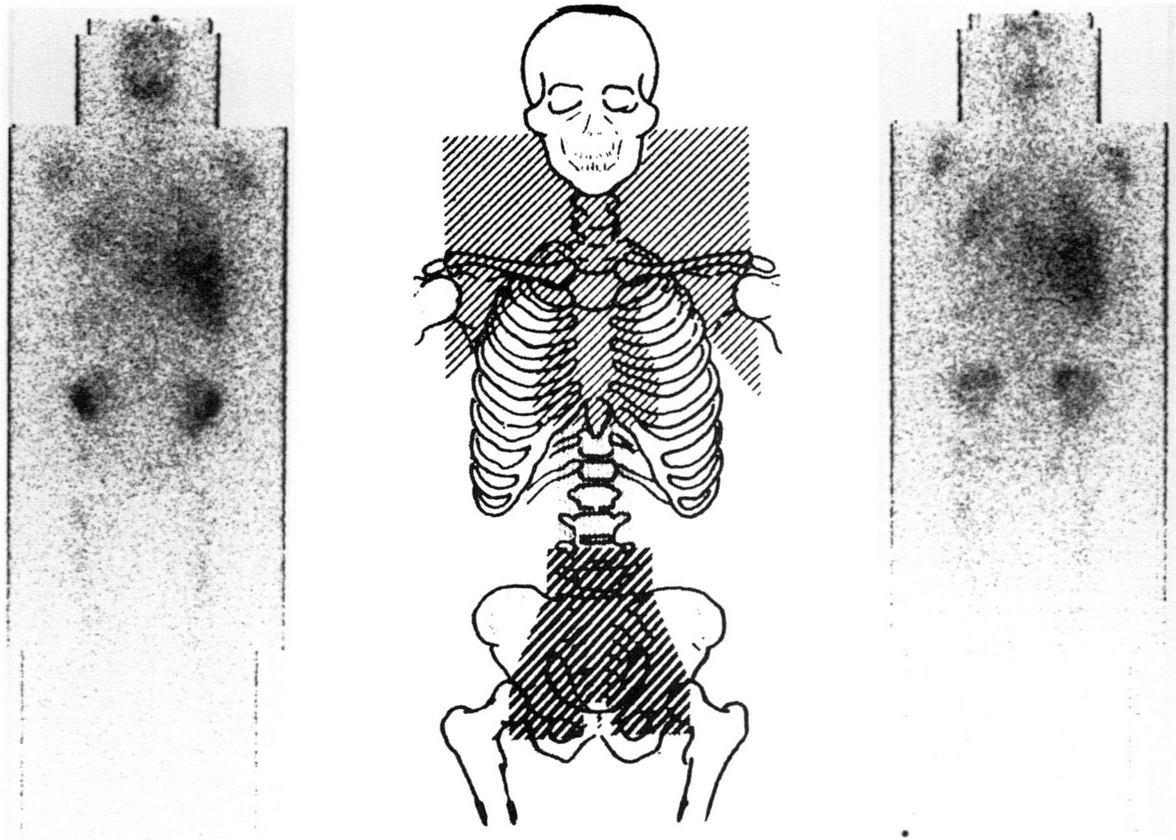

Figure 10 ^{52}Fe marrow scan 4-6 months after completion of total nodal irradiation showing marked suppression of erythropoiesis within the treatment fields. Radiation dose was 40 Gy. From Ref. 60.

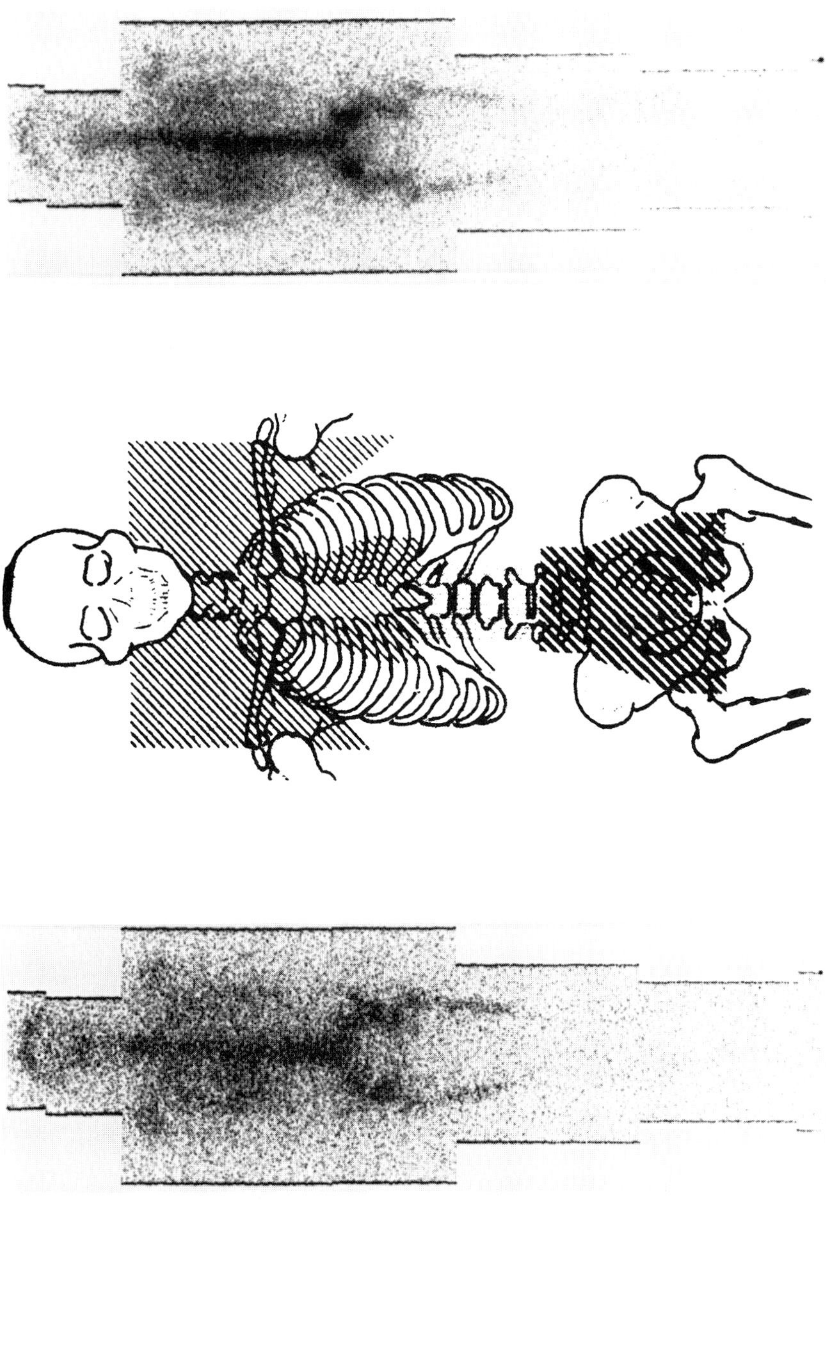

Figure 11 ^{52}Fe marrow scan 12-14 months after completion of total nodal irradiation showing good but patchy recovery in all fields. Radiation dose was 40-50 Gy. From Ref. 60.

These results were similar to our studies of single-exposure irradiation injury in the rat. In the human studies initial suppression of hemopoiesis occurred 1-12 months after irradiation, followed by regeneration of marrow 12 months after completing radiation therapy. The results differed from the experimental studies of the rat in that we failed to define a marrow ablative dose up to 46 Gy. These results do not indicate that human marrow is more radioresistant than rodent marrow but rather that fractionated radiation is less injurious than single-exposure doses, with greater opportunity for repair after fractionated exposure (60).

The nature of the stimulating or activating effects of localized radiation upon the inactive yellow marrow of the peripheral skeleton is unknown but presumably mediated by a humoral mechanism. This effect may be similar to the stimulating effect of injury to marrow following marrow curettage reported by Van Dyke and Harris (61) and Knospe et al. (62).

Rubin et al. reported similar results in human patients with Hodgkin's disease receiving localized radiation therapy. He studied inhibition and recovery of marrow within irradiated fields as well as activation of marrow in the inactive peripheral skeleton outside the irradiated fields. He used a technique of whole body marrow imaging using ^{99m}Tc-sulfur colloid to study the distribution and activity of reticuloendothelial marrow. Regeneration of marrow occurred after intervals of 1-2 years in 85% of the marrow sites. Expansion of marrow into normally inactive sites of the peripheral skeleton occurred in 15 of 27 patients during the same period, 1-2 years after irradiation (63).

There has been some question about the equivalence of ^{52}Fe and ^{99m}Tc-sulfur colloid for the study of marrow. The similar results of our studies, which used ^{52}Fe, and those of Rubin, who used ^{99m}Tc-sulfur colloid, indicate that both isotopes define the active hemopoietic marrow. In over 50 patients studied at our institution in whom concurrent scanning with these two isotopes was done, identical distributions of marrow were observed. Thus, widely available ^{99m}Tc-sulfur colloid imaging of the whole body bone marrow accurately defines the extent and activity of the active hemopoietic marrow as well as the distribution and activity of the reticuloendothelial marrow (62,63).

Sacks et al. reported studies using ^{111}In as a marrow-scanning agent of bone marrow regeneration in humans following large-field irradiation. They found that radiation dose, age of the patient, and total amount of marrow irradiated were important factors determining extent of regeneration. Time effects did not appear to be important except that most regeneration occurred within the first 12 months following irradiation. The most striking finding was the effect of the irradiation volume. Small volumes failed to regenerate, particularly compared to the greater regeneration observed with larger irradiated volumes. The authors suggested that the stimulus to regeneration might be related to a humoral factor derived from the irradiated tissue (64).

Morardet et al. reported reduced numbers of GM-CFCs in adult patients with Hodgkin's disease for up to 9 years after local irradiation therapy (65 and Chapter 13).

B. Delayed Effects of Irradiation in Accidental Whole Body Exposures

LeRoy reviewed hematological data obtained from atomic bomb casualties in Japan. Exposed persons were classified according to distance from the explosion hypocenter or ground zero and also to the degree of shielding they received from buildings, tunnels, bomb shelters, and so on. Radiation injury was classified as very severe, severe, moderately severe, and mild. All of these groups showed significant depressions in leukocytes, hemoglobin, and platelets during the acute postexposure period lasting 1-2 months. Leukocytes began to recover after 1 month and returned to normal levels (7000/mm^3) 10 weeks after exposure. Those with specific signs of radiation injury had somewhat lower leukocyte counts, but even these had normal levels (6000/mm^3) after 10 weeks. These subjects sustained radiation doses that were of median lethal size or greater. Hemoglobin levels also returned to normal in 50% of persons in these groups by 13 weeks and in over 90% of persons exposed by 17 weeks after exposure. Long-term (greater than 8 weeks) platelet data were not given (66).

Fliedner et al. performed serial cytologic studies on bone marrow cells on 8 men accidentially exposed to mixed neutron-gamma irradiation in a nuclear reactor accident at Oak Ridge, Tennessee. Studies were done early (12 hr to 23 days) and late (3.5 years after exposure). Early after exposure, a wave of "mitotically connected" abnormalities was observed: nuclear fragments in cytoplasm of erythroblasts, granulocytic precursors, and lymphocytes; bi- and multinucleated cells and giant cells. The peak of abnormalities in the erythropoietic precursors occurred after 2 days, the granulocytic precursors after 4 days, and a dose-dependent difference was observed between the high-dose group (2.36-3.65 Gy) and the low-dose group (22-68 cGy). Studies of bone marrow smears of exposed men 3½ years after exposure showed similar distributions for the high-dose and low-dose groups. However, a number of the mitoses in the high-dose group and a smaller number of mitoses in the low-dose exposure group were abnormal (aberrant mitoses excluded from further cell division) or clearly visible single or multiple chromosome bridges in late anaphase or telephase. It was not determined what the frequency of such abnormal mitoses was in healthy persons (67).

Vorder Bruegge reviewed the effects of radiation injury in victims of the atomic bombings of Japan in World War II. He stated that during the third and fourth months most of the late fatal patients exhibited marrow hyperplasia with fewer maturation defects and more neutrophils in the blood. However, in occasional patients dying more than 4 months after exposure, the marrow remained pink and gelatinous and aplasia remained prominent. Dilatation of small blood vessels caused some hypoplastic marrows to appear hyperplastic on gross examination. These patients presumably sustained lethal doses of whole body irradiation but not so severe that some marrow recovery did not occur (68).

Liebow et al. described the marrow in patients dying 6 weeks after exposure to whole body irradiation (mixed neutron-gamma) as usually showing focal myeloid regeneration and marked myeloid hyperplasia. Occasionally patients showed hypoplasia of the marrow and occasionally reticulum hyperplasia. Most patients dying 6 weeks after exposure were severely anemic, and this was noted to be in part associated with omnipresent severe infections. Most patients were not leukopenic (69).

Conrad et al. studied 290 Marshall Islanders accidentally exposed to radioactive fallout in 1954. Estimated whole body gamma doses varied from 0.14 to 1.75 Gy. The most heavily exposed group included 64 people. Exposure also included ingestion or absorption of various internally emitting isotopes including ^{89}Sr. These decayed fairly rapidly to less than 10% of the initial activities by day 82 and may have made some contribution to bone marrow injury. Leukocytes were frequently less than 1000 and platelets less than 75,000 per cubic millimeter in the more heavily exposed persons at nadirs between 24 and 45 days. Recovery to normal levels occurred by 60 days after exposure. No infections or hemorrhagic effects could be attributed to the cytopenias. The authors noted that a slight lag in complete recovery of peripheral blood elements in the exposed people compared to that of the unexposed population occurred up until 11 years postexposure (70).

C. Delayed Effects of Irradiation on Hemopoiesis Following Total Body Irradiation for Bone Marrow Transplantation

Li et al. studied blood counts and myeloid progenitor cells derived from bone marrow in 29 patients who had received bone marrow transplants 2 months to 8.5 years previously. Two of these patients received syngeneic grafts; three, autografts; and 24, allogeneic grafts. Conditioning was variable, with 22 receiving total body irradiation (3-10 Gy) and cyclophosphamide 120-200 mg/kg. Three received only TBI (13.5-15 Gy). Allograft recipients received methotrexate 15 mg/kg on day 1, 10 mg/m^2 on days 3, 6, and 11, and then weekly to day 102 for graft-versus-host prophylaxis. Leukocyte counts were minimally decreased in 4 and low in 5 patients. Hemoglobin was less than 10.0 g/dl in 3 patients, and thrombocytopenia occurred in 11 patients. Bone marrow cellularity varied from 25 to 60% (median 40%) and M:E ratios from 1:1 to 10:1 (median 2:1). The numbers of blood- and marrow-derived GM-CFCs were markedly reduced compared to normal controls, even at long intervals after transplantation. The authors removed E^+ rosette-forming cells from marrow samples in some of these patients and noted an increase in GM-CFCs. No effect was noted on erythroid progenitors (BFU-E).

They could not determine whether such an abnormality was present in vivo in these patients but speculated that this effect might account for the increased sensitivity to chemotherapy. (These results will be reviewed in more detail in Chapter 15.)

These results suggest that the reduced levels of GM-CFCs in transplant recipients result, at least in part, from an abnormal in vitro interaction between GM-CFCs and E rosette-forming cells. Whether such an abnormality is present in vivo in these patients is unknown but is suggested by the increased sensitivity of transplant recipients to chemotherapy (71).

The authors cited a variety of experimental studies of marrow transplantation in animals as well as in humans to support a hypothesis that after marrow transplantation there is an increased demand on stem cells for differentiation that takes precedence over self-renewal of stem cells and leads to progressive stem cell depletion (72-79).

Several other reports have described decreased GM-CFCs in transplant patients and also in patients with hematological disorders who were not transplanted but received various forms of cytotoxic chemotherapy or immunotherapy such as corticosteroids or antilymphocyte globulin (see Chapters 11-14). Many of these patients appeared to have persistent abnormalities of T lymphocyte function (80-89).

These studies suggest that marrow transplantation or cytotoxic chemotherapy can result in varying amounts of abnormal hemopoiesis, in part attributable to dysregulation involving T lymphocytes and perhaps regulatory factors. Such abnormal hemopoiesis may sometimes be subclinical and exist in the presence of normal peripheral blood counts. In the complex situation of pretransplant conditioning and posttransplant recovery in the face of cytotoxic drugs such as methotrexate or other immunosuppressive drugs, it is impossible to identify the specific role and contribution of radiation. However, radiation alone in the lethal range was associated with these changes (71). It is possible that the abnormal hemopoiesis commonly present in posttransplant patients could represent in part delayed effects on hemopoietic stroma that may induce these dysregulatory changes (see Chapter 17).

III. OVERVIEW OF DELAYED EFFECTS OF RADIATION INJURY ON HEMOPOIETIC TISSUES

The major effect of delayed radiation injury on hemopoietic tissues is on the hemopoietic stroma. HSCs are exquisitely sensitive to radiation. Lethal exposure for mammals begins around 4 Gy, and LD_{100} levels of exposure occur at doses of 8-10 Gy (single exposure). Acute lethality after whole body exposure occurs within 2-4 weeks from failure of HSCs in the marrow.

Whole body exposures in humans are incompatible with survival at doses over 8 Gy. Survival is possible if rescue is accomplished with a bone marrow transplant to replace the injured HSCs, but disturbances in hemopoietic regulation may be a late effect of marrow transplantation.

Survival following larger doses of partial body exposure is possible. Examples of such exposure include radiation therapy for cancer and accidental exposures such as may occur after radiation accidents involving reactors or radiation laboratories.

The studies reviewed indicate that hemopoietic stromal cells are sensitive to doses as low as 2.5-5 Gy. However, injury at this level of exposure can be detected only with in vitro systems or assays involving disruption and transplantation of stromal cells, which may distort or amplify the amount of injury. Radiation injury in vivo may be similarly sensitive, but stromal cells in vivo have a large capacity for repair. Consequently, single exposures of 20 Gy in vivo can be repaired, although the repair process is prolonged and requires 6-12 months and is only partial even after 1 year. Single exposures in vivo to doses of 40 Gy or greater results in irreparable injury to the stroma and permanent aplasia. Fractionated radiation of the type delivered in cancer therapy is less injurious to the stroma, and significant repair occurs with doses of 40-50 Gy although 6-12 months or

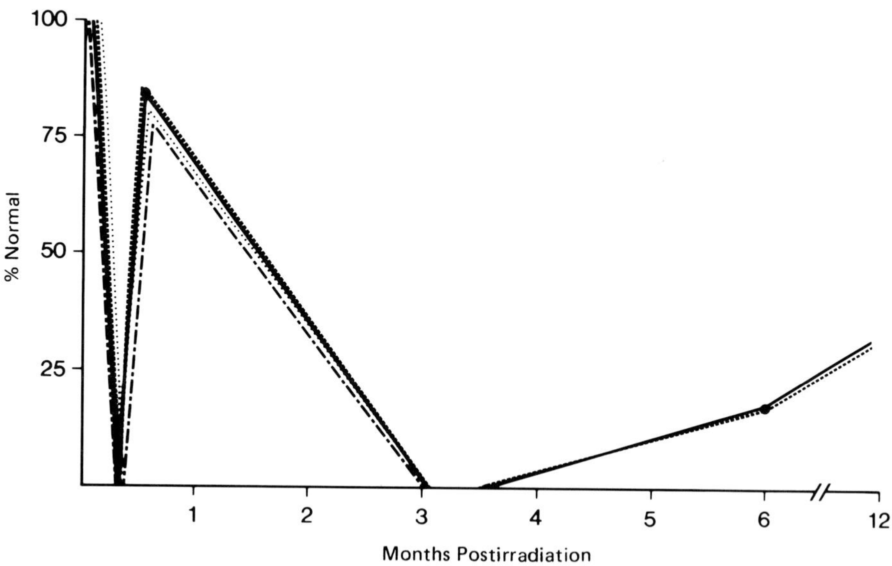

Figure 12 Interrelation of radiation-induced marrow sinusoidal injury, marrow aplasia, and hemopoietic regeneration in totally irradiated marrow. (---) Hemopoiesis, 40-100 Gy; (···) sinusoidal injury, 40-100 Gy; (—) sinusoidal injury, 20 Gy; (—) hemopoietic activity, 20 Gy.

Table 1 Effects of Local Irradiation—In Situ and In Vivo

Species	Dose (Gy)	Time after irradiation	Evolution	Ref.
Rat	20[a]	4 days	Aplasia with extensive sinusoidal injury	8
		14 days	Hemopoietic regeneration	
		30-90 days	Progressive aplasia with sinusoidal atrophy and disappearance	
		180 days	Sinusoidal regeneration and early scattered hemopoietic regeneration	
		1 year	Sinusoidal regeneration and progressive hemopoietic regeneration	
	40[a]	4 days	Aplasia with extensive sinusoidal injury	
	100[a]	14 days	Regeneration of hemopoiesis and repair of sinusoids	
		90 days - 1 year	Progressive loss of cellularity to total aplasia; progressive loss of sinusoidal structure; increasing fibrosis	
Rabbit	20-30[b]	2 days	Aplasia	
		2 months	Aplasia	13
		15 months	Regeneration (up to 50%; many areas aplastic)	
	40-50[b]	6 months	Less than 50% of control; greater regeneration of hemopoiesis with fractionated irradiation	14

(Table 1 *continues*)

Table 1 (*continued*)

Species	Dose (Gy)	Time after irradiation	Evolution	Ref.
Man	10-20[b]	15-142 months	Regeneration variable–2 patients aplastic, 5 hypoplastic, 3 normal	59
	24[b]	2-5 months	Partial regeneration	55
	30-65[b]	2-18 months	Aplasia	56
	29-60[b]	4 months	Partial regeneration (25% of normal)	57 58
	40-50[b]	3-6 months	Aplasia to hypoplasia	60
		1-2 years	Regeneration but with hypoplasia	63 64

[a]Single exposure.
[b]Fractionated exposure.

Table 2 Effects of In Vitro Irradiation[a] on Stromal Function

Source of stroma	Dose (Gy)	Interval	Effect	Ref.
Sl/Sl[d] mouse marrow	9.5	8 weeks	30-50% regeneration	16
	25	8 weeks	0% regeneration	
CBA mouse marrow	9.5	6 weeks	1% regeneration	17, 19, 20
	7.5	6 weeks	20% regeneration	
Rat marrow	10	6 weeks	10-25% regeneration	18
	20	6 weeks	0% regeneration	
Mouse marrow stroma	10	6 months	0% regeneration	29
Mouse bone stroma	10	6 months	100% regeneration	29
	20	6 months	25-50% regeneration	
	40	6 months	0% regeneration	
Mouse marrow stroma	5	—	Completely aborted the development of a supportive stromal layer in long-term cultures	24

[a]Single exposure.

longer is required. Even after several years repair may be only partial. Injury to the hemopoietic stroma after extensive radiotherapy such as total nodal irradiation for Hodgkin's disease may result in diminished hemopoietic reserve capacity and lowered peripheral blood counts for longer periods after completion of radiotherapy—up to a year or longer. Such reduction of hemopoietic reserve may be particularly important if combination cytotoxic chemotherapy is given in concert with radiotherapy. Low blood counts may require that chemotherapy be stopped or delayed or that reduced doses be given. Reduced hemopoietic reserve capacity following radiation in Hodgkin's disease or malignant lymphoma is associated with poor engraftment when an autologous transplant is done for relapsed disease or for bad risk categories of lymphoma.

Radiation injury to the hemopoietic stroma is mediated, at least in part, through effects on vascular sinusoidal cells, which in vivo turn over slowly. Radiation injury to marrow endothelium is biphasic, with initial injury rapidly repaired, followed by a secondary wave of injury requiring 1-3 months to express itself maximally. However, even this delayed injury can be repaired up to fractionated doses of 50 Gy. The role of the marrow fibroblasts in hemopoietic stromal injury is less well defined. Most of the studies of radiation effects on fibroblasts have been in vitro. Cloned marrow fibroblasts are sensitive to doses of 5 Gy or less in vitro. Long-term studies in vivo show residual effects after accumulated x-ray doses of at least 4.5 Gy (22). Phagocytic cells remain functionally active up to 30 Gy exposure as a single dose and up to 50 Gy in fractionated exposures (Tables 1 and 2).

In summary, delayed effects of radiation are expressed primarily through effects on the hemopoietic stroma. Hemopoietic stromal cells are sensitive to radiation, perhaps as sensitive as hemopoietic stem cells. The effects of single-exposure doses of 20 Gy or less or fractionated doses up to 50 Gy to stromal cells are repaired in vivo. Repair may be progressive up to 2 years or longer after exposure. Sublethal doses of irradiation consistent with long-term survival may reduce or damage stem cell pools and proliferative capacity, and cytopenias may occur.

ACKNOWLEDGMENTS

The author thanks the following publishing companies for granting permission to reproduce figures that originally appeared in the respective journals which they published: Grune and Stratton, Inc., *Blood 28,* 398-415 (1966); and J. B. Lippincott Co., *Cancer 37,* 1432-1442 (1976).

REFERENCES

1. Casarett, G. W. Histopathology of alpha irradiation from internally administered polonium. *University of Rochester Atomic Energy Commission Report* UR-201 (1952).

2. Bauer, R. Untersuchungen über die einwirkung unterscheidlich verabfolgter roentgenstrahlung auf das knochenmark und seine zellelemente, zugleich ein beitrag zum zeitfaktorproblem. *Strahlentherapie 67,* 424-501 (1940).
3. Wunsche, H. W. Fortlaufende untersuchungen über den einfluss der roentgenstrahlen auf das knochenmark. Naunyn schmeidebergs. *Arch. Exp. Pathol. 189,* 581-599 (1938).
4. Casati, A. Experimentelle untersuchungen über die roentgenwirkung auf das knochenmark. *Strahlentherapie 32,* 721-738 (1929).
5. Lingley, J. R. Gall, E. S., Hilcken, J. A. Comparative experimental studies of 200 kilovolt and 1000 kilovolt roentgen rays. II. The biological effects on the bone marrow of the albino rat. *Am. J. Pathol. 16,* 845-854 (1940).
6. Denstad, T. The radiosensitivity of the bone marrow. *Acta Radiol. Suppl. 42,* 7-176 (1943).
7. Crosby, W. H. Personal communication.
8. Knospe, W. H., Blom, J., Crosby, W. H. Regeneration of locally irradiated bone marrow. I. Dose dependent, long-term changes in the rat, with particular emphasis upon vascular and stromal reaction. *Blood 28,* 398-415 (1966).
9. Bloom, W. (Ed.). *Histopathology of irradiation from external and internal sources.* National Nuclear Energy Series, Manhattan Project Technical Section, Division IV, Plutonium Project Record, Vol. 221. McGraw-Hill, New York (1948).
10. Knospe, W. H., Blom, J., Crosby, W. H. Regeneration of locally irradiated bone marrow. II. Induction of regeneration in permanently aplastic medullary cavities. *Blood 31,* 400-405 (1968).
11. Steinberg, B., Martin, R. A. Permanent ablation of bone marrow in long bones of living rabbits. *Proc. Soc. Exp. Biol. Med. 63,* 390-391 (1946).
12. Steinberg, B., Hufford, V. Development of bone marrow in adult animals. *Arch. Pathol. 43,* 117-126 (1947).
13. Nelp, W. B., Gohil, M. N., Larson, S. M., Bower, R. E. Long-term effects of local irradiation of the marrow on erythron and red cell function. *Blood 36,* 617-622 (1970).
14. Rubin, P. Regeneration of bone marrow in rabbits following local, fractionated irradiation. *Cancer 32,* 847-852 (1973).
15. Maloney, M. A., Lamela, R. A., Patt, H. M. Decrease in hematopoietic stem cell domains as a delayed effect of x-irradiation. *Int. J. Cell Cloning 1,* 206-215 (1983).
16. Fried, W., Chamberlin, W., Knospe, W. H., Husseini, S., Trobaugh, F. E., Jr. Studies on the defective haematopoietic microenvironment of Sl/Sl^d mice. *Brit. J. Haematol. 24,* 643-650 (1973).
17. Fried, W., Husseini, S., Knospe, W. H., Trobaugh, F. E., Jr. Studies on the source of hematopoietic tissue in the marrow of subcutaneously implanted femurs. *Exp. Hematol. 1,* 29-35 (1973).
18. Maniatis, A., Tavassoli, M., Crosby, W. H. Origin of osteogenic precursor cells in extramedullary marrow implants. *Blood 38,* 569-575 (1971).
19. Chamberlin, W., Barone, J., Kedo, A., Fried, W. Lack of recovery of murine hematopoietic stromal cells after irradiation-induced damage. *Blood 44,* 385-392 (1974).

20. Fried, W., Chamberlin, W., Kedo, A., Barone, J. Effects of radiation on hematopoietic stroma. *Exp. Hematol. 4,* 310-314 (1976).
21. Wilson, F. D., O'Grady, L., McNeill, C. J., Munn, S. L. The formation of bone marrow derived fibroblastic plaques in vitro: preliminary results contrasting these populations to CFU-C. *Exp. Hematol. 2,* 343-354 (1974).
22. Xu, C. X., Hendry, J. H., Testa, N. G. The response of stromal progenitor cells in mouse marrow to graded repeated doses of x rays or neutrons. *Radiat. Res. 96,* 82-89 (1983).
23. Dexter, T. M., Allen, T. D., Lajtha, L. G. Conditions controlling the proliferation of haemopoietic stem cells in vitro. *J. Cell. Physiol. 91,* 335-344 (1977).
24. Tavassoli, M. Radiosensitivity of stromal cells responsible for in vitro maintenance of hemopoietic stem cells in continuous, long-term marrow culture. *Exp. Hematol. 10,* 435-443 (1982).
25. Zuckerman, K. S., Rhodes, R. K., Sparks, B., Chenier, B. Radioresistance of stromal cells supportive of hematopoiesis in murine long term bone marrow cell cultures. *Exp. Hematol. 13,* 372 (1985) (abstr.).
26. Naparstek, E., Donnelly, T., Kase, K., Greenberger, J. S. Biologic effects of in vitro x-irradiation of murine long-term bone marrow cultures on the production of granulocyte-macrophage colony-stimulating factors. *Exp. Hematol. 13,* 701-708 (1985).
27. Naparstek, E., Pierce, J., Metcalf, D., Shadduck, R., Ihle, J., Leder, A., Sakakeeny, M. A., Wagner, K., Falco, J., FitzGerald, T. J., Greenberger, J. Induction of growth alterations in factor-dependent hematopoietic progenitor cell lines by cocultivation with irradiated bone marrow stromal cell lines. *Blood 67,* 1395-1403 (1986).
28. Naparstek, E., Donnelly, T., Shadduck, R. K., Waheed, A., Wagner, K., Kase, K. R., Greenberger, J. S. Persistent production of colony-stimulating factor (CSF-1) by cloned bone marrow stromal cell line D2XR11 after x-irradiation. *J. Cell. Physiol. 126,* 407-413 (1986).
29. Knospe, W. H., Husseini, S. G. Hematopoiesis on cellulose ester membranes (CEM). X. Effects of in vitro irradiation of stromal cells prior to application on CEM. *Exp. Hematol. 14,* 975-980 (1986).
30. Friedenstein, A. J., Petrakova, K. V., Kurolesova, A. I., Frolova, G. P. Heterotopic transplants of bone marrow. *Transplantation 6,* 230-247 (1968).
31. Friedenstein, A. J., Latzinik, N. W., Grosheva, A. G., Gorskaya, U. F. Marrow microenvironment transfer by heterotopic transplantation of freshly isolated and cultured cells in porous sponges. *Exp. Hematol. 10,* 217-227 (1982).
32. Chertkov, J. L., Drize, N. J., Gurevitch, O. A. Hemopoietic stromal precursors in long-term culture of bone marrow. II. Significance of initial packing for creating a hemopoietic microenvironment and maintaining stromal precursors in the culture. *Exp. Hematol. 11,* 243-248 (1983).
33. Reincke, U., Hannon, E. C., Hellman, S. Residual radiation injury exhibited in long-term bone marrow cultures. *J. Cell. Physiol. 112,* 345-352 (1982).
34. Baum, S. J., Wyant, D. E. Hematopoietic recovery in irradiated dogs. *Radiat. Res. 44,* 531-544 (1970).

35. Gong, J. K., MacVittie, T. J., Vertalino, J. E. A method for determining residual injury in the hematopoietic system of the x-irradiated rat. *Radiat. Res. 37,* 467-477 (1969).
36. Baum, S. J. Erythrocyte stem cell kinetics in the postirradiation rat. *Radiat. Res. 30,* 316-324 (1967).
37. Valentine, W. N., Pearce, M. L., Lawrence, J. S. Studies on the radiosensitivity of bone marrow. II. The effect of large, repeated, whole body irradiation exposure on hematopoiesis. *Blood 7,* 14-19 (1952).
38. Testa, N. G., Hendry, J. H., Molineux, G. Long-term bone marrow damage in experimental systems and in patients after radiation or chemotherapy. *Anticancer Res. 5,* 101-110 (1985).
39. Dexter, T. M., Schofield, R., Hendry, J. H., Testa, N. G. Congenital and induced defects in haemopoietic environments. Stem cell proliferation and differentiation. In: *Aplastic anemia: pathophysiology and approaches to therapy.* Heimpel, H., Gordon Smith, E. C., Heit, W., Kubanek, B. (Eds.). Springer-Verlag, Berlin, pp. 73-78 (1979).
40. Hendry, J. H., Testa, N. G., Lajtha, L. G. Effect of repeated doses of x-rays or 14 MeV neutrons on mouse bone marrow. *Radiat. Res. 59,* 645-652 (1974).
41. Hendry, J. H., Xu, C. X., Testa, N. G. A cellular analysis of residual hemopoietic deficiencies in mice after 4 repeated doses of 4.5 gray x rays. *Int. J. Radiat. Oncol. Biol. Phys. 9,* 1641-1646 (1983).
42. Carsten, A. L., Bond, V. P. Colony-forming units in the bone marrow of partial-body irradiated mice. *Recent Results Cancer Res. 17,* 21-27 (1969).
43. Xu, C. X., Hendry, J. H., Testa, N. G. Residual deficiencies in hemopoietic precursor cell populations after repeated irradiation of mice with x-rays or neutrons: dose-response relationships. *Exp. Hematol. 14,* 230-233 (1986).
44. Schofield, R., Dexter, T. M. Studies on the self-renewal ability of CFU-S which have been serially transferred in long-term culture or in vivo. *Leuk. Res. 9,* 305-313 (1985).
45. Calvo, W., Fliedner, T. M., Steinbach, I., Alcober, V., Nothdurft, W., Fache, I. Development of fibrosis in dogs as a late consequence of whole-body x-irradiation. In: *Late biological effects of ionizing radiation. Proceedings of the symposium on the late biological effects of ionizing radiation,* Vol. II, held by the International Atomic Energy Agency, Vienna, March 13-17, 1978. International Atomic Energy Agency, Vienna, pp. 127-136.
46. Seed, T. M., Tolle, D. V., Fritz, T. E., Devine, R. L., Poole, C. M., Norris, W. P. Irradiation-induced erythroleukemia and myelogenous leukemia in the beagle dog: hematology and ultrastructure. *Blood 50,* 1061-1079 (1977).
47. Seed, T. M., Cullen, S. M., Kaspar, L. V., Tolle, D. V., Fritz, T. E. Hemopathologic consequences of protracted gamma irradiation: alterations in granulocyte reserves and granulocyte mobilization. *Blood 56,* 42-51 (1980).
48. Seed, T. M., Fritz, T. E., Tolle, D. V., Poole, C. M., Lombard, L. S., Doyle, D. E., Kaspar, L. V., Cullen, S. M., Carnes, B. A. Survival patterns and hemopathological responses of dogs under continuous gamma irradiation. In: *Response of different species to total body irradiation.* Broerse, J. J., MacVittie, T. J. (Eds.). Martinus Nijhoff, Boston, pp. 137-159 (1984).

49. Seed, T. M., Kaspar, L. V., Fritz, T. E., Tolle, D. V. Cellular responses in chronic radiation leukemogenesis. In: *Carcinogenesis,* Vol. 10. Huberman, E., Barr, S. H. (Eds.). Raven Press, New York, pp. 363-379 (1985).
50. Moore, M. A. S. Marrow cultures in polycythemia vera and myelofibrosis. *INSERM 42,* 167-168 (1975).
51. Moore, M. A. S. Embryologic and phylogenetic development of the hematopoietic system. In: *Myelofibrosis-osteosclerosis. Advances in the biosciences.* Burkhardt, R., Conley, C. L., Tennert, K., Adler, A. A., Pincus, T., Till, J. E. (Eds.). Pergamon Press, Viewat, pp. 87-101 (1975).
52. Nothdurft, W., Braasch, E., Calvo, W., Carbonell, F., Grilli, G., Fliedner, T. M. Studies on granulocyte/macrophage progenitor cells (CFU-GM) in different organs of dogs during fetal development. *Exp. Hematol. 9* (*Suppl. 9*), 163 (1981) (abstr.).
53. Brecher, G., Brambel, C. E., Brambel, F. D. Patterns of hemopoietic response to continuous whole-body irradiation. *Ann. NY Acad. Sci. 114,* 549-556 (1964).
54. Knospe, W. H., Adler, S. S., Husseini, S., Fritz, T., Wilson, F. D. Effects of chronic continuous low level γ radiation exposure (CCLLR) on hematopoiesis in the mouse. In: *Experimental hematology today–1982.* Baum, S. J., Ledney, G. D., Thierfelder, S. (Eds.). S. Karger, Basel, Chapter 30, pp. 251-259 (1982).
55. Hutaff, L. W., Belding, H. W. The effects of irradiation of the pelvis in patients with carcinoma of the cervix uteri on the iliac and sternal marrow and on the peripheral blood. *Am. J. Roentgenol. 73,* 251-258 (1955).
56. Sykes, M. P., Chu, F. C. H., Wilkerson, W. G. Local bone-marrow changes secondary to therapeutic irradiation. *Radiology 75,* 919-924 (1960).
57. Goswitz, F. A., Andrews, G. A., Kniseley, R. M. Effects of local irradiation (Co^{60} teletherapy) on the peripheral blood and bone marrow. *Blood 21,* 605-619 (1963).
58. DeGowin, R. L., Chaudhuri, T. K., Christie, J. H., Callis, M. N., Mueller, A. L. Marrow scanning in evaluation of hemopoiesis after radiotherapy. *Arch. Intern. Med. 134,* 297-303 (1974).
59. Stewart, J. W., Dische, S. Effect of radiotherapy on bone-marrow in ankylosing spondylitis. *Lancet 2,* 1063-1069 (1956).
60. Knospe, W. H., Rayudu, V. M. S., Cardello, M., Friedman, A. M., Fordham, E. W. Bone marrow scanning with ^{52}iron (^{52}Fe). Regeneration and extension of marrow after ablative doses of radiotherapy. *Cancer 37,* 1432-1442 (1976).
61. Van Dyke, D., Harris, N. Bone marrow reactions to trauma. Stimulation of erythropoietic marrow by mechanical disruption, fracture or endosteal curettage. *Blood 34,* 257-275 (1969).
62. Knospe, W. H., Gregory, S. A., Fried, W., Trobaugh, F. E., Jr. Stimulation of hematopoiesis by femoral marrow curettage in sublethally irradiated mice. *Blood 41,* 519-527 (1973).
63. Rubin, P., Landman, S., Mayer, E., Keller, B., Ciccio, S. Bone marrow regeneration and extension after extended field irradiation in Hodgkin's disease. *Cancer 32,* 699-711 (1973).

64. Sacks, E. L., Goris, M. L., Glatstein, E., Gilbert, E., Kaplan, H. S. Bone marrow regeneration following large field radiation. Influence of volume, age, dose, and time. *Cancer 42,* 1057-1065 (1978).
65. Morardet, N., Parmentier, C., Hayat, M., Charbord, P. Effects of radiotherapy on the bone marrow granulocytic progenitor cells (CFU_C) of patients with malignant lymphomas. II. Long-term effects. *Int. J. Radiat. Oncol. Biol. Phys. 4,* 853-857 (1978).
66. LeRoy, G. V. Hematology of atomic bomb casualties. *Arch. Intern. Med. 86,* 691-710 (1950).
67. Fliedner, T. M., Andrews, G. A., Cronkite, E. P., Bond, V. P. Early and late cytologic effects of whole body irradiation on human marrow. *Blood 23,* 471-487 (1964).
68. Vorder Bruegge, C. F. Radiation injury following an A-bomb explosion. *Ann. Intern. Med. 36,* 1444-1458 (1952).
69. Liebow, A. A., Warren, S., DeCoursey, E. Pathology of atomic bomb casualties. *Am. J. Pathol. 25,* 853-1027 (1949).
70. Conrad, R. A., Cronkite, E. P., Bond, V. P., Robertson, J. S., Cohn, S. H. Fallout radiation: effects on Marshallese people. In: *Atomic medicine,* 5th ed. Behrens, C. F., King, E. R., Carpender, J. W. J. (Eds.). Williams and Wilkins, Baltimore, Chapter 12, pp. 308-339 (1969).
71. Li, S., Champlin, R., Fitchen, J. H., Gale, R. P. Abnormalities of myeloid progenitor cells after "successful" bone marrow transplantation. *J. Clin. Invest. 75,* 234-241 (1985).
72. Siminovitch, L., Till, J. E., McCulloch, E. A. Decline in colony-forming ability of marrow cells subjected to serial transplantation into irradiated mice. *J. Cell. Comp. Physiol. 64,* 23-31 (1964).
73. Vos, O., Dolmans, M. J. A. S. Self-renewal of colony forming units (CFU) in serial bone marrow transplantation experiments. *Cell Tissue Kinet. 5,* 371-385 (1972).
74. Harrison, D. E. Normal function of transplanted mouse erythrocyte precursors for 21 months beyond donor life spans. *Nature 237,* 220-222 (1972).
75. Hellman, S., Botnick, L. E., Hannon, E. C., Vigneulle, R. M. Proliferative capacity of murine hematopoietic stem cells. *Proc. Natl. Acad. Sci. USA 75,* 490-494 (1978).
76. Morley, A., Trainor, K., Blake, J. A primary stem cell lesion in experimental chronic hypoplastic marrow failure. *Blood 45,* 681-688 (1975).
77. Boggs, D. R., Boggs, S. S. Possible pathogenic mechanisms in aplastic anemia. *Transplant. Proc. 10,* 125-130 (1978).
78. Harrison, D. E., Astle, C. M. Loss of stem cell repopulating ability upon transplantation. Effects of donor age, cell number and transplantation procedures. *J. Exp. Med. 156,* 1767-1779 (1982).
79. Raghavachar, A., Prummer, O., Fliedner, T. M., Steinbach, K. H. Functional studies on myeloid progenitor cell reconstitution after autologous stem cell transplantation. *Exp. Hematol. 11* (*Suppl. 14*), 71 (1983) (abstr.).
80. Haak, H. L., Goselink, H. M., Veenhof, W., Pellinkhof-Stadelmann, S., Kleiverda, J. K., te Velde, J. Acquired aplastic anaemia in adults. IV. Histological

and CFU studies in transplanted and non-transplanted patients. *Scand. J. Haematol. 19,* 159-171 (1977).

81. Barrett, A. J., Adams, J. A proliferative defect of human bone marrow after transplantation. *Brit. J. Haematol. 49,* 159-164 (1981).
82. Atkinson, K., Norrie, S., Chan, P., Biggs, J. Bone marrow cellularity and blood and marrow myeloid and erythroid stem cell colony growth during the first three months after allogeneic marrow transplantation for severe aplastic anemia or acute leukemia. *Exp. Hematol. 10* (*Suppl. 11*), 34 (1982) (abstr.).
83. Faille, A., Maraninchi, D., Gluckman, E., Devergie, A., Balitrand, N., Ketels, F., Dresch, C. Granulocyte progenitor compartments after allogeneic bone marrow grafts. *Scand. J. Haematol. 26,* 202-214 (1981).
84. Arnold, R., Schmeiser, T., Heit, W., Frickhofen, N., Pabst, G., Heimpel, H., Kubanek, B. Hemopoietic reconstitution after bone marrow transplantation. *Exp. Hematol. 14,* 271-277 (1986).
85. Bacigalupo, A., Podesta, M., Mingari, M. C., Moretta, L., Van Lint, M. T., Marmont, A. Immune suppression of hematopoiesis in aplastic anemia: activity of T-gamma lymphocytes. *J. Immunol. 125,* 1449-1453 (1980).
86. Layward, L., Levinsky, R. J., Butler, M. Long-term abnormalities in T and B lymphocyte function in children following treatment for acute lymphoblastic leukaemia. *Brit. J. Haematol. 49,* 251-258 (1981).
87. Weiner, R. S., Oblon, D. J., Gross, M. A. Stem cell defects after intensive cytoreductive therapy for AML. *Exp. Hematol. 11* (*Suppl. 14*), 41 (1983) (abstr.).
88. Peschel, C., Konwalinka, G., Geissler, D., Tomaschek, B., Grunewald, K., Huber, H., Odavic, R., Braunsteiner, H. Studies of myelopoiesis in vitro on blood and bone marrow cells of patients with acute leukemia in long-term remission. *Leuk. Res. 7,* 397-406 (1983).
89. Gale, R. P., Li, S., Fitchen, J. H. Hematopoietic reconstitution following bone marrow transplantation: absent or decreased myeloid progenitor cells (CFU-C). *Exp. Hematol. 10* (*Suppl. 11*), 31 (1982) (abstr.).

6

Drugs and Chemicals as Agents of Bone Marrow Failure

NEAL S. YOUNG
Cell Biology Section, Clinical Hematology Branch, National Heart, Lung, and Blood Institute, National Institutes of Health, Bethesda, Maryland

Chemicals, some in the form of drugs, are commonly viewed as agents of bone marrow failure, yet a critical reader can only be dissatisfied with the literature on this subject. The cause-and-effect relationship between many chemicals and bone marrow failure is speculative, and in most cases little is known of the mechanism(s) of drug-induced aplastic anemia. Practical tests are not available to predict individual susceptibility, and the public health implications of exposure of populations to low concentrations of potentially toxic chemicals are unknown. This chapter represents a selective, synthetic summary; readers are referred to the traditional "blacklists" of drugs and chemicals in hematology textbooks and comprehensive reviews (1-6).

I. CLINICAL OBSERVATIONS

A. Classification

The usual division between agents that regularly produce marrow depression and those that rarely do so appropriately emphasizes the idiosyncratic nature of some drug reactions. Myelosuppression is the expected effect of many drugs used in cancer chemotherapy; in commonly employed doses, these drugs always produce pancytopenia and temporary marrow aplasia. These drugs have been selected for their inhibitory effect on (malignant) cell proliferation, and as a consequence they are usually active in animal models and in tissue culture. Activity across species boundaries results from action at some fundamental cellular process common to higher organisms such as DNA replication and also from RNA transcription, protein synthesis, and the mechanics of cell division. In contrast, agents that rarely act to produce disease usually have no effect in animals, partly because of limitations in the number of animals that can be tested but also because of fundamental differences in drug metabolism between other species of mammals, especially rodents and primates. Idiosyncratic agents may be suppressive in cell culture, but usually at extraordinarily high concentrations that are difficult to relate to therapeutic doses.

Although convenient, this division is not absolute. There are genetically based individual variations in hematological susceptibility to chemotherapeutic agents (see below). Some agents, at least in the doses to which humans are exposed, appear to be intermediate in their effect; the great majority of benzene workers do not develop aplastic anemia, although this agent is sufficiently consistent a myelosuppressive that it was once employed as therapy in acute leukemia (7). While most drugs linked to bone marrow failure appear only very occasionally to precede a hematological catastrophe, careful observation may disclose milder, more regular hematopoietic effects, such as mild leukopenia in chronic users of phenothiazine (8) and the alterations in erythropoiesis due to chloramphenicol (9).

B. Case Reports

Rare drug reactions are inferred from association, usually in the form of case reports of individual patients or registries of toxic events in patients taking drugs. Case reports are most convincing when not only the outcome, but also the exposure is very rare. Case reporting is cumulative—a single case report inspires others, and negative relationships are, of course. difficult to document. Case reporting is highly selective and varies with the climate of suspicion surrounding the individual agent and drugs in general, the perceived legal consequences, and the peculiarities of the subspecialty employing the drug. And case reporting has its aesthetic facet; some associations acquire tacit acceptance because they are memorable, like that of aplastic anemia with hair dyes or glue sniffing. The cumulative effect of case histories implicating hair dyes published in the 1930s and 1940s, and especially the casual quotation of earlier reports to support causal relationships, has been contrasted to the paucity of cases recently reported, despite markedly increased product use (10,11). Six cases of aplastic anemia secondary to glue sniffing, a popular activity in the 1960s, would seem a convincing cohort, especially given the aromatic hydrocarbon base of the presumed toxin (12). However, five of the cases were patients with sickle cell disease and transient aplastic crisis, in retrospect recognized as a specific viral illness (13).

C. Epidemiology

Case reports can suggest, but epidemiology can establish, an association between drug and toxic event. Epidemiologic studies are much more difficult to perform, of course, and, especially for rare associations, require herculean efforts at data collection to attain statistical power. Improperly performed, epidemiologic studies can be misleading and obfuscatory. Unfortunately, the crucial details of design—subject selection, data acquisition and processing, stratification, statistical analyses—may not be adequately described in the final publication to allow an assessment of quality. Commonly, for subtle effects such as very rare drug reactions, several studies of the same problem arrive at conflicting conclusions; the mutual canceling effect of contradictory studies, while natural, may be unfair.

While the strength of medical case reports is clinical detail, most large surveys rely on secondary sources of information. Of necessity, the definition of disease is often adapted to the material available, such as hospital records, death certificates, or official statistics. The nosology of bone marrow failure syndromes presents a further confounding factor. Distinctions among aplastic anemia, hypoplastic anemia, refractory anemia, and panctyopenia, even if properly made, may or may not be meaningful. Low blood counts also may be the consequence of treatment of other, primary diseases. Adequate tissue for diagnosis, particularly bone marrow biopsies in asplastic anemia, often is not obtained.

D. Association and Causality

Causality cannot be inferred from case reports but commonly is, partly because these data become imbedded in reference tables and partly because confirmatory studies are so much more difficult to perform. But even a strong association demonstrated in analyses of series of patients or of epidemiologic surveys does not establish a mechanism for a relationship between drug or chemical and hematological syndrome. Patients often receive drugs (an antibiotic for fever, for example) at the onset of their hematological disease but prior to diagnosis; 24 patients of 138 exposed persons received chloramphenicol *after* diagnosis of a blood dyscrasia in one study (14). Occult virus infection has been linked to generalized bone marrow failure (13). A commonly employed drug that is administered for symptoms of a virus infection (an anti-inflammatory for polyarthralgia or antibiotic for fever) might then falsely appear to be associated with the subsequent marrow disease. A history of drug or chemical exposure is routinely obtained in patients with aplastic anemia; when control populations are subjected to a serious interrogation they may have equally impressive records of drug exposure (15).

II. THREE EXAMPLES

A. Benzene

1. Benzene Poisoning (16,17)

Benzene is the chemical most convincingly linked to bone marrow failure. Benzene bone marrow poisoning was first described by Santesson at the end of the last century in Germany, an ironic but not surprising coincidence given the central position of benzene in the chemical industry and the role of the aniline dyes as stains for the study of bone marrow morphology. A "typical clinical picture" in benzene workers was described by an early observer as "progressive anemia with malaise, epistaxis, then rapid decline, petechiae, hemorrhage [from many organs] . . . fever more or less intense, sometimes chills, eventually disturbances of the nervous system and death" (18). In fact, the clinical pattern of marrow failure is more variable, ranging from mild depression of one hemopoietic lineage to frank, severe aplasia (18-23). About half of the patients who develop pancytopenia will recover spontaneously (23). Leukemia as well as aplastic anemia can result from benzene exposure, although it is probably five or six times less common than aplasia (24,25). The two diagnoses may be made in the same individual, as benzene-associated leukemia commonly develops in patients with preexisting pancytopenia (24,26). Conversely, it is not uncommon for patients to present with cellular bone marrows before development of aplastic anemia, and a cellular bone marrow is a favorable prognostic sign (24). Onset of bone marrow failure or aplasia can occur months to years after exposure has been discontinued.

Benzene was (and is) used extensively in industry: as a profitable by-product in coal burning and petroleum refining; in the preparation of polymers, detergents, pesticides, and aromatic intermediates of drugs and chemicals; and as a solvent, degreasing agent, or thinner in printing and the manufacture of cements and adhesives, shoes, and rubber products (16,27). Benzene is one of the most frequently produced chemicals; in the United States in 1983, benzene production was estimated at 11-12 billion pounds. Although regulation of benzene exposure has become routine in the West, benzene exposures in some industrialized third world nations like China may continue to be extremely high (Professor Ying Songnian, personal communication). Benzene exposure also occurs through common solvents: rubber solvent (1.5% benzene), varnish makers' and painters' naphtha (0.1%), and Stoddard solvent (0.1-0.7%) (Ref. 28; NIOSH Criteria Document: Recommendations for an Occupational Exposure Standard for Refined Petroleum Solvents). Benzene is present in crude oil and is also generated during motor fuel refining processes, ultimately averaging from less than 2% (United States) to as high as 8% (Europe) by volume in gasoline; as organic antiknock additives have been reduced, the proportion of benzene in recent gasoline blends has been increased (27). While industrial workers endure the highest exposures, benzene is ubiquitous. Benzene, presumably derived from biological sources, can be detected in the atmosphere even in remote regions. However, much higher levels of benzene (and other volative organic compounds) have been measured in ambient air and water in the vicinity of roadways, refineries, and chemical plants (27) and in the breath of normal New Jersey subjects (29). Methodologic difficulties in establishing the existence of a threshold effect, similar to the dilemma of low dose exposure to gamma irradiation, underlie the scientific and legal controversy over permissible benzene exposure.

Variability of work environments, imprecision in measuring benzene exposure, and the commonly delayed onset of disease make accurate incidence figures difficult to obtain. Anemia, leukopenia, and pancytopenia are frequent among workers exposed to benzene at concentrations above 50 ppm for extended periods or 100 ppm intermittently (15). In the early large series, the majority of benzene workers showed aberrations in blood counts (19,21,22). In a more recent prospective and controlled examination of heavily exposed Turkish workers who appeared healthy, hematological abnormalities were present in 24% and almost 3% were pancytopenic (23). The risk of leukemia correlates strongly with cumulative exposure to benzene (30). Cumulative exposure almost certainly is the single most important variable in determining bone marrow failure, consistent with the common clinical observation that short periods of high exposure or chronic low-dose exposure are equivalent in increasing the risk of aplastic anemia.

2. Benzene Metabolism (17,31).

Despite abundant data, the role of benzene metabolism in bone marrow toxicity is only vaguely defined. Benzene and its metabolites are potent antimetabolites, presumably due to covalent binding to macromolecules, especially DNA. Benzene is lipophilic and accumulates at high concentrations in the fat of bone marrow (32). Benzene metabolism proceeds by oxidation, through potentially toxic intermediates, to water-soluble conjugated compounds (31). Cytochrome P-450 activity is present in bone marrow (33), and phenolic metabolites of benzene accumulate and persist in the marrow (33); administered benzene (34) and its phenolic intermediates (35) covalently bind to bone marrow DNA. Nonetheless, the primary role of the liver in benzene metabolism is suggested by the partial abrogation of marrow toxicity in hepatectomized animals (36).

Animals treated with benzene regularly show bone marrow depression (37-42). Considerable variability results from differences in species, regimens and routes of administration, and length of treatment. Even with long-term studies, it has been difficult to reproduce in animals the typical course of chronic exposure in human workers. Pathologically, pancytopenia with marrow hypercellularity may be more common in some experimental animals than the acellularity that characterizes symptomatic patients. Nevertheless, by many criteria—marrow cellularity, thymidine or iron incorporation, colony formation—benzene administered to animals suppresses marrow cell proliferation. Acutely, the more mature (and cycling) precursor cells appear to be most sensitive, reflected in changes in marrow cellularity; BFU-E, CFU-E, and GM-CFC numbers decline and may rebound to variable degrees with relatively limited periods of exposure to high concentrations of benzene. However, effects on more primitive hemopoietic stem cells are more difficult to measure, especially important functions like self-renewal or repopulation capacity. Rats exposed intermittently to benzene can maintain their circulating white cell number but show marked decreases in CFU-S numbers; with continuous exposure, white cell number falls but CFU-S are maintained (39), suggesting progressive marrow depletion of stem cells. Benzene exposure also may affect the marrow stroma. Marrow from exposed mice does not sustain hemopoiesis in long-term culture; the decline in CFU-S in the nonadherent fraction has been associated with a stroma devoid of fat cells (42).

In vitro, low concentrations of benzene increase GM-CFC-derived colonies, but benzene metabolites (phenol, hydroquinone, benzenetriol, toluene) inhibit colony formation without stimulation at any concentration (43), consistent with the observation of hyperplasia in some benzene workers early in the course of disease and leukocytosis and increased colony numbers in animals with relatively short periods of exposure. In vitro systems, both clonal and long-term cultures, would be helpful in distinguishing a mechanism of stem cell depletion from direct toxicity for the stem cell.

3. Other Aromatic Hydrocarbons

The clinical evidence relating benzene to bone marrow failure in humans is unequivocal. The clinical data concerning other hydrocarbon chemicals are much more ambiguous. Although the implicated molecules are more or less closely related in formula to benzene (Fig. 1), others of equally frightening structure have not been associated with bone marrow syndromes. Very large populations are exposed to this heterogeneous group of chemicals, not only in their use as gardening aids but also as residues in food from their massive employment in agriculture. these substances are present in the ambient environment (44) and ultimately in humans, in the body (45) and bone marrow fat (46). Differences in exposure to insecticides have been proposed to underlie geographic variation in the incidence of aplastic anemia (47,48). Studies are complicated by the high background exposure and the diversity of implicated compounds.

The first case report of aplastic anemia may follow an accidental, particularly heavy, or unusual exposure to a chemical in the form of pesticide or herbicide [for example, chlorinated hydrocarbons (47-55)], in industry [production of explosives with trinitrololuene (56)], and even occasionally as therapy [dinitrophenol for obesity (57)]. Case reports of other associations, often with much briefer exposures to very commonly employed chemicals, then follow. In contrast to benzene, exposure to other hydrocarbons represents a very minor proportion of the toxin exposures of aplastic anemia patients; these data are especially difficult to interpret because of ubiquitous agents in the community (insecticides or hairspray) and the bias of history-taking from aplastic anemia patients.

Population surveys of industry workers exposed to pesticides during manufacture of application have not shown increased risk of aplastic anemia (58-61); these studies are often performed by the industry. One study suggested an increased risk of acute leukemia (61). The occupational risks of farming have been repeatedly assessed. Farming does not appear with unusual frequency on the death certificates of patients with aplastic anemia (62,63). Some (64-66) but not all (67) studies have suggested an increased mortality from acute leukemia among farmers.

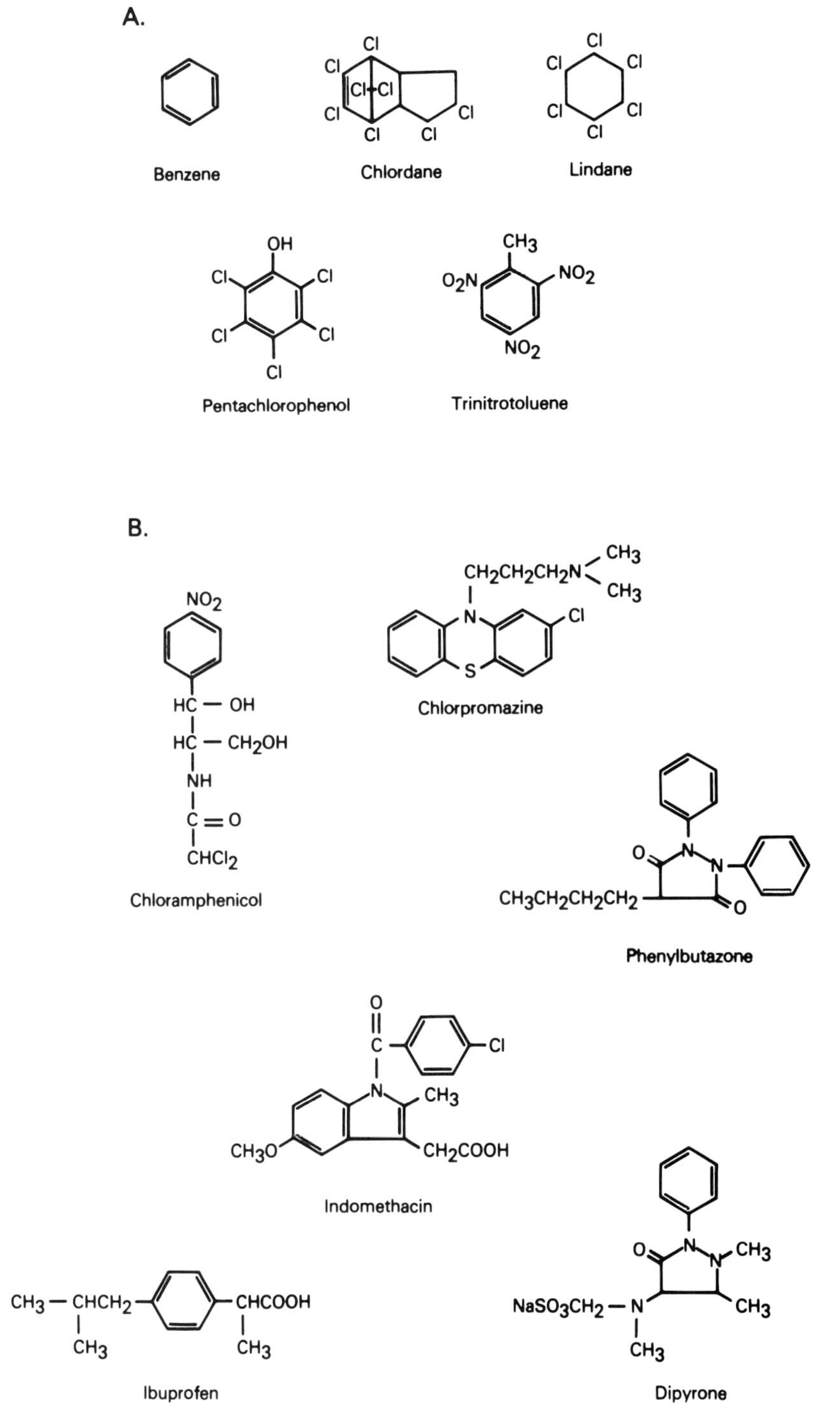

Figure 1 Structures of some chemicals (*A*) and drugs (*B*) associated with bone marrow failure.

However, analysis of death certificates of farmers in British Columbia showed an increased mortality from aplastic anemia (proportional mortality ratio 174) and leukemia (PMR 122), with the aplastic anemia deaths most increased during a single decade (66). In one study of the effects of insecticide use on apple growers, a greater incidence of neutropenia was found among those with chemical contact than in local residents without contact (68). Clinical and laboratory studies of workers who manufactured insecticides also have been negative (69, 70), although some toxin-exposed workers have shown decreased cellularity in bone marrow with normal blood counts (71). Peripheral blood counts are an insensitive indicator of bone marrow function, but histologic interpretation of the marrow is subjective and progenitor assays are not applicable to population surveys. In total, these studies suggest a weaker relationship between aromatic hydrocarbons and bone marrow failure than exists for benzene, but in some populations and, more important, with some compounds, exposure may increase the risk of aplastic anemia and leukemia.

B. Chloramphenicol

1. Clinical Data

Reports of fatal aplastic anemia following chloramphenicol appeared shortly after the introduction of this popular antibiotic in 1949 (72). Delay in recognizing this association was a major motivation in the establishment of a national registry on blood dyscrasias; between 1953 and 1960, chloramphenicol use was reported to the registry in over half the patients (53 of 97) who developed pancytopenia (73, 74). Many of these studies suffered from serious selection bias, and the methods

Table 1 Chloramphenicol-Associated Aplastic Anemia

Geographical area	Date	% Drug-related	% Total	Source
California	1957-1961	78	29	Death certificates (14)
California	1963-1964	59	17	Death certificates (75)
Sweden	1966-1971	17	6	Hospital discharges (76)
Europe	1971-1977	22	8	Registry (15)
	1980-1983	6	2	Registry (15)
Israel	1961-1965	56	25	Hospital survey (77)
Japan	1958-1974	30	3	Autopsies (78)
Japan	1973	45	8	Hospital survey (79)
Korea	1958-1974	37	10	Personal series (80)

for determining denominators were crude. In some instances, chloramphenicol use preceded disease by only a few days. Chloramphenicol has appeared prominently among the drugs taken by aplastic anemia patients in many subsequent large series (Table 1). In one small case control study, patients with aplastic anemia or leukemia were queried as to drug use prior to onset of their disease; 14 of 28 patients with aplasia had received chloramphenicol in the year preceding presentation with their disease compared to only 1 of 16 patients with acute leukemia (79). From the frequency of chloramphenicol use among patients who later develop bone marrow failure, an appreciable effect on the incidence of disease would be expected with changes in prescribing habits. Significant variation in the incidence of fatal aplastic anemia with sales of chloramphenicol was reported for California and the United States as a whole (14), but aplastic anemia rates surprisingly have not declined for Sweden (76) or Japan (79) despite dramatic changes in antibiotic usage.

Aplastic anemia is a rare complication of chloramphenicol; estimates have been based on the number of cases divided by the computed number of therapeutic courses, and therefore dependent on the presumed average dose of chloramphenicol, ranging from 1 in 46,000 (75) to 1 in 60,000 (14) (dose 4 g) to 1 in 25,000 (7.5 g) (75). Pancytopenia is a far more common late complication of chloramphenicol than either isolated cytopenias or acute leukemia. The appearance of aplastic anemia is delayed usually 2-3 months after treatment with chloramphenicol (81). There is no dose relationship, some patients having received only a few grams of chloramphenicol orally, and exposure has even been limited to ophthalmic solutions (82) or skin contact (83). The relatively trivial indications for treatment in affected patients were stressed in early reports (14). Residual chloramphenicol in quantities exceeding concentrations associated with aplasia in humans has been found in food animals (84).

As interest in the hematological effects of chloramphenicol grew, a milder, more consistent, and dose-related effect on bone marrow was recognized. Patients would develop stereotypical changes with therapy: increased serum transferrin saturation, reticulocytopenia, and decreased numbers and vacuolization of bone marrow erythroid precursors (9,85). Decreased iron clearance on ferrokinetic study of some patients (86) is consistent with ineffective erythropoiesis, but patients usually do not become anemic. Decreases in platelet and white blood cells were less consistent and can be observed with other antibiotic regimens. Some, but not all, patients treated with very large doses of chloramphenicol have developed more profound hemopoietic depression of all cell lines (9,87), usually reversible but occasionally fatal (88). No clinical relationship has been established between the immediate effects of chloramphenicol and later development of bone marrow failure in individual patients, and patients in Europe treated with an analog, thiamphenicol, develop dose-related but not idiosyncratic hematological effects (89).

2. Chloramphenicol Chemistry and Hemopoietic Effects (90,91)

Chloramphenicol contains a nitrobenzene ring, unusual for an antibiotic. Thiamphenicol, in which the *para*-nitro group is replaced by a sulfonylmethyl group, has been used extensively in Europe. Chloramphenicol acts as an antibiotic by inhibiting bacterial ribosomal protein translation. Chloramphenicol does not bind to mammalian ribosomes, but at therapeutic concentrations it inhibits mitochondrial protein synthesis. Mitochondrial protein includes enzymes like ferrochelatase, which catalyzes the insertion of iron into protoprophyrin. The dose-dependent effects on erythropoiesis of chloramphenicol (and thiamphenicol, which has similar activity on protein synthesis) have been related to this mechanism of action (92).

Thiamphenicol use has not been associated with aplastic anemia in any significant frequency (89). Some in vitro data have also implicated the nitro group and in particular the generation of more toxic nitroreductive products of chloramphenicol (Fig. 2). Chloramphenicol and thiamphenicol behave similarly in assays like inhibition of hemopoietic colony formation (93) and degradation of isolated or cellular DNA (94-96), but only chloramphenicol can be metabolized to the more reactive nitroso derivatives that have much higher activity in these assays. Although nitrosochloramphenicol is not produced in the bone marrow and has a very short half-life, other related gut bacteria metabolites (such as dehydrochloramphenicol) are both more stable and more active inhibitors of GM-CFC growth, are more cytotoxic to marrow cells in suspension, and are better DNA strand breakers (97). How gut bacteria would produce sufficient toxic metabolites to induce bone marrow failure after intravenous (98) or local (82,83) therapy with cloramphenicol has not been explained. In an alternative model (99), dehalogenation of chloramphenicol by P-450 cytochrome microsomal oxidases produces a reactive oxamic acid derivative. The metabolite can acylate proteins. Chloramphenicol analogs such as thiamphenicol are not activated by this enzyme system to reactive intermediates. A hydroxylamine metabolite of chloramphenicol that forms stable free radicals can also be generated by microsomal enzymes (99). The low incidence of aplasia with chloramphenicol therapy could be explained by a combination of unusual metabolic defects—increased formation of an oxamic acid derivative, decreased detoxification of a hydroxylamine—that generate reactive metabolites.

The potency of chloramphenicol metabolites clouds the interpretation of experiments performed with chloramphenicol alone in vitro or in animals with metabolic systems different from man's. In contrast to benzene or cytotoxic agents, chloramphenicol is not an inhibitor of cell proliferation. In low doses, chloramphenicol can stimulate myeloid progenitor-derived colony formation in vitro (100), and it increases GM-CFC and CFU-S numbers in treated mice (101). One child with neutropenia has improved with cloramphenicol therapy (102). Chloramphenicol perturbation of the hemopoietic microenvironment has been inferred from delayed hemopoietic recovery following irradiation in

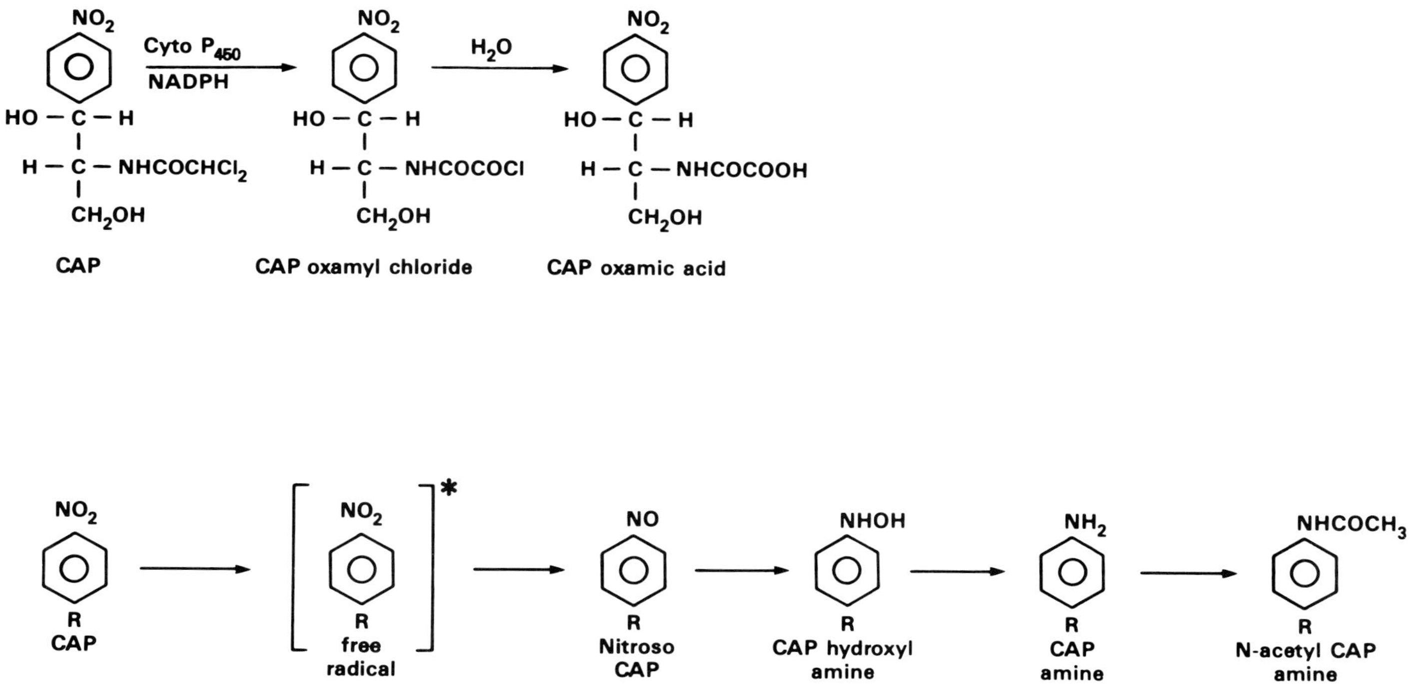

Figure 2 Chloramphenicol metabolism. Two pathways that have been associated with production of toxic intermediates are shown.

chloramphenicol-treated animals (103) and the greater chloramphenicol sensitivity of long-term bone marrow culture compared to clonal assays (104).

C. Nonsteroidal Anti-Inflammatory Drugs

1. Clinical and Epidemiologic Patterns (105,106)

Nonsteroidal anti-inflammatory drugs have replaced chloramphenicol on recent lists of incriminated drugs. Compared to chloramphenicol, the pace of case reporting of adverse drug reactions was slower with phenylbutazone, 6 years elapsing between the market introduction and the first association with aplastic anemia (107), possibly due to concomitant explanations for neutropenia such as underlying disease or therapy with gold salts. The true incidence of aplastic anemia associated with nonsteroidal drugs may be low, as estimates have ranged from 1 in 50,000 to 1 in a million treatment courses (106,108,109). Horses given massive doses of phenylbutazone more commonly become neutropenic (110) (doses in humans also may have been large when the drug was first introduced). A recent massive multicenter epidemiologic survey measured the relationship of analgesic drug use to agranulocytosis and aplastic anemia in Europe (111). For agranulocytosis, increased risk was associated with dipyrone (risk ratio = 24, based on use in the week before onset of illness), indomethacin (rr 9), and phenylbutazone (rr 4). For aplastic anemia, similar data were obtained: indomethacin (rr 13), diclofenac (rr 9), and phenylbutazone (rr 9).

2. Mechanisms

The difficulty of inferring a mechanism from in vitro data is even greater for the nonsteroidal agents than for chloramphenicol, due to the extreme infrequency of the complication, the variety of drugs cited, and the absence of a consistent bone marrow effect of nonsteroidal drugs. The butazones have been shown to be cytotoxic in a dose-dependent relationship to myeloid progenitors in vitro (112). In other studies of amidopyrine (113) and ibuprofen (114), inhibition of hemopoietic colony formation has depended on the presence of the patient's serum plus drug, implying an antibody-mediated mechanism (see below). A mechanism common to all nonsteroidal anti-inflammatories is their inhibition of cyclooxygenase activity. However, the anticipated effects on prostaglandins (decreased synthesis) and leukotrienes (increased synthesis) would be expected to stimulate rather than inhibit hemopoiesis.

III. PATHOGENIC MECHANISMS

A. Metabolic

Many drugs and chemicals, especially if they have limited water solubility, must be enzymatically degraded before conjugation and excretion (Fig. 3). Degradative

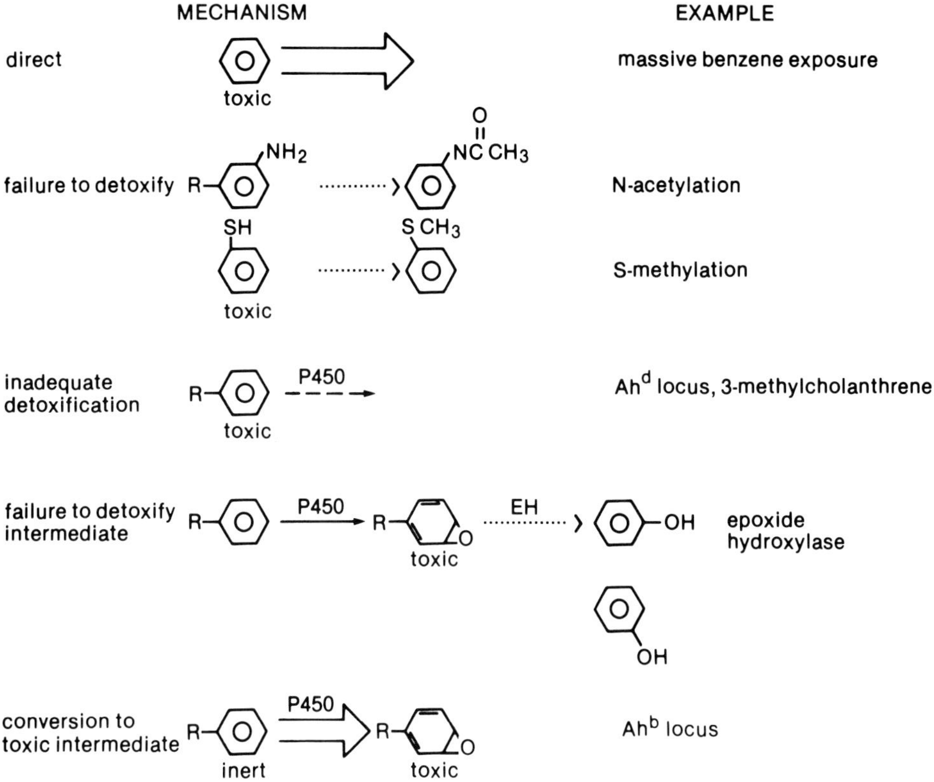

Figure 3 Some mechanisms of chemical- or drug-mediated marrow cytotoxicity.

pathways for xenobiotics like drugs and chemicals are specific, redundant, and interrelated (Table 2). For some aromatic hydrocarbons, polar groups are added by phase I enzymes, part of the cytochrome P-450 mitochondrial system; these moieties are then the targets of attachment of phase II enzyme systems that add glucuronide, sulfate, acetate, and glycine molecules to increase solubility and allow excretion. Other xenobiotics are directly metabolized by addition of methyl or acetyl groups. Intermediate compounds in drug metabolism, especially arene oxides, are often highly reactive with macromolecules because of their electrophilic properties (115); one group of diol epoxide metabolites of benzo[c]phenanthrene binds to deoxyadenosine in DNA (116). Toxic intermediate compounds often are unstable, and they may represent only a minor branch on the metabolic tree. Their production in a specific tissue may result in local organ damage, but because of their low concentration or brief half-life the presence of the compounds themselves may have to be deduced from indirect evidence rather than

Table 2 Detoxifying Enzyme Systems

Enzyme	Substrate	Genetics	Clinical examples
Arylhydrocarbon hydroxylase	Aromatic hydrocarbons	Single allelle	Strain-specific murine aplastic anemia
Epoxide hydroxylase	Arene oxides	Complex	Phenytoin aplastic anemia
N-Acetylation	Sulfa compounds	Polymorphic (50% slow)	Procainamide SLE, leukopenia
S-Methylation	Thiiopurines	Single allelle ($TPMT^L$ = 0.059)	Thiopurine leukopenia (propylthioracil?)

physical measurement. The mechanisms discussed below have been chosen because they are directly applicable to bone marrow failure resulting from drug or chemical exposure and because they demonstrate genetic variability (Table 2).

1. Arylhydrocarbon Hydroxylase and the Ah Locus (117a,117b)

This enzyme is one of the P-450 cytochrome hemoproteins that constitute a microsomal catalytic system of monooxygenases. P-450 activity can be induced by exposure to specific substrates. One form of P-450 activity, aryl hydrocarbon hydroxylase, can readily be induced by polycyclic aromatic compounds in wild mice. Wild mice have the Ah^b genetic locus, and unresponsive mice are homozygous for the Ah^d gene; Ah encodes a cytosolic receptor for the aromatic hydrocarbon. Enzyme inducibility in mice is associated with local tumor formation in response to application of a hydrocarbon to skin or trachea; high activities have also been associated with lung cancer in humans.

In contrast, mice with low enzyme activity who ingest an aromatic polycyclic hydrocarbon such as benzo[*a*]pyrene develop aplastic anemia more rapidly and consistently than do animals with inducible enzymes, who are not susceptible to bone marrow depression with this chemical. Phenobarbital administration is protective, presumably by inducing drug-conjugating enzyme activities, as is concomitant α-naphthoflavone administration, which inhibits P-450 metabolism. In vitro, myeloid cells and progenitors from Ah^b/Ah^b animals (wild type) are more sensitive than marrow from low-activity animals, because more toxic metabolites are generated locally by the more responsive enzyme system (118). In the intact animal, high enzyme activity is protective at the level of intestine and liver, where benzo[*a*]pyrene is detoxified in Ah^b animals; in contrast, large quantities of unaltered hydrocarbon reach the bone marrow in Ah^d/Ah^d animals. The magnitude of enzyme inducibility of bone marrow in the two types of animals is dependent on the concentration of inducer present in that tissue and whether the animal has a high-affinity (Ah^b) or poor-affinity (Ah^d/Ah^d) receptor. Large quantities of inducer can overwhelm low-affinity receptor and affect AHH induction. Therefore, the likelihood of myelotoxicity in these genetic strains with systemic toxin administration is a function of the ability of the major detoxification organs for "first-pass" elimination.

Most of the chemicals and drugs implicated in causing human aplastic anemia contain cyclical aromatic hydrocarbon structures and must be metabolized by similar P-450 enzyme systems. Measurement of aryl hydrocarbon hydroxylase activity is technically difficult, especially because of the magnitude of day-to-day variation and the limited degree of inducibility. Genetic variation in metabolizing and detoxifying chemicals in organs like liver and gut or in generating toxic metabolites in the marrow itself will probably correlate with hemopoietic susceptibility.

2. Detoxification of Intermediates by Epoxide Hydrolases (119,120)

Monooxygenase enzymes catalyze formation of arene oxides from aromatic hydrocarbons. These electrophilic, highly reactive and unstable intermediates are the substrates of enzymes that convert epoxides to phenols. Epoxide hydrolase activity is a property of a large and poorly defined enzyme system that shows marked substrate specificity and considerable individual and racial variation.

A convenient assay for epoxide hydrolase detoxification employs rat microsomes and NADPH to generate reactive intermediates from a specific drug or chemical (120-122). As arene oxides themselves cannot be readily quantitated because of their instability, cytotoxicity can be used as a measure of their presence. Cells, usually lymphocytes, from the patient serve both as a source of detoxifying enzymes and as indicators of arene oxide cell killing. In this assay, normal cells will die in the presence of an inhibitor of epoxide hydrolase, and cells can be rescued by exogenous enzyme. Used retrospectively, this system has identified individuals susceptible to phenytoin hepatotoxicity (121) and birth defects (122). In a patient with phenytoin-associated aplastic anemia, application of this assay showed dose-dependent cytotoxicity for the patient's lymphocytes in the presence of the drug's metabolites, no toxicity for normal cells, and intermediate toxicity for cells from the patient's mother (123). The patient's cells were not killed by phenytoin alone nor did the metabolites of other drugs injure them.

3. S-Methylation of Thiopurines (124)

Methylation is an important step in the metabolism of many drugs, chemicals, and neurotransmitters. Thiopurine methyltransferase catalyzes the S-methylation of drugs such as 6-mercaptopurine, 6-thioguanine, and azathioprine. Enzyme activity can be measured in red blood cells, and population and family studies are consistent with the inheritance of enzyme activity at a single genetic locus, with estimated gene frequencies of 94% for high enzyme activity ($TPMT^H$) and 6% for low ($TPMT^L$). The majority of individuals have high (89%) or intermediate (11%) levels of enzyme activity. Patients homozygous for $TPMT^L$, about 0.3% of the population, have undetectable enzyme levels; on treatment with azathioprine or 6-mercaptopurine, they accumulate intracellular 6-thioguanine, a purine analog that can be incorporated into DNA (125). 6-Thioguanine levels are elevated in the erythrocytes of patients with thiopurine-induced myelosuppression [neutropenia (126) and megaloblastic anemia (127)]. In three dermatologic patients with severe hematological complications of azathioprine therapy, the enzyme activity was undetectable in two, and the level was in the intermediate range in the third (125).

4. N-Acetylation (128)

N-Acetyltransferase activity is a polymorphic activity; its genetics are consistent with an autosomal recessive trait. Acetylation can be easily assayed by the administration of a test dose of caffeine and measurement of urinary metabolites. Acetylation rates vary greatly among races, with fast acetylation much more frequent among Orientals than among Caucasians. The rapid acetylation phenotype has been associated with isoniazid failure in tuberculosis; the slow phenotype has been associated with drug-induced lupus and increased risks of leprosy and bladder cancer. In 6 out of 6 patients with sulfonamide reactions, a slow acetylation phenotype was present (expected frequency 0.56); all six also showed abnormal lymphocyte toxicity in the presence of sulfa and microsomal oxidase enzymes (120). These results are consistent with shunting of sulfa away from an acetylation arm of detoxification to a cytochrome P-450-mediated pathway, with generation of a toxic intermediate, likely a hydroxylamine. Slow acetylation protects against procainamide-induced lupus (129), and procainamide also can be metabolized to a hydroxylamine intermediate (130). The interaction of procainamide or a metabolite with nucleoproteins resulting in production of antinuclear antibodies has not been defined. Procainamide is also associated with agranulocytosis.

B. Immunologic

As suggested by the practical example of procainamide, metabolic pathways are not independent of immunologic responses; the complexity of detoxification enzyme systems rivals that of the immune system, and both serve as host defenses against foreign molecules (117b). Drugs, chemicals, and their metabolites might induce reactivity to a similar membrane epitope, function as a hapten when bound to cell surfaces, or directly affect the immune system. Chloramphenicol administered to animals alters the B cell response (131), and phenytoin in humans can induce T suppressor cell activity (132).

Table 3 Drug-Dependent, Antibody-Mediated Bone Marrow Suppression In Vitro

Drug	Syndrome	Inhibitor	C'	Specificity	Ref.
Diphenylhydantoin	Agranulocytosis	Ig	No	GM-CFC, PMN, PBL	135
Quinidine	Pancytopenia	Acute serum	No	GM-CFC, CFU-E; not PMN	136
Quinidine	Agranulocytosis	Acute serum	No?	GM-CFC[a]; not PMN	137
Diphenylhydantoin	Red cell aplasia	Acute IgG	No	CFU-E[b]; not GM-CFC	138
Ibuprofen	Agranulocytosis	Acute IgG	Yes	GM-CFC, Mix-CFC; not erythroid	115
Chlorpropamide	Agranulocytosis	Acute IgG	Yes	GM-CFC; not BFU-E, Mix-CFC, PMN	139

PBL = peripheral blood lymphocytes; PMN = polymorphonuclear cells; GM-CFC = granulocyte-macrophage colony forming cells; Mix-CFC = multipotential colony forming cells; CFU-E = colony forming units, erythroid.

[a]Inhibitory of autologous but not allogeneic bone marrow.

[b]Inhibitory but not cytotoxic.

Humoral mediation of drug-associated bone marrow depression was first suggested by studies in humans. Readministration of small amounts of a suspect drug after recovery from agranulocytosis (133) or infusion of plasma from agranulocytic patients into normal volunteers (134) precipitates leukopenia. An immune mechanism has been studied with hemopoietic colony formation in vitro as a test system for the presence of antibody to progenitor or precursor cells. As summarized in Table 3, in a few well-studied individual cases an antibody with specificity for the presumed marrow target cell has been demonstrated in vitro. Antibodies clearly have pathogenic roles in peripheral destruction of blood cells; they may also be present in nonimmune cases, presumably secondary reactants to disease-associated membrane alterations. Prompt disappearance of inhibitory activity with hematological improvement and the dependence on the presence of drug for cytotoxicity are evidence of a primary role in these cases, however.

IV. CONCLUSION: ANOMALIES

Some marked variations in the incidence of drug reactions over time and place have not been adequately explained. Agranulocytosis was common in Finnish trials of Cloazapine (140) and in New Zealand with mianserin (106), but these results were not reproduced elsewhere. A prominent feature of the recent epidemiologic survey of agranulocytosis and aplastic anemia in Europe was the very high rate of variability in incidence figures and risk ratios with associated drugs (111). For dipyrone, the relative risk was 24 for Ulm, Berlin, and Barcelona, but there was no associated risk for Israel and Budapest; such discrepancies are not readily explained by racial differences. Even more puzzling is the changing incidence of drug-associated agranulocytosis in patients treated with phenothiazines (Ref. 8, and Pisciotta, personal communication). When first described, agranulocytosis occurred in about 1 out of 300 treated patients and "benign" neutropenia was present in 1 in 11; in vitro studies suggested cytotoxicity for marrow progenitors. In follow-up studies in the same mental hospital only a few years later, cases of leukopenia were rare.

Chloramphenicol occurrence in twins suggested a genetic basis for bone marrow failure in humans (141). Rare variants of enzymes are not uncommon: if a large enough population is studied, rare allelles (frequency < 0.005) can probably be detected for all enzymes, even those without polymorphic loci (142). Measurements of average heterozygosity/locus for rare allelles have ranged from 1 to 3/1000 individuals; some rare variants may have very low gene frequencies (< 0.001). Homozygous recessive individuals for such variant enzymes in detoxification pathways genes would constitute the susceptible population for idiosycratic events due to drug or chemical exposure. The interrelated and redundant nature of metabolic pathways and the immune system provides a further level of complexity. Elimination of rare susceptible individuals by fatal sequelae when a drug is introduced would explain the apparent decline in hematological complications with drug use over time.

Individual susceptibility also might be based on genetic differences in hemopoietic function. In mice, a single genetic locus controls the proportion of BFU-E in cell cycle and susceptibility to Friend virus effects (143). Hemopoietic progenitor number in normal human bone marrow and blood has very wide variation, but heterogeneity of stem cell and progenitor function in humans has not been addressed experimentally in a systematic way. An abnormal response of hemopoietic cells from some individuals to drugs has been inferred for chlorpromazine (144) and chloramphenicol (145) but the inference is usually based on experiments using cells from patients who have recovered from a marrow insult.

Finally, viruses may interact with drugs (13,146): infectious mononucleosis and ampicillin combine to effect a high frequency of cutaneous eruption, and influenza and aspirin to increase the risk of Reye's syndrome (146). Not only may a drug be administered for a symptom of a virus infection, but viruses have significant effects on both immune reactivity and drug metabolism. Some viruses and vaccines can alter hepatic metabolism of drugs (147,148); enzymatic induction and depression may occur as an interferon effect (149,150).

ACKNOWLEDGMENTS

The author is thankful for careful reading of the manuscript and helpful comments of Stephen Spielberg (Toronto Childrens Hospital), Samuel Shapiro (Boston University), and Daniel Nebert (National Institute of Child Health and Human Development).

REFERENCES

1. Vincent, P. C. Drug-induced aplastic anemia and agranulocytosis. Incidence and mechanisms. *Drugs 31,* 52-63 (1986).
2. Heimpel, H., Wolfgang, H. Drug-induced aplastic anemia: clinical aspects. *Clin. Haematol. 9,* 641-662 (1980).
3. Benestad, H. B. Drug mechanisms in marrow aplasia. In: *Aplastic anemia.* Geary, C. G. (ed.). Bailliere Tindall, London, pp. 26-42 (1979).
4. Pisciotta, A. V. Immune and toxic mechanisms in drug-induced agranulocytosis. *Semin. Hematol. 10,* 279-310 (1973).
5. Williams, D. M., Lynch, R. E., Cartwright, G. E. Drug-induced aplastic anemia. *Semin. Hematol. 10,* 195-223 (1973).
6. Bithell, T. C., Wintrobe, M. M. Drug-induced aplastic anemia. *Semin. Hematol. 4,* 194-221 (1967).
7. Selling, L. Benzol as a leucotoxin. Studies on the degeneration and regeneration of the blood and haematopoietic organs. *Johns Hopkins Hosp. Rep. 17,* 83- (1916).
8. Pisciotta, A. V. Agranulocytosis induced by certain phenothiazine derivatives. *JAMA 308,* 1862-1868 (1969).
9. Volini, I. F., Greenspan, I., Ehrlich, L., Gonner, J. A., Felsenfeld, O., Schwartz, S. O. Hemopoietic changes during administration of chloramphenicol (chloromycetin). *JAMA 142,* 1333-1335 (1950).
10. Burnett, C. M., Corbett, J. F., Lanman, B. M. Hair dyes and aplastic anemia. *Drug Chem. Toxicol. 1,* 45-61 (1977-1978).
11. Hopkins, J. E., Manoharan, A. Severe aplastic anemia following the use of hair dye: report of two cases and review of literature. *Postgrad. Med. J. 61,* 1003-1005 (1985).
12. Powars, D. Aplastic anemia secondary to glue sniffing. *New Engl. J. Med. 273,* 700-702 (1965).
13. Young, N., Mortimer, P. Viruses and bone marrow failure. *Blood 63,* 729-737 (1984).
14. Smick, K. M., Condit, P. K., Proctor, R. L., Sutcher, V. Fatal aplastic anemia. An epidemiological study of its relationship to the drug chloramphenicol. *J. Chronic Dis. 17,* 899-914 (1964).
15. The Cooperative Study Group for Aplastic and Refractory Anemias. Toxic etiology of aplastic anemia. *Sex. Transmit. Dis. 11,* 343-346 (1984).
16. Fishbein, L. An overview of environmental and toxicological aspects of aromatic hydrocarbons. I. Benzene. *Sci. Total Environ. 40,* 189-218 (1984).
17. Snyder, R., Kocsis, J. J. Current concepts of chronic benzene toxicity. *CRC Crit. Rev. Toxicol. 3,* 265-288 (1975).

18. Hamilton, A. General review. Benzene (benzol) poisoning. *Arch. Pathol. 11,* 434-454 (1931).
19. Hunter, F. T. Chronic exposure to benzene (benzol). II. The clinical effects. *J. Ind. Hyg. 21,* 331-354 (1939).
20. Erf, L. A., Rhoads, C. P. The hematological effects of benzene (benzol) poisoning. *J. Ind. Hyg. Toxicol. 21,* 421-435 (1939).
21. Goldwater, L. J. Disturbances in the blood following exposure to benzol. *J. Lab. Clin. Med. 26,* 957-973 (1941).
22. Oldfelt, C. O. Benzene poisoning; clinical considerations. *Acta Med. Scand. 119,* 380-425 (1944).
23. Aksoy, M., Koray, D., Akgun, T., Erdem, S., Dincol, G. Haematological effects of chronic benzene poisoning in 217 workers. *Brit. J. Ind. Med. 28,* 296-302 (1971).
24. Aksoy, M., Erdem, S. Followup study on the mortality and the development of leukemia in 44 pancytopenic patients with chronic exposure to benzene. *Blood 52,* 285-291 (1978).
25. Vigliani, E. C., Saita, G. Benzene and leukemia. *New Engl. J. Med. 271,* 872-876 (1964).
26. DeGowin, R. L. Benzene exposure and aplastic anemia followed by leukemia 15 years later. *JAMA 185,* 748-751 (1963).
27. Brief, R. S., Lynch, J., Bernath, T., Scala, R. A. Benzene in the workplace. *Am. Ind. Hyg. Assoc. J. 41,* 616-623 (1980).
28. Elkins, H. B., Pagnotto, L. D. Benzene content of petroleum solvents. *A. M.A. Arch. Ind. Health 13,* 51-54 (1956).
29. Wallace, L. A., Pellizzari, E., Hartwell, T., Rosenzweig, M., Erickson, M., Sparacino, C., Zelon, H. Personal exposure to volatile organic compounds. I. Direct measurements in breathing-zone air, drinking water, food, and exhaled breath. *Environ. Res. 35,* 293-319 (1984).
30. Rinsky, R. A. Benzene and leukemia: an epidemiologic risk assessment. *New Engl. J. Med. 316,* 1044-1050 (1987).
31. Sawahata, T., Rickert, D. E., Greenlee, W. F. Metabolism of benzene and its metabolites in bone marrow. In: *Toxicology of the blood and bone marrow.* Irons, R. D. (Ed.). Raven Press, New York, pp. 141-148 (1985).
32. Sato, A., Nakajima, T., Fujiware, Y., Hirosawa, K. Pharmacokinetics of benzene and toluene. *Int. Arch. Arbeitsmed. 33,* 169-182 (1974).
33. Moeschlin, S., Speck, B. Experimental studies on the mechanism of action of benzene on the bone marrow (radioautographic studies using ^{3}H-thymidine). *Acta Haematol. 38,* 104-111 (1967).
34. Irons, R. D., Dent, J. G., Baker, T. S., Rickert, D. E. Benzene is metabolized and covalently bound in bone marrow in situ. *Chem. Biol. Interact. 30,* 241-245 (1980).
35. Greenlee, W. F., Sun, J. D., Bus, J. S. A proposed mechanism of benzene toxicity: formation of reactive intermediates from polyphenol metabolites. *Toxicol. Appl. Pharmacol. 59,* 187-195 (1981).
36. Sammett, D., Lee, E. W., Kocsis, J. J., Snyder, R. Partial hepatectomy reduces both metabolism and toxicity of benzene. *J. Toxicol. Environ. Health 5,* 785-792 (1979).

37. Gerarde, H. W. Toxicological studies on hydrocarbons. II. A comparison study of the effect of benzene and certain mono-*n*-alkylbenzenes on hemopoiesis and bone marrow metabolism in rats. *AMA Arch. Ind. Health 13,* 468-474 (1956).
38. Uyeki, E. M., Ashkar, A. E., Shoeman, D. W., Bisel, T. U. Acute toxicity of benzene inhalation to hemopoietic precursor cells. *Toxicol. Appl. Pharmacol. 40,* 49-57 (1977).
39. Gill, D. P., Jenkins, V. K., Kempen, R. R., Ellis, S. The importance of pluripotential stem cells in benzene toxicity. *Toxicology 16,* 163-171 (1980).
40. Green, J. D., Snyder, C. A., LoBue, J., Goldstein, B. D., Albert, R. E. Acute and chronic dose/response effects of inhaled benzene on multipotential hematopoietic stem (CFU-S) and granulocyte/macrophage protenitor (GM-CFU-C) cells in CD-1 mice. *Toxicol. Appl. Pharmacol. 58,* 492-503 (1981).
41. Hilderbrand, R. L., Murphy, M. J. The effects of benzene inhalation on murine hematopoietic precursor cells (CFU-e, BFU-e and CFU-gm). *Int. J. Cell Cloning 1,* 240-253 (1983).
42. Garnett, H. M., Cronkite, E. P., Drew, R. T. Effect of in vivo exposure to benzene on the characteristics of bone marrow adherent cells. *Leuk. Res. 7,* 803-810 (1983).
43. Bostrom, B., Smith, K., Ramsay, N. Low concentrations of benzene stimulate CFU/GM. *Blood 66,* 119a (1985).
44. Richards, R. P., Kramer, J. W., Baker, D. B., Krieger, K. A. Pesticides in rainwater in the northeastern United States. *Nature 327,* 129-131 (1987).
45. Dale, W. E., Quinby, G. E. Chlorinated insecticides in the body fat of people in the United States. *Science 142,* 593-595 (1963).
46. Anselstetter, V., Ballschmiter, K., Dmochewitz, S., Heimpel, H. Aplastic anemia: residue analysis of chlorinated hydrocarbons in human bone marrow biopsy specimens by high resolution gas chromatography. *Acta Haematol. 73,* 6-10 (1985).
47. Sanchez-Medal, L., Castanedo, J. P., Garcia-Rojas, F. Insecticides and aplastic anemia. *New Engl. J. Med. 269,* 1365-1367 (1963).
48. Young, N. S., Issaragrasil, S., Chieh, C. W., Takaku, F. Aplastic anemia in the orient. *Brit. J. Haematol. 62,* 1-6 (1986).
49. Loge, J. P. Aplastic anemia following exposure to benzene hexachloride (lindane). *JAMA 193,* 110-114 (1965).
50. West, I. Lindane and hematologic reactions. *Arch. Environ. Health 15,* 97-101 (1967).
51. Council on Pharmacy and Chemistry. Toxic effects of technical benzene hexachloride and its principal isomers. *JAMA 147,* 571-574 (1951).
52. Infante, P. F., Epstein, S. S., Newton, W. A. Blood dyscrasias and childhood tumors and exposure to chlordane and heptachlor. *Scand. J. Work Environ. Health 4,* 137-150 (1978).
53. Council on Pharmacy and Chemistry. The present status of chlordane. *JAMA 158,* 1364-1367 (1955).
54. Council of Pharmacy and Chemistry. Pharmacologic and toxicologic aspects of DDT (chlorophenothane U.S.P.). *JAMA 145,* 728-733 (1951).

55. Roberts, H. J. Aplastic anemia due to pentachlorophenol and tetrachlorophenol. *South. Med. J. 56,* 632-635 (1963).
56. Crawford, M. A. D. Aplastic anaemia due to trinitrotoluene intoxication. *Brit. Med. J. 3,* 430-437 (1954).
57. Imerman, S. W., Imerman, C. P. Dinitrophenol poisoning with thrombocytopenia, granulopenia, anemia and purpura complicated by lung abscess. *JAMA 106,* 1085-1088 (1936).
58. Ditraglia, D., Brown, D. P., Namekata, T., Iverson, N. Mortality study of workers employed at organochlorine pesticide manufacturing plants. *Scand. J. Work Environ. Health 7,* 140-146 (1981).
59. Stein, W. J., Hayes, W. J. Health survey of pest control operators. *Ind. Med. Surg. 33,* 549-555 (1964).
60. Wang, H. H., MacMahon, B. Mortality of pesticide applicators. *J. Occup. Med. 21,* 741-744 (1979).
61. Wang, H. H., MacMahon, B. Mortality of workers employed in the manufacture of chlordane and heptachlor. *J. Occup. Med. 21,* 745-748 (1979).
62. Blair, A., Grauman, D. J., Lubin, J. H., Fraumeni, J. F. Lung cancer and other causes of death among licensed pesticide applicators. *JNCI 71,* 31-37 (1983).
63. Wang, H. H., Grufferman, S. Aplastic anemia and occupational pesticide exposure: a case-control study. *J. Occup. Med. 23,* 364-366 (1981).
64. Blair, A., Thomas, T. L. Leukemia among Nebraska farmers: a death certificate study. *Am. J. Epidemiol. 110,* 264-273 (1979).
65. Burmeister, L. F., Van Lier, S. F., Isacson, P. Leukemia and farm practices in Iowa. *Am. J. Epidemiol. 115,* 720-728 (1982).
66. Gallagher, R. P., Threlfall, W. J., Jeffries, E., Band, P. R., Spinelli, J., Coldman, A. J. Cancer and aplastic anemia in British Columbia farmers. *JNCI 72,* 1311-1315 (1984).
67. Linos, A., Kyle, R. A., O'Fallon, W. M., Kurland, L. T. A case-control study of occupational exposures and leukaemia. *Int. J. Epidemiol. 9,* 131-135 (1980).
68. Davignon, L. F., St-Pierre, J., Charest, G., Tourangeau, F. J. A study of the chronic effects of insecticides in man. *Can. Med. Assoc. J. 92,* 597-602 (1965).
69. Alvarez, W. C., Hyman, S. Absence of toxic manifestations in workers exposed to chlordane. *Arch. Ind. Hyg. Occup. Med. 8,* 480-483 (1953).
70. Frinci, F., Spurbeck, G. H. A study of workers exposed to the insecticides chlordan, aldrin, dieldrin. *Arch. Ind. Hyg. Occup. Med. 3,* 64-72 (1951).
71. Cullen, M. R., Rado, T., Waldron, J. A., Sparer, J., Welch, L. S. Bone marrow injury in lithographers exposed to glycol ethers and organic solvents used in multicolor offset and ultraviolet curing printing processes. *Arch. Environ. Health 38,* 347-354 (1983).
72. Lewis, C. N., Putnam, L. E., Hendricks, F. D., Kerlan, I., Welch, H. Chloramphenicol (chloromycetin) in relation to blood dyscrasias with observations of other drugs. A special study. *Antibiot. Chemother. II,* 601-609 (1952).
73. Huguley, C. M., Erslev, A. J., Bergsagel, D. E. Drug-related blood dyscrasias. *JAMA 177,* 23-26 (1961).

74. Best, W. R. Chloramphenicol-associated blood dyscrasias. *JAMA 201*, 99-106 (1967).
75. Wallerstein, R. O., Condit, P. K., Kasper, C. K., Brown, J. W., Morrison, F. R. Statewide study of chloramphenicol therapy and fatal aplastic anemia. *JAMA 208*, 2045-2050 (1969).
76. Bottiger, L. E. Drug-induced aplastic anaemia in Sweden with special reference to chloramphenicol. *Postgrad. Med. J. 50*, 127-131 (1974).
77. Modan, B., Segal, S., Shani, M., Sheba, C. Aplastic anemia in Israel: evaluation of the etiological role of chloramphenicol on a community-wide basis. *Am. J. Med. Sci. 270*, 441-445 (1975).
78. Shimamine, T., Ishihara, K., Imamura, T. Pathological findings in aplastic anemia. In: *Aplastic anemia.* Hibino, S., Takaku, F., Shahidi, N. T. (Eds.). University Park Press, Baltimore, MD, pp. 3-18 (1976).
79. Aoki, K., Ohtani, M., Shimizu, H. Epidemiological approach to the etiology of aplastic anemia. In: *Aplastic anemia.* Hibino, S., Takaku, F., Shahidi, N. T. (Eds.). University Park Press, Baltimore, MD, pp. 155-170 (1976).
80. Whang, K. S. Aplastic anemia in Korea: a clinical study of 309 cases. In: *Aplastic anemia.* Hibino, S., Takaku, F., Shahidi, N. T. (Eds.). University Park Press, Baltimore, MD, pp. 225-242 (1976).
81. Polak, B. C. P., Wesseling, H., Schut, D., Herxheimer, A., Meyler, L. Blood dyscrasias attributed to chloramphenicol. A review of 576 published and unpublished cases. *Acta Med. Scand. 192*, 409-414 (1972).
82. Issaragrisil, S., Piankijagum, A. Aplastic anemia following topical administration of ophthalmic chloramphenicol: report of a case and review of the literature. *J. Med. Assoc. Thailand 68*, 309-312 (1985).
83. Del Giacco, G. S., Petrini, M. T., Jannelli, S., Carcassi, U. Fatal bone marrow hypoplasia in a shepherd using chloramphenicol spray. *Lancet 1*, 945 (1981).
84. Settepani, J. A. The hazard of using chloramphenicol in food animals. *J. Am. Vet. Med. Assoc. 184*, 930-931 (1984).
85. Scott, J. L., Finegold, S. M., Belkin, G. A., Lawrence, J. S. A controlled double-blind study of the hematologic toxicity of chloramphenicol. *New Engl. J. Med. 272*, 1137-1142 (1965).
86. Rubin, D., Weisberger, A. S., Botti, R. E., Storaasli, J. P. Changes in iron metabolism in early chloramphenicol toxicity. *J. Clin. Invest. 37*, 1286-1292 (1958).
87. Krakoff, I. H., Karnofsky, D. A., Burchenal, J. H. Effects of large doses of chloramphenicol on human subjects. *New Engl. J. Med. 253*, 7-10 (1955).
88. Daum, R. S., Cohen, D. L., Smith, A. L. Fatal aplastic anemia following apparent "dose-related" choloramphenicol toxicity. *J. Pediatr. 94*, 403-406 (1979).
89. Ferrari, V. Salient features of thiamphenicol: review of clinical pharmacokinetics and toxicity. *Sex. Transmit. Dis. 11*, 336-339 (1984).
90. Yunis, A. A. Mechanisms underlying marrow toxicity from chloramphenicol and thiamphenicol. In: *The year in hematology*. Silber, R., LoBue, J., Gordon, A. S. (Eds.). Plenum, New York, pp. 143-170 (1978).

91. Yunis, A. A., Miller, A. M., Salem, Z., Arimura, G. K. Chloramphenicol toxicity: pathogenetic mechanisms and role of the p-NO_2 in aplastic anemia. *Clin. Toxicol. 17,* 359-373 (1980).
92. Samir, A.-K., Salem, Z., Yunis, A. A. Mitochondrial metabolism in normal, myeloid, and erythroid hyperplastic rabbit bone marrow: effect of chloramphenicol. *Am. J. Hematol. 8,* 71-79 (1980).
93. Ratzan, R. J., Moore, M. A. S., Yunis, A. A. Effect of chloramphenicol and thiamphenicol on the in vitro colony-forming cell. *Blood 43,* 363-369 (1974).
94. Murray, T., Downey, K. M., Yunis, A. A. Degradation of isolated deoxyribonucleic acid mediated by nitroso-chloramphenicol. Possible role in chloramphenicol-induced aplastic anemia. *Biochem. Pharmacol. 31,* 2291-2296 (1982).
95. Murray, T. R., Downey, K. M., Yunis, A. A. Cloramphenicol-mediated DNA damage and its possible role in the inhibitory effects of chloramphenicol on DNA synthesis. *J. Lab. Clin. Med. 102,* 926-932 (1983).
96. Yunis, A. A., Arimura, G. K., Isildar, M. DNA damage induced by chloramphenicol and its nitroso derivative: damage in intact cells. *Am. J. Hematol. 24,* 77-84 (1987).
97. Isildar, M., Jimenez, J. J., Arimura, G. K., Yunis, A. A. Aplastic anemia from chloramphenicol may be mediated by its bacterial metabolites. *Clin. Res. 35,* 650A (1987).
98. Alavi, J. B. Aplastic anemia associated with intravenous chloramphenicol. *Am. J. Hematol. 15,* 375-379 (1983).
99. Kirshna, G., Aykac, I., Siegel, D. Recent studies on the mechanisms of chloramphenicol activation responsible for aplastic anemia. In: *Safety problems related to chloramphenicol and thiamphenicol therapy.* Najean, Y., et al. (Eds.). Raven Press, New York, pp. 5-16 (1981).
100. Bostrom, B., Smith, K., Ramsay, N. K. C. Stimulation of human committed bone marrow stem cells (CFU-GM) by chloramphenicol. *Exp. Hematol. 14,* 156-161 (1986).
101. Firkin, F. C., Sumner, M. A., Bradley, T. R. The influence of chloramphenicol on the bone marrow haemopoietic stem cell compartment. *Exp. Hematol. 2,* 264-268 (1974).
102. Adams, G. R., Pearson, H. A. Chloramphenicol-responsive chronic neutropenia. *New Engl. J. Med. 309,* 1039-1041 (1984).
103. Nara, N., Bessho, M., Hirashima, K., Momo, H. Effects of chloramphenicol on hematopoietic inductive microenvironment. *Exp. Hematol. 10,* 20-25 (1982).
104. Sawada, H., Tezuka, H., Kamamoto, T., Nishikori, M., Yoshida, Y., Uchino, H., Kirikae, T., Tsurusawa, M., Mori, K. J. Effects of chloramphenicol on hemopoietic cells and their microenvironment in vitro. *Acta Haematol. Jpn. 48,* 1323-1331 (1985).
105. Miescher, P. A., Pola, W. Haematological effects of non-narcotic analgesics. *Drugs 32,* 90-108 (1986).
106. Chaplin, S. Bone marrow depression due to mianserin, phenylbutazone, oxyphenbutazone, and chloramphenicol. Part I. *Adverse Drug React. Acute Poisoning Rev. 5,* 97-101 (1986).

107. Venning, G. R. Identification of adverse reactions to new drugs. II (continued). How were 18 important adverse reactions discovered and with what delays? *Brit. Med. J. 286,* 365-368 (1983).
108. McCarthy, D. D., Chalmers, T. M. Hematological complications of phenylbutazone therapy: review of the literature and report of two cases. *Can. Med. Assoc. J. 90,* 1061-1067 (1964).
109. Inman, W. H. W. Study of fatal bone marrow depression with special reference to phenylbutazone and oxyphenbutazone. *Brit. Med. J. 1,* 1500-1505 (1977).
110. MacKay, R. J., French, T. W., Nguyen, H. T., Mayhew, I. G. Effects of large doses of phenylbutazone administration to horses. *Am. J. Vet. Res. 44,* 774-780 (1983).
111. International Agranulocytosis and Aplastic Anemia Study. Risks of agranulocytosis and aplastic anemia. A first report of their relation to drug use with special reference to analgesics. *JAMA 256,* 1749-1757 (19xx).
112. Smith, C. S., Chinn, S., Watts, R. W. E. The sensitivity of human bone marrow granulocyte/monocyte precursor cells to phenylbutazone, oxyphenbutazone and gamma-hydroxyphenylbutazone in vitro, with observations on the bone marrow colony formation in phenylbutazone-induced granulocytopoenia. *Biochem. Pharmacol. 26,* 847-852 (1977).
113. Barrett, A. J., Weller, E., Rozengurt, N., Longhurst, P., Humble, J. G. Amidopyrine agranulocytosis: drug inhibition of granulocyte colonies in the presence of patient's serum. *Brit. Med. J. 2,* 850-851 (1976).
114. Mamus, S. W., Burton, J. D., Groat, J. D., Schulte, D. A., Lobell, M., Zanjani, E. D. Ibuprofen-associated pure white-cell aplasia. *New Engl. J. Med. 314,* 624-625 (1986).
115. Jerina, D. M., Daly, J. W. Arene oxides: a new aspect of drug metabolism. *Science 185,* 573-582 (1974).
116. Dipple, A., Pigott, M. A., Agarwal, S. K., Yaki, H., Sayer, J. M., Jerina, D. M. Optically active benzo[*c*]phenanthrene diol epoxides bind extensively to adenine in DNA. *Nature 327,* 535-536 (1987).
117a. Nebert. D. W. Genetic differences in susceptibility to chemically induced myelotoxicity and leukemia. *Environ. Health Perspect. 39,* 11-22 (1981).
117b. Nebert, D. W., Gonzalez, F. J. P450 genes: structure, evolution and regulation. *Ann. Rev. Biochem. 56,* 945-993 (1987).
118. Legraverend, C., Harrison, D. E., Ruscetti, F. W., Nebert, D. W. Bone marrow toxicity induced by oral benzo[*a*]pyrene: protection resides at the level of the intestine and liver. *Toxicol. Appl. Pharmacol. 70,* 390-401 (1983).
119. Spielberg, S. P. Acetaminophen toxicity in human lymphocytes in vitro. *J. Pharmacol. Exp. Ther. 213,* 395-397 (1980).
120. Shear, N. H., Spielberg, S. P., Grant, D. M., Tang, B. K., Kalow, W. Differences in metabolism of sulfonamides predisposing to idiosyncratic toxicity. *Ann. Intern. Med. 105,* 179-184 (1986).
121. Spielberg, S. P., Gordon, G. B., Blake, D. A., Goldstein, D. A., Herlong, H. F. Predisposition to phenytoin hepatotoxicity assessed in vitro. *New Engl. J. Med. 305,* 722-727 (1981).

122. Strikler, S. M., Dansky, L. V., Miller, M. A., Seni, M.-H., Andermann, E., Spielberg, S. P. Genetic predisposition to phenytoin-induced birth defects. *Lancet 2,* 746-749 (1985).
123. Gerson, W. T., Fine, D. G., Spielberg, S. P., Sensenbrenner, L. L. Anticonvulsant-induced aplastic anemia: increased susceptibility to toxic drug metabolites in vitro. *Blood 61,* 889-893 (1983).
124. Weinshilboum, R. Pharmacogenetics of methyl conjugation and thiopurine drug toxicity. *Prog. Clin. Biol. Res. 135,* 167-181 (1983).
125. Lennard, L., VanLoon, J. A., Lilleyman, J. S., Weinshilboum, R. M. Thiopurine pharmacogenetics in leukemia: correlation of erythrocyte thiopurine methyltransferase activity and 6-thioguanine nucleotide concentrations. *Clin. Pharmacol. Ther. 41,* 18-25 (1987).
126. Lennard, L., Rees, C. A., Lilleyman, J. S., Maddocks, J. L. Childhood leukaemia: a relationship between intracellular y-mercaptopurine metabolites and neutropenia. *Brit. J. Clin. Pharmacol. 16,* 359-363 (1983).
127. Lennard, L., Murphy, M. F., Maddocks, J. L. Severe megaloblastic anaemia associated with abnormal azathioprine metabolism. *Brit. J. Clin. Pharmacol. 17,* 171-172 (1984).
128. Price, D. A. Acetylation. In: *Ethnic differences in reactions to drugs and xenobiotics.* Kalow, W., Goedde, H. W., Agarwal, D. P. (Eds.). Alan R. Liss, New York, pp. 209-242 (1986).
129. Woosley, R. L., Roden, D. M. Importance of metabolites in antiarrhythmic therapy. *Amer. J. Cardiol. 52,* 3C-7C (1983).
130. Uetrecht, J. P., Sweetman, B. J., Woosley, R. L., Oates, J. A. Metabolism of procainamide to a hydroxylamine by rat and human hepatic microsomes. *Drug. Metab. Dispos. 12,* 77-81 (1984).
131. Couderc, J., Perrodon, Y., Ventura, M., Liacopoulos, P., Danchin, A. Specification of the immune response: its suppression induced by chloramphenicol in vitro. *Biosci. Rep. 3,* 19-29 (1983).
132. Dosch, H.-M., Jason, J., Gelfand, E. W. Transient antibody deficiency and abnormal T suppressor cells induced by phenytoin. *New Engl. J. Med. 306,* 406-409 (1982).
133. Madison, F. W., Squier, T. L. The etiology of primary granulocytopenic (agranulocytic angina). *JAMA 102,* 755-759 (1934).
134. Moeschlin, S., Wagner, K. Agranulocytosis due to the occurrence of leukocyte agglutinins. *Acta Haematol. 8,* 29- (1952).
135. Taetle, R., Lane, T. A., Mendelsohn, J. Drug-induced agranulocytosis: in vitro evidence for immune suppression of granulopoiesis and a cross-reacting lymphocyte antibody. *Blood 54,* 501-512 (1979).
136. Kelton, J. G., Haung, A. T., Mold, N., Logue, G., Rosse, W. F. The use of in vitro technics to study drug-induced pancytopenia. *New Engl. J. Med. 301,* 621-624 (1979).
137. Ascensao, J. L., Flynn, P. J., Slungaard, A., Wachsman, W., Zanjani, E. D., Jacob, H. S. Quinidine-induced neutropenia: report of a case with drug-dependent inhibition of granulocyte colony generation. *Acta Haematol. 72,* 349-354 (1984).

138. Dessypris, E. N., Redline, S., Harris, J. W., Krantz, S. B. Diphenylhydantoin-induced pure red cell asplasia. *Blood 65,* 789-794 (1985).
139. Levitt, L. J. Chlorpropamide-induced pure white cell aplasia. *Blood 69,* 394-400 (1987).
140. Anderman, B., Griffith, R. W. Clozapine-induced agranulocytosis: a situation report up to August 1976. *Eur. J. Clin. Pharmacol. 11,* 199-201 (1977).
141. Nagao, T., Mauer, A. M. Concordance for drug induced aplastic anemia in identical twins. *New Engl. J. Med. 281,* 7-11 (1969).
142. Vogel, F., Motulsky, A. G. *Human genetics.* Springer-Verlag, New York (1986).
143. Suzuki, S., Axelrad, A. A. Fv-2 locus controls the proportion of erythropoietic progenitor cells (BFU-E) synthesizing DNA in normal mice. *Cell 19,* 225-236 (1980).
144. Pisciotta, A. V. Studies on agranulocytosis. IX. A biochemical defect in chlorpromazine-sensitive marrow cells. *J. Lab. Clin. Med. 78,* 435-448 (1971).
145. Howell, A., Andrews, T. M., Watts, R. W. Bone marrow cells resistant to chloramphenicol in chloramphenicol-induced aplastic anemia. *Lancet 1,* 65 (1975).
146. Levy, M. The combined effect of viruses and drugs in drug-induced diseases. *Med. Hypoth. 14,* 293-296 (1984).
147. D'Arcy, P. F. Vaccine-drug interactions. *Drug. Intell. Clin. Pharmacol. 18,* 697-700 (1984).
148. Meredith, C. G., Christian, C. D., Johnson, R. F., Troxell, R., Davis, G. L., Schenker, S. Effects of influenza virus vaccine on hepatic drug metabolism. *Clin. Pharmacol. Ther. 37,* 396-401 (1985).
149. Deloria, L., Abbott, V., Gooderham, N., Mannering, G. J. Induction of xanthine oxidase and depression of cytochrome P-450 by interferon inducers: genetic difference in the responses of mice. *Biochem. Biophys. Res. Commun. 131,* 109-114 (1985).
150. Peterson, T. C., Renton, K. W. The role of lymphocytes, macrophages and interferon in the depression of drug metabolism by dextran sulfate. *Immunopharmacology 11,* 21-28 (1986).

7

Induced Chromosome Damage After Irradiation and Cytotoxic Drugs

NIEL WALD and MARY K. CONNER
Graduate School of Public Health, University of Pittsburgh, Pittsburgh, Pennsylvania

I. INTRODUCTION

This chapter reviews those aspects of induced chromosome damage that are produced by therapeutic agents used in the treatment of blood dyscrasias and other neoplastic or nonmalignant diseases. The nature and mechanisms of induced damage to chromosomes from cytotoxic drugs and ionizing radiation are discussed, with emphasis on regimens and dose ranges in clinical use. Evidence for long-term or late cytogenetic effects is reviewed. The relationship of therapy-related cytogenetic damage to the subsequent development of additional hematological neoplasia is considered.

II. CYTOGENETIC STUDIES IN PERIPHERAL BLOOD LYMPHOCYTES

A. Methodology

Cytogenetic studies in humans were facilitated by the recognition by Moorehead and colleagues (1) that the circulating peripheral blood lymphocyte (PBL) was a readily accessible cell that could be stimulated to divide in short-term culture. As a consequence of their quiescent (G_0) state during in vivo exposure and their relatively long life span, PBLs permit repeated and/or long-term assessment of chromosomal damage.

The utilization of cytogenetic analysis for assessment of cytotoxic exposure has relied on several different end points (2). The classical methodology enumerates chromosomal aberrations (numerical and/or morphological), and more recent methods assess sister chromatid exchanges (SCE). Chromosomal aberrations reflect chromosome breakage events and are observed as gaps, breaks, terminal or interstitial deletions, acentric fragments, and such chromosomal interchanges or rearrangements as dicentrics, rings, and translocations. Morphological alterations that are confined to one chromatid are termed chromatid aberrations, whereas those that occur at identical loci in both chromatids are called chromosome aberrations. Chromatid and chromosome aberrations are gross structural abnormalities that are relatively easy to detect.

Smaller and more subtle changes such as inversion of a small segment of the chromosome may be detected by banding techniques, but since these are related to the previous lesions in frequency, they are rarely scored directly. SCEs are visualized following differential staining of cells that have incorporated 5-bromo-2'-deoxyuridine (BrdUrd) during culture (3,4). SCEs are recognized as apparent reciprocal exchanges of chromatin between sister chromatids.

It is important to recognize that there are certain appropriate modifications of the common cytogenetic study procedure utilized in diagnostic studies of in utero or neonatal infants for genetic diagnostic purposes or adults with endocrine, hematological, and other neoplastic diseases. These include the use of 48-hr peripheral blood cell cultures, the scoring of 100-200 or more metaphase cells, and the use of simultaneous control samples. The fact that radiation and chemical damage occur at random and are dose-related in magnitude makes the scoring of large numbers of cells essential if small changes are to be detected.

There have been several attempts to avoid the labor-intensive technique of classical aberration scoring. One approach is to use modern automated technology to facilitate the method. The procedural steps for which digital image processing techniques have been used include metaphase location as well as karyotyping. The latter procedure is not really suitable for aberration scoring, and more direct approaches to software development for this specific purpose are in progress. Success has already been reported in metaphase location by such methodology (5). Several commercial organizations have advertised equipment for one or both of these functions. A second approach is through flow system technology. Here the aberration scoring involves the extremely rapid assessment of individual chromosomes. The frequency of deviation from the standard size distribution peaks in the histogram of the normal chromosome complement serves indirectly to assess the aberration frequency (6,7).

Another approach is to utilize a less specific end point by scoring the frequency of interphase PBL micronuclei (8). The micronucleus is considered to be the result of chromosome fragmentation, with the acentric fragment being left in the cytoplasm after the first mitosis following the injury has taken place. Since a fragment may result from a deletion as well as from dicentric or ring formation, the scoring of these fragments as micronuclei does not provide information as to the specific lesion from which they originate. However, the ease of scoring makes this technique a more practical approach to population screening.

B. Evidence for Chromosome Damage

1. Radiation-Induced Damage

Evidence for the production of chromosome damage by ionizing radiation has been accumulating since Muller's discovery that radiation exposure produced genetic abnormalites in *Drosophila* (9).

Sax (10) reported cytogenetic dose-response relationships in *Tradescantia.* Intensive studies of other variables such as dose rate, linear energy transfer (LET), oxygen concentration, and temperature provided Lea (11) with a basis for a mechanistic hypothesis involving the production of chromosome aberrations by interactions with the ionizing events evoked by the energy deposited along the pathway of a radiation particle.

The fact that relatively uniform whole body radiation exposure in humans produces the same results as the in vitro exposure of human blood (12) make it possible to use many of the in vitro dose-response relationships and other data in the assessment of human exposure. Various forms of aberration detection and quantitation have therefore been utilized in evaluating irradiated individuals or populations.

The first application was in the evaluation of individual radiation workers inadvertently exposed to relatively high irradiation. This use as a supplement to, or substitute for, physical means of exposure assessment was facilitated by the ability to calibrate the cytogenetic test system by exposing human blood cells in vitro to known exposures from a comparable radiation source for calibration purposes. Not only does this assessment facilitate therapeutic decision making and planning as well as prognostic evaluation in actual overexposures, but it also serves to relieve unwarranted anxiety in uncertain exposure situations where physical dosimetry is absent or does not correspond to the actual patient exposure. Lloyd et al. have reported on studies of almost 700 such individuals in the United Kingdom since 1972 (13,14).

A second use of the cytogenetic methodology has been in the assessment of populations whose occupational activities or general environment is thought to provide some increase in long-term low-level radiation exposure. Studies of this kind on radiation workers have been reported (15-17). The environmental or geographic studies involve populations with long-term exposure to low-level radiation backgrounds higher than those generally found. An example is an epidemiologic investigation in China where the location of the study population had a natural radioactivity level three times higher than that of the control population (18).

In addition to the classical aberration scoring, other indices of chromosome damage have been used. Fliedner et al. observed micronuclei in the circulating blood and marrow cells of 8 men irradiated in a criticality accident at Oak Ridge

National Laboratory (19). In an effort to facilitate the performance of large numbers of cytogenetic studies in populations at low doses and at low dose rates, the possible use of the frequency of micronucleus formation as an end point representative of chromosomal aberration frequency has been proposed. It offers the benefits that interphase nuclei are scored and the analysis of results of these preparations is relatively simple (8,20). Unfortunately, Krepinsky and Heddle (21) reported that an in vitro calibration curve suggests that this is a useful measure only for doses greater than 25 cGy. This is probably due to the relatively high spontaneous level of chromatid aberrations, which can produce micronuclei but would be excluded from scoring in the standard metaphase chromosome analysis. They did suggest, however, the possible future application of the method for the evaluation of lymphocyte radiosensitivity in radiation workers.

Sister chromatid exchange scoring was applied to the study of the effects of radiation as well as those of chemicals when the BrdUrd technique facilitated its use (22). It was soon recognized that radiation, although a powerful mutagen, is a relatively poor inducer of SCE (23). A partial explanation was suggested by Gundy et al. (24) in their finding that there was a dose-related increase but that it was notable only at relatively low doses. Because of the many known and unknown extraneous variables in studies using SCE, the relationship of radiation exposure to SCE frequency is not yet clear.

2. Damage Induced by Cytostatic Agents

Numerous studies have documented the cytogenetic effects of cytostatic chemicals. The cytogenetic consequences of cytostatic agents are diverse and depend on the specific mode of action of the individual agents. Table 1 classifies various cytostatic agents according to broad categories of chemical reactivity and genotoxic activity as indicated by production of chromosomal aberrations and SCE in PBLs and evidence of carcinogenicity in treated patients. With regard to SCE-inducing activities, the cytostatic agents in Table 1 can be classified into four categories: potent, weak, questionable, and negative SCE-inducing agents.

Potent SCE-Inducing Agents. As a class, the alkylating agents are consistently the most potent SCE-inducing agents. Cisplatin is also included in this class; although it is not a true alkylating agent, it mimics bifunctional alkylating agents in its ability to form intra- and interstrand DNA cross-links (57). Two members of the diverse class of antitumor antibiotics are also strong SCE inducers: mitomycin C, a cross-linking agent, and adriamycin, an intercalating agent. In general, the agents classified as strong SCE inducers are also clastogenic (chromosome-damaging) and carcinogenic.

Weak SCE-Inducing Agents. The antitumor antibiotics actinomycin D and daunomycin react with DNA via intercalation and are weakly effective as SCE inducers. Likewise, the antimetabolites methotrexate and azathioprine are weakly

Table 1 Cytogenetic and Carcinogenic Effects of Commonly Used Cytostatic Agents[a]

Class/agent	Number[b] of cases	Cytogenetic aberrations	Effect on SCE[c]	Ref.	Carcinogenicity	Ref.[d]
Alkylating Agents						
Busulfan (myleran)	>48	+	+	25-28	+	53,54
Chlorambucil (leukeran)	>109	+	+	28-34	+	53,54
Cyclophosphamide	>239	+	+	25-29, 35-37	+	53,54
L-PAM (melphalan)	>144	+	+	26-28, 38-40	+	53,54
ACNU, BCNU, CCNU, MeCCNU	>57	+	+	26-28,41	+	54
Procarbazine	>2	+	(+)	26,42	(+)	55
Cisplatin	7		+	43	+	55,56
Antitumor Antibiotics						
Adriamycin	>14	+	+	22,25,27, 44		
Actinomycin D	>13	±	±	25,27,44		
Bleomycin	>12	+	±	26,27,44, 45	(+)	55
Daunomycin	22	±	+	26,27		
Mitomycin C	>25		+	26,27, 46-48	(+)	55

(Table 1 *continues*)

Table 1 (*continued*)

Class/agent	Number[b] of cases	Cytogenetic aberrations	Effect on SCE[c]	Ref.	Carcinogenicity	Ref.[d]
Antimetabolites						
Ara-C	>63	+	(±)	27,28,30		
Azathioprine (imuran)	>100	(±)	(±)	27,28,49	+	42
5-FU	>65	±	±	25-28		
6-MP	36	+	±	26-28,50		
Methotrexate (amethopterin)	>100	(±)	(±)	27,36,45, 51		
Spindle Poisons						
Colchicine	>40		–	27		
Vincristine	>59	(±)	–	27,28,52		

[a]Updated from Ref. 27.
[b]Total number of cases studied for aberrations and/or SCE: +, positive; (+), weakly positive; – negative; ± conflicting results.
[c]Generally the results are in PBL of exposed patients. Some cases may also include bone marrow responses.
[d]Carcinogenicity data are given only for those positive or suspect agents.
Abbreviations used: L-PAM, 1-phenylalanine mustard; ACNU, acetyl chloroethyl nitrosourea; BCNU, bischloroethyl nitrosourea; CCNU, cyclohexyl chloroethyl nitrosourea; MeCCNU, methyl cyclohexyl chloroethyl nitrosourea; ara-C, cytosine arabinoside; 5-FU, 5-fluorouracil; 6-MP, 6-mercaptopurine.

active in producing SCEs. This class is also weakly clastogenic and, at most, of questionable carcinogenic activity.

Questionable SCE-Inducing Agents. Conflicting reports have been published on the SCE-inducing activities of the antimetabolites ara-C, 5-FU, and 6-MP and the antitumor antibiotic bleomycin. Much of this inconsistency arises from the fact that different studies examined cytogenetic parameters at various times after patient treatment. Positive effects were observed when the analysis was carried out during or immediately after treatment (see Section II.D on evidence for long-term effects of cytostatic damage). In particular, the antimetabolites are S-phase-dependent, and in order to elicit an SCE response in lymphocytes, the agent per se must persist in sufficiently high intracellular concentration to produce a response at the time of lymphocyte culturing. Negative or questionable results in PBLs should not be taken to imply that antimetabolites do not produce genotoxic damage in bone marrow cells that are in a proliferative state during therapeutic exposure. The chromosome-damaging activities of this group of SCE inducers range from weakly to strongly (bleomycin) clastogenic. Their carcinogenicity is, at most, questionable (bleomycin).

Negative SCE Inducing Agents. The mitotic spindle poisons colchicine and vincristine have not been shown to be SCE-inducing agents. They are, at most, weakly active clastogens and do not appear to be carcinogenic.

Raposa (28) recently reported a striking correlation between SCE-inducing activities of cytostatic agents and the induction of iatrogenic leukemias. Of 164 cases of secondary acute nonlymphocytic leukemia (S-ANLL) associated with monochemotherapy (L-PAM, 84 cases; chlorambucil, 48 cases; cyclophosphamide, 18 cases), 151 (92%) cases involved treatment with a positive SCE-inducing agent and only 13 (8%) by agents that do not produce a positive SCE response in human PBLs. In 616 cases of S-ANLL associated with combined modality therapy, 523 cases (85%) involved therapies that included positive SCE inducers whereas 85 (14%) and 8 (1%) of the cases involved questionable or negative, respectively, SCE inducers. Raposa's data strongly support the use of SCE to assess the potential carcinogenic risk of cytostatic agents.

C. Mechanisms of Radiation and Chemically Induced Chromosomal Aberrations and SCEs

Many different research approaches have led to a general acceptance that damage to DNA is a major general reason for cell killing by ionizing radiation and cytostatic agents. Specific cytogenetic consequences of physical and chemical agents are determined by the type(s) of DNA lesions produced by the particular agent and the accuracy of mechanisms involved in repair of induced lesions.

The nature of the chemical modifications produced in DNA by radiation may be classified into four types: single-strand breaks, double-strand breaks, base damage, and DNA-protein cross-links. Of the commonly used cytostatic agents, bleomycin is uniquely effective in producing single- and double-strand breakage of DNA. By contrast, the majority of cytostatic agents react directly with specific nucleophilic sites on DNA (mono- or bifunctional alkylating agents), distort the structure of DNA (inercalating agents), or interfere with the replication of DNA (antimetabolites).

Single-strand breaks are readily repaired via a replication-like process that utilizes the intact strand as a template. The continuity of the strand is restored by a ligase. Radiation and chemically induced base damage, either localized or cross-linked to protein in other base sites, is repaired by a stepwise excision repair process. Initially, excision repair enzymes catalyze removal of a segment of DNA containing the damaged site. The resulting single-stranded region is repaired as previously described. Repair of double-strand breaks is more problematic because of the absence of an intact template strand. Consequently, double-strand breakage initiates misrepair processes and the formation of chromosome aberrations. The importance of DNA repair in the production of chromosome aberrations was recognized almost 50 years ago (10) and has since been the focus of a number of books and review articles (58-61).

Which DNA lesion(s) is or are the important alteration(s) involved in the origin of specific cytogenetic responses is not yet entirely clear. In the past decade assiduous application by numerous investigators using a classic biochemical approach to complex systems—the inhibition of specific steps in a sequence of reactions—has begun to narrow down the numerous possibilities. Specifically, the inhibition of DNA repair by a variety of agents acting on different parts of the repair process in a variety of cells at different stages in their life cycle has been employed.

1. Formation of Chromosome Aberrations During G_1 or G_0

Chromosome aberrations have long been recognized as a visible manifestation of DNA damage. Chromsome-type aberrations are produced as the result of misrepair during G_1 or G_0, are replicated during the subsequent S phase, and are evident at the first metaphase following their formation. The best-supported hypotheses appear to be that DNA double-strand breaks and DNA base damage are the most likely lesions involved in the production of chromosomal aberrations during G_1 or G_0 (60,61).

Virsik-Peuckert and Harder (62) suggest that although it is very probable that double-strand damage of DNA is a final necessary step in the formation of chromosome aberrations, it may not necessarily be directly induced but could be the result of a process of incomplete repair of other types of lesions such as base damage, as suggested by Preston (60). The publications of Natarajan et al. (63) and Holmberg and Gumauskas (64) add support to the importance of radiation-induced short-lived DNA strand breaks in the formation of chromosome aberrations. Those agents (e.g., radiation and bleomycin) that directly induce primarily double- and single-strand DNA breakage are most effective in producing chromosome-type aberrations. However, low frequencies of chromosome-type aberrations have also been observed in the first mitosis following exposure of cells to chemical agents that do not directly produce DNA strand breakage. The origin of such aberrations is most likely the indirect production, during G_1 or G_0, of single- or double-strand breaks associated with incomplete repair processes. The frequency of chromosome-type aberrations is expected to depend upon the rate of G_1 repair processes and the duration of G_1. If the rate of G_1 repair is slow, the probability of formation of coincident breaks capable of interacting to produce chromosome aberrations will be low (65). However, because the potential for production of G_1 repair-dependent strand breakage increases with the duration of interphase, caution must be exercised in extrapolating from a population with slow turnover to a rapidly proliferating cell population (66). Modulation of chromosome aberration frequency is also expected if G_1 repair is inhibited so as to extend the lifetime of strand gaps (65). The latter may contribute to enhancement of chromosome aberrations in combined modality protocols.

2. S-Phase-Dependent Cytogenetic Processes

Those agents that interact directly, particularly covalently, with DNA are the most potent inducers of chromatid aberrations and SCEs. Although exact mechanisms have not been elucidated, several scenarios have been proposed for production of chromatid aberrations and SCEs.

The types of lesions produced via direct interaction of cytostatic agents with DNA are, with the exception of cross-links, single-stranded damage. Such lesions do not lead directly to DNA strand breakage but may be repaired (e.g., excision repair) or remain intact until the cell enters the subsequent S phase. Chromatid aberrations originate during S phase as a result of misreplication at or near the site of unrepaired damage (66-69). In addition, single-strand breaks generated indirectly, via incomplete excision repair just prior to S phase, may also initiate misreplication and the formation of chromatid aberrations (70). Irrespective of the cell cycle stage during which chemical damage is induced in DNA, chromatid-type aberrations predominate in the first mitosis following their formation (69).

Neither the exact relationship between chromosomal aberrations and SCEs nor the nature of DNA damage culminating in the two phenomena is known. Nevertheless, it is generally accepted that chromatid aberrations and SCEs arise by unique mechanisms and are produced by different lesions (69). SCE frequencies are not markedly increased, as are chromosomal aberrations, by agents such as radiation and bleomycin that produce extensive single- and double-strand damage. Rather, high frequencies of SCEs are produced by chemicals at dose levels that do not effectively produce chromosomal aberrations (22).

SCE is an S-phase-dependent process that occurs in response to unrepaired damage able to persist at least until the first of two replication cycles in the presence of BrdUrd (71) and is not evident until metaphase of the second replication cycle. Unlike chromatid-type aberrations, which are a manifestation of misreplication, SCEs are apparent in both sister chromatids and are evidence of successful replication. Although SCE is obviously representative of a replication bypass mechanism, controversy exists as to whether the SCE occurs at or adjacent to the actual lesion or, alternatively, at the junction site of replicon clusters (72,73).

Those agents capable of forming cross-links between the two strands of the DNA duplex are among the most potent SCE inducers. However, the exact role of cross-links per se in the production of SCE is controversial (74). The replication bypass model of Shafer (72) predicts that in order for a cell to survive replication past an interstrand cross-link, an SCE must occur and the cross-link be preserved. On the other hand, the Painter model (73) proposes that cross-links may be effective SCE inducers by virtue of their ability to block chain elongation and, presumably, permit more time for partial repair to occur and initiate the exchange event.

In constrast to alkylating agents, antimetabolites are at most weakly effective at producing SCEs and chromosomal aberrations in PBLs. Because they do not covalently or otherwise bind to DNA, but rather interefere with its synthesis, antimetabolites per se must be present during S phase if they are to produce an elevated SCE or aberration response. The presence of antimetabolites during S phase enhances the misincorporation of bases into DNA during synthesis (75). Misincorporation of bases may inhibit chain elongation and thereby evoke SCE production. Alternatively, frequent episodes of repair following misincorporation of bases may generate single-strand breaks or gaps and, consequently, chromatid aberrations. The fact that antimetabolites must be present in the cell at sufficiently high concentrations to direct misincorporation of bases during S phase severely limits the time interval between treatment and analysis during which cytogenetic effects are expected to be observed (27).

Regardless of the cytogenetic parameter being evaluated, assessment of chemically induced cytogenetic damage inherently presents more difficulties than that of radiation damage because:

1. Many chemicals are not direct-acting per se but require biotransformation to produce an electrophilic agent capable of reacting directly with DNA. Consequently, in vitro data are not always predictive of in vivo responses. In addition, considerable interindividual diversity exists in the enzymes involved in metabolic activation and detoxification processes.
2. Different alkylating agents vary dramatically in their preferred sites of reaction with DNA (76) and consequently in their persistence or rates of repair.

Expression of the S-phase-dependent processes of SCEs and chromatid aberrations as primary cytogenetic indicators of DNA damage is expected to reflect the heterogeneous nature of cytostatic agents and to decrease over time as a consequence of repair and cell population turnover. In addition, interindividual variations in these cytogenetic responses parallel genetic diversities inherent in pharmacokinetic processes involved in biotransformation and repair in exposed populations.

A large body of studies have developed meaningful relationships between doses and dose rates and the frequency of chromosome alterations. It is clear that induced chromosome aberrations, therefore, are of fundamental importance to our understanding of the effects of radiation and cytostatic agents on cells and are a major concern in individual protection and therapy.

D. Evidence for Long-Term Effects

In considering the evidence for long-term effects of radiation and chemicals in producing chromosome damage, two types of studies will be considered. One involves the findings of chromosome studies in exposed individuals and populations. The other focuses on distinctive cytogenetic features of patients who have developed exposure-related hematological neoplasms as presumed late effects of therapy.

1. Persistent Damage Following Irradiation

The evidence for the long-term persistence of radiation-exposure-related cytogenetic damage in humans stems from observations in several exposure situations. These include humans accidentally exposed to high levels of radiation from industrial sources, patients receiving external or internal exposure for medical reasons, and members of the Japanese populations exposed to atomic bomb radiation in World War II. Included as well are populations receiving chronic or intermittent low levels of occupational or environmental radiation exposure.

The development in 1960 of a practical method for studying chromosome aberrations in peripheral blood cells (1) made it possible to apply such examinations to patients who had suffered potential radiation overexposure. In addition to their use promptly after exposure to evaluate the reality and magnitude of biological effects as well as to draw inferences on the quantity and distribution of the radiation exposure, longer-term follow-up studies have been performed. Bender and Gooch (77) observed that overexposure induced the persistent presence of dose-related chromosome aberrations 2½ years after the Y-12 accident of 1958. Further follow-up studies performed after 7, 8, 10½ (78) and 16 (79) years continued to reveal the presence of dose-related levels of cytogenetic abnormalities. Similar follow-up results were found 19 years after a criticality accident in a reactor in Vinca, Yugoslavia (80).

It must be borne in mind that the physical dosimetry of persons exposed accidentally involves uncertainties related to the unplanned nature of the events. On the other hand, studies involving radiation therapy administered to patients have the benefit that the radiation exposure is planned in advance and carefully monitored. Unfortunately, the life expectancy of such patients, who are usually being treated for cancer, has been somewhat limited. Norman et al. (81,82) determined the rate of elimination of lymphocyte aberrations in women given radiation therapy for cervical carcinoma. Assuming the presence of radiation-induced acentric chromosome fragments to indicate the first mitosis following exposure, they found an upper limit of 29 months and a mean life span of about 18 ± 2 months for the cells containing an acentric fragment on first division.

In another study, the cytogenetic effects of radiation exposure for a nonneoplastic disease, ankylosing spondylitis, were studied by Court Brown and colleagues (83). They noted that cells with both stable and unstable radiation-induced aberrations persisted 8 years and possibly 20 years after exposure, the latter being the longest period then studied. Further studies of this population have shown persistence for longer than 30 years (84).

Cytogenetic changes have been sought and found in the circulating blood cells of Japanese atomic bomb survivors (85). The dose-response relationship of the aberrations was described in 1971 (86), confirming the work of Sasaki and Miyata (87). Kamada and co-workers noted that the aberrations were increased in both B lymphocytes (88) and T lymphocytes (89). They also noted a nonrandom distribution of break points with high incidences in some regions in which leukemic cells also show alterations. A review of the cytogenetic findings in both normal and leukemic A-bomb survivors and a discussion of the significance of the aberrations in relation to malignant transformation were provided by Kamada and Tonaka (90).

More recently, the preliminary results of a reevaluation of A-bomb radiation air doses (91,92) were utilized by Awa and colleagues to reanalyze the cytogenetic information (93). The major change in the new dosimetry results is that the relative magnitude of the neutron component in Hiroshima is much lower. The previously observed consistently higher frequency of aberrant cells in every dose range in Hiroshima compared to Nagasaki had been explained as the effect of the supposed greater neutron exposure in Hiroshima with its greater efficacy for chromosome damage. Awa's new analysis using the new dosimetry shows that the difference between the two cities, particularly in the dose range below 2 Gy, is virtually nonexistent (93).

Another study carried out by Awa (94) has revealed that thus far there is no statistically significant increase in the frequency of offspring with chromosomal abnormalities as a result of parental irradiation.

Inadvertent human exposures to atomic bomb fallout occurred in 1954 in the course of a nuclear weapons test at Bikini Atoll in the Marshall Islands. Cytogenetic studies 10 years later revealed chromosome aberrations in 23 of 43 exposed persons (95). In the course of the same event, members of a Japanese fishing boat crew were also exposed to the fallout. They have been studied cytogenetically from 13 to 28 years after the exposure (96). Despite a gradual decrease with the passage of time, the incidence of dicentric chromosomes and rings 27-28 years after exposure was still about three times as high as the frequency in an unexposed control population. Again the incidence of stable aberrations was more constant and significantly higher, about 45 times higher than the frequency in controls. It is of interest that no late effects of radiation exposure on health have been observed in this small group.

A rapid falloff in the frequency of unstable aberrations has recently been observed in 5 individuals involved in an unusual radiation overexposure resulting from the unwitting opening of a ^{60}Co teletherapy unit with resultant dispersion of the 6000 pellets of ^{60}Co in a community in Juarez, Mexico (97). Twenty-one months later, the unstable aberrations had fallen by 70% on the average in these individuals (98).

Littlefield has also reported on the cytogenetic findings over a 6-year period following the skin and internal contamination with ^{241}Am of a nuclear chemical plant worker as a result of a chemical explosion of an ion exchange column (99). Americium-241 is an alpha-radiation source, which accounts for the observed overdispersion of two-break chromosome lesions. Vigorous chelation therapy with DTPA reduced this individual's body burden over the period of several years during which it was administered. The frequency of radiation-damaged metaphase cells was observed to fall gradually for the first 3 years and then increase again. This unusual pattern may be associated with the continued presence of a residuum of the original contamination. The more usual long-term pattern in patients following receipt of internal radioisotopes, including ^{131}I and ^{32}P, for therapeutic purposes has been a continuous decline over a number of years (100).

From the standpoint of information relating to continuing or late radiation-induced cytogenetic changes, it must be recognized that the magnitude of exposure was relatively high and its duration relatively brief in the previously discussed observations, whereas in the ones now to be considered the magnitude of the exposure is relatively low and its duration relatively long on a continuous or frequent intermittent basis prior to and during the period of cytogenetic studies. Because the aberration frequency in such studies is much lower than in those previously discussed, they require large numbers of observations and are therefore difficult to perform. Considerations in the successful performance of such studies were reviewed by Conner and Wald (101), and the status and results of such cytogenetic screening were reviewed by Wald (102). Bloom edited a manual of consensus guidelines for the performance of population studies of this type, including the cytogenetic methodology (103). The results of such studies were recently reviewed by Evans (68).

The first such prospective study was initiated by Evans and his colleagues in a group of 197 dockyard workers in 1968. These men were studied annually over the succeeding 10 years during which they were exposed to neutron and gamma radiation while servicing nuclear submarines. The cumulative exposures acquired below the regulatory limit over the 10-year period ranged from 1 to 30 rem, and there was a significant increase in aberrations with increasing exposure in a linear relationship (15). The rate of production of dicentric aberrations, 1.4×10^{-4} dicentrics per cell per rem, was influenced by the worker's age and the time relationship between the most recent exposures and the blood sampling. The dicentric frequency per cell per rem increased from 1.53×10^{-4} at age 25 years to 2.6×10^{-4} at age 55. Also, the recent exposures had a greater influence on the aberration frequencies than the more remote exposures.

At about the same time Lloyd and co-workers (16) carried out a retrospective study of about 200 workers including 50 unexposed controls at the National Radiological Protection Board in England. The exposures here were to beta and gamma radiation, all within permissible exposure limits over a 4-12-year period with the cumulative doses ranging from 6 to 50 rem. The NRPB survey showed a very similar linear response of dicenteric frequency to dose with a mean of $2.22 \pm 0.94 \times 10^{-4}$ per cell per rem, which compares very well with that of Evens's "recent" dose effect of $2.32 \pm 0.91 \times 10^{-4}$ dicentrics/rem. The frequency was about threefold higher than that of the control group. Because of the very low dose required to double the frequency of aberrations in these studies, Lloyd inferred that the incidence of aberrations per unit dose was much higher than any observed incidence of radiation-induced cancer and therefore that the cytogenetic results would not be of direct prognostic value in assessing the cancer risk.

Another retrospective study of 57 German nuclear power plant employees was reported by Bauchinger et al. (17). There were variations in the radiation conditions and dose distributions in the various plants. Significantly higher aberration frequencies for rings and dicentrics and acentric chromosomes were found in the radiation workers than in an 11-person control group. However, the correlation between aberration frequency and dose was not present in this study. This may have resulted from the small number of subjects, particularly in the higher end of the dose range (15-25 cGy).

A similar study was carried out on 6 power plant workers and 6 controls (104). The exposed workers had higher than normal amounts of ^{210}Pb in their urine, from 69.9 to 535.4 mBq/liter, and chromosome aberrations in 6-10% of their metaphases as compared to the controls with an average of 38.5 mBq/liter and 1.5-4% of cells with aberrations that consisted of chromatid deletions only and no structural chromosome aberrations.

Another recent study involved 59 fossil fuel power plant workers, 89 nuclear power plant workers, and 23 controls (165). The frequency of cells with fragments and dicentrics was higher in the fossil fuel workers (0.66%) than in the nuclear plant workers (0.54%), with adjustments for an average 3-year half-life of lymphocytes and the length of exposure. The fossil fuel workers had 3 times the dicentric frequency (1.24%) of the nuclear plant workers (0.44%), and the acentrics were 2.53% and 1.02%, respectively. The control frequencies for dicentrics (0.11%) and acentric fragments (0.23%) were significantly less than for either of the two power plant worker groups.

Considering all of these studies, it does appear that cytogenetic analyses of worker populations receiving x- or gamma irradiation from external sources, even within the permissible exposure limits, do show a small but consistent increase in aberration frequencies over a working lifetime. The relationship of this finding to the risk of developing a radiation-induced cancer is not clear.

There have been few studies of chromosome aberration frequencies in workers occupationally exposed to internal radionuclide deposition since Boyd et al. first reported a cytogenetic investigation of luminous-dial painters in 1966 (105). The self-luminous paint incorporated radium sulfate and sometimes mesothorium. Measurement of the ingested material was made by radon breath measurements and whole body counting. Sixty-two women were studied who had ceased their luminizing work 17-19 years before the study of their chromosomes was carried out. They showed a frequency of cells with chromosome aberrations ranging from 3.6% in the group with radium body burdens up to 0.04 mCi to 6.76% in the group with from 0.10 to 0.56 mCi. The general population had a frequency of 2.81%. There was a gradient in keeping with increasing body activity for both the stable and unstable aberrations. The inhalation of radon from external sources has also been shown to result in an increased aberration frequency in uranium miners (106).

More recently the relatively small population of workers who have acquired plutonium body burdens has come under study. Brandom and Bloom (107) have reviewed the limited cytogenetic observations in plutonium workers. Early studies by Dolphin (108) were interpreted as showing only aberration frequencies that could be accounted for by the workers' external radiation exposure.

A group of 26 plutonium workers exposed during World War II on the Manhattan Project have been studied after 27 and 32 years. In the 27-year follow-up study (109), no increase in chromosome aberrations was found. In the 32-year results, there was no apparent correlation between aberration yields and plutonium body burdens (110). More recent studies by Schofield, Tawn, and Brandom involving ^{239}Pu and by Deloy involving ^{238}Pu were reviewed by Brandom and Bloom (107). They demonstrated an increase in the mean frequencies of chromosome aberrations compared with control frequencies. The effect of the alpha radiation associated with plutonium was to produce an overdispersion of aberrations in relation to a Poisson distribution in all of these groups. The discrepancies in various studies were probably related to the complexities of plutonium compounds from a physicochemical and biological standpoint. More recently, Tawn and coworkers (111) reported on the cytogenetics of 54 workers with estimates of more than 296-Bq plutonium body burdens. Even when external radiation exposure was considered, it appeared that significant deposits of plutonium did increase the frequency of chromosome aberrations. In banding studies the radiation-induced break points appeared to be randomly distributed among the chromosomes, on the basis of length.

In addition to the worker population studies described above, observations have been made on subsets of the general population who live in environments where natural radiation is elevated above the overall mean values. Pohl-Ruling and Fischer (112) reviewed this subject, giving particular attention to the "radon spa" Badgastein in Austria. The area is characterized by a subsoil containing relatively high amounts of radium and thorium that provides external irradiation and thermal springs that elevate the radon content of the air indoors and outdoors within the town. Estimates of the mean alpha blood dose were made, taking into account environmental factors as well as the specific location and occupation of the inhabitants. Subjects were separated into seven groups with increasing burdens, and the chromosome aberration frequencies were determined.

At low doses and dose rates the aberration frequencies increased up to about 3 mGy/year alpha and gamma blood dose. Additional fractionally delivered doses mainly from internal alpha irradiation caused the curve to level off into a plateau. Pohl-Ruling and Fischer also reviewed the results of similar investigations in Brazil, India, Finland, Japan, The People's Republic of China, Yugoslavia, France, and the state of Colorado, U.S.A. (112). All of these investigations showed an increase in chromosome aberrations at elevated natural radiation environmental levels. However, the highest value of aberration frequency, excluding occupationally exposed workers, was not above 1.9%.

Because of the major uncertainties in many of these studies involving small numbers, cytogenetic scoring differences, population peculiarities, and variations in dose assessment, the shape of the dose-response curve relating the exposures to aberration frequencies cannot be drawn except in the Badgastein study. The authors postulate that the plateau that follows the small increase at very low dose and dose rates could be due to the action of repair enzymes triggered at higher doses, which can control the radiation damage until the dose goes beyond a certain point, after which its effects are again dose-related. The plateau appears to go from about 3 mGy to 10 cGy in the Badgastein study, and there is a suggestion of a similar effect in vitro between 4 mGy and 5 cGy in a multilaboratory investigation (113).

To summarize this section, the persistence of radiation-induced chromosome changes is evident following significant acute exposures of individuals or populations to nuclear weapons, industrial radiation accidents, and medical radiation exposure. In the case of populations of workers within occupational exposure limits and members of the general population in areas of elevated natural radioactivity background, the increases in aberration frequency are much less dramatic but appear to be present. The results of these studies are confounded by many variables and generally preclude the exact determination of a dose-response relationship. Many authors have pointed out the value of combined prospective epidemiologic and cytogenetic studies in order to obtain more useful information in the low-dose, low-dose-rate area. In particular, the search for the relationship between the persistent radiation-induced aberrations and the risk of radiation-induced cancer might thereby be facilitated.

2. Evidence for Long-Term Cytostatic Damage

Cytogenetic observations of sister chromatid exchange and chromosome aberrations have been employed to monitor patients during therapy and at various times after cessation of therapy. The following studies, categorized according to specific cytostatic agents, demonstrate that short-term and long-term effects of cytostatic agents are dependent on (1) specific cytostatic agents, (2) duration of treatment, and (3) individual responses to the cytostatic agent.

Adriamycin–Alone and in Combination with Cisplatin. SCE levels in the peripheral blood lymphocytes (PBLs) of a patient given a single intravenous dose of adriamycin were elevated within 10 min after treatment, remaining at >2X baseline levels at 24 hr, but decreased to baseline levels 1 month after treatment (114). Following a higher acute dose (800 mg, IV), the SCE and chromosome aberration (mainly exchange figures) rates in the PBLs of a patient increased in parallel (25). Peak SCE elevations of 2X baseline were apparent with little change over a 3-month period, but baseline levels were observed at 5 months. By contrast, peak aberration rates of 4X baseline decreased rapidly over 1 month and returned to normal levels within 2 months after treatment.

SCE and chromosome aberration rates in PBLs were examined in patients 1 month following the previous course and 5 hr after a subsequent course of adriamycin/cisplatin together or in combination with cyclophosphamide (115). In the 1-month posttreatment samples, 1 of 3 patients on adriamycin/cisplatin alone and 2 of 2 patients on adriamycin/cisplatin/cyclophosphamide had increased SCE levels, whereas none of the patients had increased chromosomal aberration rates. At 5 hr posttreatment, all patients exhibited SCE increases but extremely variable aberration rates that ranged from no increase (1 patient, adriamycin/cisplatin) to highly increased (1 patient, adriamycin/cisplatin; 1 patient, adriamycin/cisplatin/cyclophosphamide).

Azathioprine (Imuran). PBLs of multiple sclerosis patients who were currently on azathioprine therapy (150 mg/day; 2 weeks to 6 months), who had previously received azathioprine (total dose 14-288 g; 3-60 months; 7 months to 4 years previously), or who did not receive any azathioprine were evaluated for chromosomal aberrations (116). The only significant effect was a slightly increased incidence of chromosomal gaps in the PBLs of those patients who were currently or previously on azathioprine relative to nontreated patients and controls. In a prospective study of patients on azathioprine, Kucerova et al. (49) observed a significant time-dependent increase in chromosome aberrations in the PBLs of 1 of 4 patients over a 38-month period. A small but significant increase in SCE frequencies was apparent in nearly all patients. However, the SCE levels were not dose-dependent or cumulative. Extreme interindividual variation in cytogenetic responses was noted.

Bleomycin. Cytogenetic evaluation of bone marrow cells of patients throughout the course of bleomycin therapy revealed the presence of hypochromatic and achromatic regions; chromosome and chromatid breaks, including acentric fragments; but no unstable aberrations such as dicentrics, rings, or multiradials (117). Aberrations persisted for at least a month in bone marrow cells of 2 of 4 patients. By contrast, the most frequently observed aberrations in the PBLs of patients during the course of bleomycin therapy were dicentrics (118). These apparently conflicting results reflect the proliferative differences of bone marrow and PBLs. Unstable aberrations such as dicentrics are rapidly lost in a proliferating population such as bone marrow. However, dicentrics are induced by double-strand breaks in G_0 lymphocytes and can persist indefinitely until the cells are cultured in vitro.

Busulfan. SCE and chromosomal aberrations were studied in the PBLs of a patient who received a total dose of 150 mg of busulfan over the course of 5 weeks (25). SCE levels increased significantly during treatment, peaked at 5 weeks after termination of treatment, and were at normal levels after 5 months. No significant effect was seen in the frequency of chromosomal aberrations.

Chlorambucil. In studies of 10 Bechcet and 23 juvenile chronic arthritis patients, Palmer et al. (31,32) reported elevated SCE levels in PBLs that were dependent on daily dose and duration of chlorambucil treatment. Elevated SCE levels persisted for as long as 5 months posttreatment. In the former study, the patient who received the highest dose (total 11.6 g over 68 months) exhibited the highest SCE level and subsequently developed S-ANLL. Chlorambucil has also been reported to produce chromosome aberrations in PBLs of patients during therapy (33,50). In the study by Reeves et al. (33), the rate of breakage induced by chlorambucil was found to decrease somewhat in some uveitis patients for several months following treatment, but more complex aberrations appeared later and persisted for as long as 82 months after treatment was discontinued. Aberrations were nonclonal and included numerical and such structural aberrations as deletions and translocations. Breakage at fragile sites in 4 patients was considered to be constitutive and not the result of chlorambucil treatment.

Chloroethyl Nitrosourea Derivatives. Bifunctional chloroethyl nitrosoureas are particularly effective in producing SCE and aberrations that may persist for relatively long periods of time after therapy. For example, acetyl chloroethyl nitrosourea (ACNU; 250 mg, acute IV dose) produced SCE elevations in PBLs of >5X baseline within 1 day posttreatment, and levels of >4X were still apparent 10-27 days after treatment (26). Likewise, cyclohexyl chloroethyl nitrosourea (CCNU) has been shown to produce SCE levels that remain elevated for at least 6-8 weeks and in some cases 4 months after treatment (45,119,120). Furthermore, repeated intervals of CCNU produced continuous increases in SCE levels both immediately before and after successive courses. Complex chromosomal aberrations were observed in PBLs of all 8 of 8 patients from 6 days to 8 months following treatment with bischloroethyl nitrosourea (BCNU). One patient exhibited cells with interchanges for as long as 26 months after therapy (41).

An excellent example of the utilization of PBL cytogenetics for monitoring patients during posttherapy is provided by studies by Gebhart et al. (121-123). In cytostatic interval therapy, MeCCNU (alternate intervals only) combined with 5-FU and vincristine was administered. Chromosome aberration and SCE rates were evaluated at various times during and after therapy. Individual breakage rates varied considerably (4- to more than 30-fold) but were distinctly increased immediately after and, for the most part, at 4 weeks after therapy. Peak breakage rates occurred after courses that included MeCCNU and accumulated with successive rounds of therapy. Elevated SCEs (3-4X baseline) were observed immediately after intervals and in the latter stages of therapy were even higher at 4 weeks posttherapy than immediately following the course of therapy. Interindividual variation in SCE responses was not as great as for aberration responses. Longer-term follow-up of cytogenetic responses was not carried out.

Cisplatin. SCE levels were evaluated in PBLs of patients at intervals of 1-14 days following treatment with cisplatin (43). A greater than twofold increase in SCE levels was seen as long as 14 days after an intravenous cisplatin dose of 120 mg X 2.

Cyclophosphamide–Alone and in Combination Therapy. Following treatment of patients with cyclophosphamide, increased frequencies of SCE and/or chromosome aberrations in PBLs have been reported in numerous studies (25, 26,37,50,124-127). Dose is a major determinant of the duration of elevated SCE responses, but considerable interindividual variation is also apparent. Single oral doses of 150 mg (25) to 3500 mg (26) have been reported to produce a transient (1-2 day) increase in SCE levels followed by a rapid decline to baseline levels. A single acute dose (1-1.4 g) of cyclophosphamide produced, within 4-20 hr, peak responses that decreased relatively rapidly within 7 days and subsequently declined more slowly to baseline levels over the next 4-6 weeks (28,127). Multiple courses of cyclophosphamide resulted in accumulation of SCE levels to a plateau followed by a similar biphasic decline, with significant elevations apparent in some cases as long as 4 months after treatment (25,28,127). Similar, although in some cases more retarded, patterns of SCE decrease were reported in combination chemotherapy involving cyclophosphamide together with at least one of the following agents: daunomycin, vincristine, bleomycin, methotrexate, prednisone, actinomycin D, 5-fluorouracil, procarbazine, 6-mercaptopurine (28,35,127). Following cyclophosphamide therapy, chromosome aberrations were reported to decrease more rapidly than SCE (25).

It is also of interest to note the occurrence of clonal chromosomal abnormalities in bone marrow samples of two of five autologous bone marrow transplant patients who were in complete remission and on no maintenance therapy for at least 2-20 months (128). In one patient, 2 of 40 cells exhibited a t(1q;21q), and in another 6 of 27 cells had simultaneous del(1p), dup(1p). Neither patient exhibited chromosome abnormalities prior to transplant. The observed abnormalities may have resulted from either in vitro treatment of marrow with the cyclophosphamide derivative Asta Z 7557 or, alternatively, total body irradiation.

L-PAM. Within 2 hr after treatment of a patient with 16 mg L-PAM (IV), a peak PBL SCE response occurred, and only a slight decrease was apparent at 24 hr (39). An accumulation of SCE levels has been observed prior to and after successive courses of L-PAM, and elevated levels persist for at least 4 weeks after treatment (26,28,120). Preliminary studies in our laboratory indicate the same general trend but with considerable interindividual variation (40).

In contrast to normalization of SCE observed at 4 months posttherapy, chromosomal aberrations characterized by exchanges and multiple complex rearrangements may persist for several years in PBLs of patients following L-PAM therapy (38,129). The time course of chromosome aberrations following L-PAM therapy has been described (38). Individual aberration frequencies were at their highest levels within 10 months, and at their lowest, but still generally elevated, at 11-30 months posttherapy. Some patients (approximately 5%) exhibited significantly increased chromosome aberrations for as long as 90 months, and still other cases appeared to be increasing after 80-90 months. One patient who exhibited 18-30% aberrations in three out of four samples over 41-60 months posttherapy was later found to have gastric cancer, but none of the 50 patients developed S-ANLL during the time of the study.

In the study reported by Einhorn et al. (129), increased multiple and complex chromosome abnormalities and DNA alkaline elution patterns that suggested persistence of DNA cross-links were seen in PBLs 3 years and more after L-PAM therapy. At the same time no evidence of bone marrow aberrations was apparent. Most aberrations were of the unstable type in PBLs and would be eliminated rapidly in the proliferative bone marrow population. In the course of this study, 5 of 6 and 1 of 6 patients subsequently developed preleukemia and leukemia, respectively.

Methotrexate. Studies of patients receiving methotrexate therapy have generally reported no significant effect on SCE (51,52,126,130) or chromosome aberration (33,34,131) frequencies in PBLs at various intervals during or immediately after therapy. However, relative to immediately after treatment, higher aberration frequencies were reported in PBLs 5-9 years after termination of treatment (34). This led to suggestions that previously sequestered lymphocytes may express damage or that progeny of damaged progenitor cells may become apparent long after treatment.

Procarbazine. The SCE responses of 2 patients on procarbazine (50 or 100 mg/day; orally) were cumulative with successive doses (26), but no indication was given concerning persistence of the SCE responses.

Combined Modality Therapy. Aronson et al. (132) reported cytogenetic responses in PBLs of 12 patients who had previously received various types of chemotherapy and were currently on various combined modality therapies. Studies were generally carried from 1 week through 1 month after the last treatment. Four basic patterns of SCE responses were observed. A control-like SCE frequency distribution exhibiting normal means and ranges of SCEs was observed in one patient 1 month after administration of several cytostatic agents that are known to be ineffective SCE inducers. SCE distributions similar to control but containing a significant number of cells with high SCE levels (high-frequency cells, HFCs) were observed in samples studied more than 2 weeks following weakly or moderately effective SCE inducers. Following protocols that included cyclophosphamide, flattened distributions with a shift to moderate or high SCE levels were observed. All of the cases in which non-control-like SCE distributions were seen also exhibited chromosome aberrations, including translocations, deletions, and marker chromosomes. However, no correlation was apparent between SCE and aberration levels.

Leukemic children who were in remission and on maintenance chemotherapy had normal levels of SCEs in their PBLs. However, children on intensive therapy had elevated acute and persistent SCE responses that correlated with the specific chemotherapy regimen. Elevated SCE levels persisted for 49 days in a patient who subsequently relapsed (36). A study of 11 children at cessation of chemotherapy revealed normal SCE levels and increased rates of structural chromosomal aberrations (133).

Elevated levels of such chromosomal aberrations as translocations, dicentrics, rings, inversions, and markers have been reported to persist in PBLs for several years following chemotherapy (34,131,134,135). In some cases aberration frequencies are higher 5-9 years after than at shorter intervals posttreatment (34).

Lambert et al. (38) have suggested that the high frequency of aberrations in PBLs at extended times after cessation of therapy may reflect damaged progenitor cells from which abnormal and possibly malignant cell clones may be generated. Support of this suggestion is provided in a report of a patient who had previously been treated with cyclophosphamide, methotrexate, and CCNU and subsequently developed S-ANLL (136). At that time the patient's bone marrow demonstrated a very complex hypodiploid karyotype, and PHA-stimulated PBLs showed 10% hypodiploidy and 7.5% incidence of cells with major and minor complex aberrations.

From the previously discussed studies, it appears that SCE levels reflect cumulative toxicity throughout the course of treatment and, for some particularly effective SCE-inducing agents, several months after treatment. Population mean SCE levels decrease relatively rapidly (within several months) as a result of DNA repair and peripheral lymphocyte repopulation. The presence of HFCs in SCE frequency distributions is evidence for somewhat longer persistence of elevated SCEs in a subpopulation of PBLs (132,137). In spite of their generally shorter life span relative to chromosome-type aberrations, SCEs provide a more sensitive means of monitoring genotoxic damage produced during alkylating agent chemotherapy and for several months after cessation of treatment. It remains to be determined whether enhanced risk estimates are associated with specific patterns of SCE responses. By contrast, chromosomal aberrations may persist in PBLs for several years after treatment as a direct result of cytostatic agent damage or in progeny of previously damaged progenitor cells. However, chromosomal aberrations are not as definitive in chemical exposure as in radiation exposure, due to the great diversity in chemical activity and mechanisms of genotoxicity of cytostatic agents as well as individual responses to those agents.

III. LONG-TERM CYTOGENETIC EFFECTS ASSOCIATED WITH CYTOSTATIC THERAPY-RELATED LEUKEMIA

A. Nonrandom Chromosomal Involvement in Bone Marrow Cells in S-ANLL

1. Major Chromosomal Involvement in S-ANLL

It is widely recognized that S-ANLL may occur as a consequence of chemical and/or radiation therapy of a primary malignancy or other disease. A preleukemic phase commonly precedes S-ANLL. Therapy-related S-ANLL is most commonly expressed as acute myeloblastic leukemia (AML), erythroleukemia (EL), acute myelomonocytic leukemia (AMMoL), and acute promyelocytic leukemia (APL) (138). Cytogenetic studies of bone marrow cells from patients having S-ANLL have revealed (1) a high frequency of aneuploidy, (2) nonrandom involvement of specific chromosomes, and (3) karyotype instability and complexity.

Rowley et al. (139) were the first to draw attention to the high frequency of occurrence of clones of cells exhibiting aneuploidy—in particular, hypodiploidy—in bone marrow samples from patients with S-ANLL. In a cumulative study of 47 previous and new cases of S-ANLL, Rowley (140) observed the presence of abnormal karyotypes in 44 of the 47 (93.6%). Of the 44 cases demonstrating chromosomal abnormalities, 39 (88.6%) were aneuploid. In the 39 patients with aneuploidy, there was a consistent loss of the entire chromosome or portions of the long arm (q−) of chromosomes number 5 and/or 7. Specific chromosomal involvement included −5 (14 cases), 5q− (6 cases), −7 (24 cases), 7q− (5 cases), and both −5/5q− and −7/7q− (12 cases). Losses of other chromosomes occurred in at most 4 patients. Rarely were chromosomal gains (+8 in 2 patients) seen. Losses involving both chromosomes 5 and 7 were observed only in patients whose primary malignancies were lymphomas (13 of 32), in contrast to other malignancies (0 in 15). The highest frequency of involvement of both chromosomes 5 and 7 was seen in patients who had previously been treated for their primary malignancy with radiation and chemotherapy (9 of 24, 38%) as compared to radiation (2 of 8, 25%) or chemotherapy alone (2 of 15, 13%). These findings suggested a possible association between (1) the type of primary disease and karyotype and (2) the type of treatment of the primary disease and karyotype.

Subsequent studies confirmed the frequent involvement of −5/5q− and −7/7q− in S-ANLL (138,166). In a review of 188 previously published cases, including 25 of Rowley's cases and 18 new cases, Sandberg et al. (138) also noted that involvement of portions or all of chromosome number 3 or 7 was relatively common. Among the 206 total cases examined, they noted the following chromosomal involvement: number 7 (60 cases, 29%), 5 (38 cases, 19%), 17 (34 cases, 17%), 3 (24 cases, 12%), 21 (21 cases, 10%), and 8 (19 cases, 9%). On the basis of these data, it was suggested that chromosomes numbers 3 and 17 be added to numbers 5 and 7 as chromosomes that are commonly associated with S-ANLL. Similar conclusions were reached regarding the frequent expression of hypodiploidy and involvement of chromosomes numbers 5, 7, and 17 in an exhaustive review of secondary leukemias of childhood and young adulthood (141).

In order to further evaluate the involvement of specific chromosomes in S-ANLL, several recent studies were examined (Table 2). Rather than present an exhaustive survey of all reported cases (including individual case reports and cases selected on the basis of similar cytogenetic findings or specific treatment protocols), the only studies (including Sandberg's 18 cases) included in Table 2 are those recent studies having a cross section of patients with ANLL secondary to a variety of malignancies and treatment protocols. In addition, all of the studies in Table 2 presented banded karyotype data. Abnormal karyotypes were reported in 88.3% of the 117 total cases. In those cases (102) exhibiting abnormal karyotypes, hypodiploidy (57 cases, 56%) was more commonly observed than were hyperdiploidy (23 cases, 22.5%) and pseudodiploidy (30 cases, 29%). In agreement with previous studies, the most common chromosomal involvements were −7/7q− (47 cases, 46%) and −5/5q− (34 cases, 33%). Involvement of both −7/7q− and −5/5q− was apparent in 13 cases (13%). The frequency of loss of chromosome number 17 (15 cases, 15%) and gain of chromosome number 8 (10

Table 2 Specific Chromosomal Involvement in Cases of S-ANLL

	Number of cases with one or more clones										
	Exhibiting abnormal karyotype and chromosome numbers of:			Exhibiting involvement of chromosomes							
Total number of cases	<46	46	>46	−5/5q−	−7/7g−	−5/5q− and −7/7g−	8(+/−)[a]	3(+/−)[a]	17(+/−)[a]	Number of cases with all normal karyotypes	Ref.
18	12	1	3	4	5	0	1/2	3/2	2/4	2	138
24	10	6	2	5	12	4	2/3	1/1	2/4	6	143
55[b]	29	16	9	19	26	8	2/2	5/2	4/4	6	144
20	6	7	9	6	4	1	5/0	3/2	4/3	1	145
117	57	30	23	34	47	13	10/7	12/7	12/15	15	
Percent[c]	48.7	25.6	19.7	29	40	11.1	8.5/6	10.2/6	10.2/12/8	12.8	
Percent[d]	55.9	29.4	22.5	33.3	46	12.7	9.8/6.8	11.8/6.8	11.8/11.7		

[a] +/−, gain or translocation of chromosome or chromosomal segments/loss of all or part of chromosome or chromosomal segments.
[b] Includes only those cases involving cytostatic therapy and not occupational exposures.
[c] Percentage of total cases.
[d] Percentage of abnormal cases having the specific chromosomal abnormality.

cases, 10%) were consistent with a 1982 review (138), whereas loss of chromosome 3 (7 cases, 7%) was a considerably less frequent observation. On the other hand, gains or alterations involving chromosomes 3 (12 cases, 12%) and 17 (12 cases, 12%) were not uncommon. It is of interest to note that all four studies listed in Table 2 reported considerable interindividual karyotypic variation and complexity.

Data from the studies in Table 2 were compiled according to nature of the primary disease and prior treatment modality (Table 3) in order to examine possible associations with specific chromosomal alterations. As previously concluded by the Groupe Francais de Cytogenetique Hematologique (144), involvement of chromosome number 7, alone or together with number 5, is more common in patients with primary lymphomas or hemopoietic neoplasias than in patients with solid tumors or other diseases. On the other hand, solid tumors or other diseases are associated with a higher frequency of alteration (gain/rearrangement as well as loss) of chromosome number 17. These differences may simply reflect the relative aggressiveness of the treatment modalities employed. With regard to treatment modalities, radiation alone is considerably less effective than chemotherapy alone or combined with radiation in producing hypodiploidy, specifically involving chromosome number 7. By constrast, chemotherapy alone is less effective than radiation with or without chemotherapy in effecting losses involving chromosome number 17. Of the 36 cases involving only chemotherapy, only 2 cases (138,143) involved losses of chromosome number 17. As previously suggested by Rowley, specific primary disease therapy appears to be the primary determinant of specific karyotypic changes in S-ANLL.

Considerable evidence exists that S-ANLL and its associated nonrandom karyotypic changes are, in fact, consequences of prior mutagenic/clastogenic exposure, rather than a normal progression of a primary malignancy. Sandberg and Vuopio (147) have reported comparative cytogenetic data in secondary leukemias associated with treated and untreated neoplasia. Of 56 cases of treatment-related S-ANLL, 75% demonstrated some karyotypically abnormal bone marrow clones. The most commonly involved chromosomes were those already discussed: numbers 7 (15 cases), 5 (15 cases), and 17 (10 cases). In addition, 5 cases involving chromosome number 1 were reported. In the admittedly smaller (14 cases) control group (ANLL patients having a previous but untreated primary malignancy), chromosomal involvement generally differed from that in the therapy-related S-ANLL group. The most common chromosomal involvement included numbers 6 (4 cases); 22 (3 cases); and 3, 5, 8, and 16 (2 cases each). Although the sample size in the nontreated group is too small to draw definitive conclusions, it appears that distinctly different chromosomes are involved in karyotypic changes in secondary leukemias associated with treated and nontreated primary malignancies.

Further evidence for a mutagenic etiology of S-ANLL is provided by studies of occupational exposure and de novo ANLL. The same karyotypic changes

Table 3 Distribution, According to Primary Disease and Prior Treatment Modality, of S-ANLL Patients Who Exhibit Abnormal Bone Marrow Karyotypes. (Data compiled from literature sources in Table 2)

		Number of cases with 1 or more clones exhibiting:				
			Involvement of chromosomes:			
	Abnormal karyotype	Hypodiploidy	−5/5q−	−7/7q−	−5/5q− and −7/7q−	17(+/−)[a]
Primary disease						
Lymphoma/hemopoietic malignancy	59	33 (56%)	18 (31%)	32 (54%)	9 (15%)	5/6 (8.5%/10%)
Solid tumors/other disease	43	24 (55%)	16 (37%)	15 (35%)	4 (9%)	7/9 (16%/23%)
Treatment						
R+C[b]	52	32 (62%)	19 (36%)	26 (50%)	8 (15%)	5/10 (10%/19%)
C	36	20 (56%)	11 (31%)	19 (53%)	5 (14%)	5/2 (7%/6%)
R	14	5 (36%)	4 (29%)	2 (14%)	0 (0%)	2/3 (14%/21%)

[a]+/−, gain or translocation of chromosome or chromosomal segment/loss of chromosome or chromosomal segment.
[b]R, radiation; C, chemotherapy.

described for therapy-related S-ANLL are also seen, but at a lower frequency, in de novo ANLL and primarily in a subset of de novo ANLL cases exhibiting other potentially mutagenic exposures. In a retrospective study of 56 patients with ANLL, Mitelman et al. (148) identified 23 cases with occupational exposure to solvents, insecticides, and petroleum products and 33 cases with no identifiable occupational exposure. In the exposed group, 83% of the cases exhibited clonal karyotype abnormalities. The most frequent chromosomal involvement included: −5/5q− (5 cases), −7/7q− (5 cases), +8 (6 cases), and +21 (4 cases). Single cases of −X, t(8;21), t(9;22), −17, and −Y were seen. By contrast, clonal karyotypic abnormalities were observed in only 24% of the 33 no-exposure cases of de novo ANLL. Only single cases of −7/7q− and +21 were observed in the nonexposed group. Rather, the nonexposed group showed a greater frequency of involvement of +9 (2 cases) as well as chromosomal rearrangements (1 case each): i(17q), t(15;21), t(8;16), t(16;16).

Subsequent studies (140,144,149) have generally confirmed the enhanced frequency of karyotype abnormalities and nonrandom involvement of chromosomes −5/5q−, −7/7q−, +8, and, less consistently, −17 in exposure-associated de novo ANLL relative to non-exposure-related de novo ANLL. The latter cases are generally associated with a lower incidence of karyotype abnormalities and a higher incidence of specific chromosomal translocations. The specific chromosomal translocations, t(8;21) and t(15;17), are also more closely associated with de novo ANLL in younger patients than in older patients (140). Occupational exposure and age-related effects led Rowley to suggest that prior mutagenic exposure should be suspected in cases of de novo ANLL that exhibit nonrandom chromosomal changes similar to those in therapy-related S-ANLL, i.e., increased frequency of involvement of −5/5q−, −7/7q−, +8, and −17 (140).

Involvement of −17 in therapy- or occupational exposure-related ANLL is of notable interest. The Group Francais de Cytogenetique Hematologique (144) identified −17 as occurring more frequently following occupational hazard exposure than following chemotherapy. In 8 cases of ANLL following occupational exposure and having karyotype abnormalities, 5 exhibited karyotypes in which a number 17 chromosome was missing. Occupational exposures included benzene (2 cases), irradiation (2 cases), and nonspecific solvents (1 case). The fact that −17 was not consistently cited in the other previously discussed occupational studies may reflect a greater diversity of occupational hazard exposures in those studies. Likewise, the relatively low association of chemotherapeutic agents alone with −17 (Table 3) may reflect the nature and mechanism of action of specific chemotherapeutic agents. The two cases of chemotherapy alone associated with −17 involved multiple chemotherapeutic agents that included cyclophosphamide (138) or cyclophosphamide and BCNU (143). More recently, Wilmoth et al. (142) identified 5 cases involving −17 in a population of 20 patients with S-ANLL treated with L-PAM and suggested that a specific association may exist between monosomy 17 and L-PAM therapy. Therapeutic and chemical agents, in general, exhibit tremendous variation in reactivity and mechanism of action. Whether or not specific structure-activity relationships exist regarding chromosome 17 monosomy remains to be elucidated.

2. Minor Chromosomal Involvement in S-ANLL

In their study of 20 S-ANLL cases previously treated with L-PAM, Wilmoth et al. (142) observed in addition to the frequent involvement of −5/5q− (10 cases), −7/7q− (6 cases), and −17 (4 cases, either (1) del(12)(p11) as a simple deletion (3 cases) or a dicentric (1 case), or (2) a translocation involving 19q13.

These alterations of chromosomes 12 and 19 were speculated to be related to L-PAM, since similar occurrences of 12p− (12 cases) and translocations of 19q13 (11 cases) were rare occurrences in more than 800 patients with leukemia or preleukemia. Table 4 summarizes additional cases from the recent studies, previously considered in Table 2, having similar involvement of chromosomes 12 and 19. Further studies are required to determine wihether nonrandom involvement of chromosomes numbers 12 or 19 is associated with in S-ANLL induced by specific cytostatic agents.

Also included in Table 4 are recent data concerning suggestions of an association of chromosome number 1 with S-ANLL. The initial suggestion of chromosome number 1 involvement in preleukemia and S-ANLL associated with cytostatic exposure was presented by Scheres et al. (146,150). The latter studies presented karyotypic data on preleukemic and S-ANLL patients who specifically expressed a t(1;7) (p11;p11) abnormality (total number of cases unknown). It is of interest to note that all of these studies were of simple karyotypes that, in addition to the t(1q;7p), *always* included a missing chromosome 7; that is, all cases were monosomic for 7q and trisomic for 1q. Additional cases potentially involving chromosome number 1 are presented in Table 4. In some cases insufficient data are available to implicate specific regions of chromosome number 1, but the coincident involvement of −7/7q− and chromosome number 1 should not be overlooked. It is also important to recognize that the translocation chromosome t(1;7) replaces the missing chromosome number 7, which is of comparable size and is easily overlooked, particularly if banding is not done (146). Perhaps the importance of minor chromosomal abnormalities in S-ANLL will be clarified via further studies incorporating more refined methods of detecting chromosome aberration.

B. More Refined Methods for Cytogenetic Analysis of Bone Marrow

As recently pointed out by Rowley (151), the different frequencies reported for specific chromosomal abnormalities may be due to technical problems rather than to real differences in frequencies. Short-term (24-hr) bone marrow culture

Table 4 Minor Chromosomal Alterations Having Potential Nonrandom Association with S-ANLL

Chromosome number	Total number of cases	Karyotypic abnormality[a]	Number of cases with karyotypic abnormality	Ref.
12	20	del(12) (p11)	3	142
	(L-PAM-treated)	dic(12;20) (12qter-12 p11)	1	
	24	-12	2	143
		del(12) (p11)	1	
	55	-12	3	144
		12p-	1	
		t(13;12) (?;?)	1	
	20	-12	1	145
		t(7;12) (p15;p13)	1	
		t(11;12) (q21;p13)	1	
19	20	t(17;19) (p13;q13)	1	142
	(L-PAM-treated)	t(19;?) (q13;?)	2	
		t(17;19) (q11;q13)	1	
	18	-19	1	138
	55	-19	4	144
		t(11,19) (?;?)		
1	_[b]	-7/7q-, t(1;7) (p11;p11)	22	146
	24	-7, t(1q;7p)	2	143
	55	-7, t(1;3) (?;?)	1	144
		t(1;5) (?;?)	1	
		-7, t(1;6) (?;?)	1	
		-7, mar 1	2	
		mar 1	1	
	20	-7, +1		

[a]Specific chromosomal abnormality was generally present in a complex karyotype [with the exception of the t(1;7) study in preleukemia by Sheres et al. (146)].
[b]Unspecified number of preleukemic and leukemic patients.

rather than direct preparation may enhance the expression of karyotype abnormalities. Normal cells may divide preferentially in bone marrow, whereas in culture an admixture of cells, including leukemic cells, may be present. Dramatic evidence for the effect of cell culture is provided by studies of the t(15;17) associated with APL. Only rare instances of t(15;17) and APL as an S-ANLL have been reported (138,140). More frequently APL is associated with de novo ANLL. In summarizing the findings of the second and fourth workshops on chromosomes in leukemia, Rowley (151) related that t(15;17) was reported in only 41% of 80 cases of APL at the former workshop and in 70% of 61 cases at the latter. Bone marrow culture was considered to be an important factor in the improved detection of t(15;17).

In direct bone marrow preparations, chromosomes tend to be contracted, making it difficult to resolve of banding patterns. Recently developed synchronized cell culture and thymidine release techniques improve the mitotic yield and produce more elongated chromosomes and high-resolution banding patterns (152). Greatly improved detection of abnormal clones and precise delineation of break points are achieved with these methods.

Testa et al. (153) have detected karyotype abnormalities in 86% of 23 cases of ANLL (two cases of S-ANLL) in short-term synchronized cultures. With extended use of these techniques, perhaps most, but not necessarily all, cases of ANLL, including S-ANLL, will be found to have chromosomal abnormalities. Of course, it is possible, and in fact very likely, that some abnormalities may be of too small a magnitude to be observed cytologically even with these improved methods of detection.

Further refinements in methodology include the use of flow cytogenetic analysis wherein large numbers of specific chromosomes can be made available for DNA probe localization of small genomic regions (154,155).

C. Cytogenetic Evolution and Progression of Leukemia

S-ANLL is frequently preceded by a preleukemic phase with later progression to frank leukemia. Clonal karyotype abnormalities frequently appear during the preleukemic phase and subsequently evolve in parallel with the progression of the disease. An excellent example of karyotype evolution has been presented by Tomonaga et al. (156). One patient initially exhibited the clonal karyotype 45, XY, −7. Within 2 years the patient developed progressive neoplasia and subsequently AMMoL. The clonal karyotype evolved to 45, XY, −7, t(1q−;Bq+), Bq−, 12p− in parallel with disease progression. Similar karyotype evolution is apparent in the studies presented here, in spite of the fact that individual patients were studied at various stages in disease progression. In the study by Scheres et al. (146) of t(1;7) in preleukemia, abnormal clonal karyotypes were generally simple and characterized by −7, t(1;7). In addition, some clones exhibited more than 1 extra chromosome. Multiple clones were present in some cases but only one complex karyotype was reported. This is in contrast to the high incidence of complex and unstable clones reported in patients with S-ANLL (138; Table 2). The various cases were most likely at different stages of the disease wherein clonal evolution was occurring without a stable karyotype characterizing a major population of cells. Presumably, in time a dominant stable clone may be established.

Bone marrow aplasia induced by cytostatic agents may allow an initially only slightly altered clone to begin expansion. A variety of mechanisms may be responsible for additional progressive mutational events (157). The original clone may have acquired a DNA-repair defect or defective mitotic apparatus causing further mutational events to occur more frequently than normal. These progressive alterations may be accompanied by selection of more deviant cytogenetic subpopulations. Obviously, host genotype is a predominant factor in the initiation and evolution of genetic and/or cytogenetic abnormalities.

D. Chromosomal Mechanisms of Oncogenesis

Mechanisms of oncogenesis at the chromosomal level may be related to alteration in number (aneuploidy) or morphology (breakage events). Considerable excitement has been generated by the realizations that (1) a limited number of chromosomal sites are involved in the chromosomal rearrangements consistently associated with a variety of cancers (158) and (2) chromosomal break points frequently associated with cancer coincidentally reside in the same band regions as certain cellular oncogenes (151). Gene activation via chromosomal rearrangement is illustrated by the now classic case of activation of the c-myc oncogene on chromosome 8q24 associated with t(8;14)(q24;q32) in Burkitt's lymphoma (159). Similar rearrangements may be pertinent to activation of oncogenes in certain leukemias (151). With respect to S-ANLL, Scheres et al. (146) have suggested that t(1;7) may have minor association (particularly in the early stages) with S-ANLL and, perhaps, with activation of N-ras-1. In general, chromosomal breakage disrupts the genomic continuity and may thereby activate previously latent genes by interfering with controlling (suppressing) regions (160). Such mechanisms might be relevant to gene activation in S-ANLL associated with 5q− or 7q−. Alternatively, hemizygous expression of recessive genes may be a more relevant mechanism in those cases exhibiting monosomy for entire chromosomes or portions of chromosomes numbers 5 and 7. Mechanisms relating to trisomic situations (e.g., +8) are more difficult to envision other than simply via a gene dosage effect. In this respect, it has been noted that cellular oncogenes on chromosome 8 (c-mos and c-myc) have not, to date, been shown to be activated in ANLL (161).

Recently, increased attention has been directed to the possible association of heritable fragile sites and susceptibility to neoplasia. Fragile sites are sites of chromosomal gaps or breaks that are expressed at metaphase following cell culturing in specific media. A significant association exists between fragile sites and cancer break points (162-164). Rowley (140) has identified 2 cases of chemical carcinogen-related cancer break points associated with constitutional fragile sites: (1) 3p14, in heavy smokers exhibiting small-cell cancer of the lung, and (2) 7q31, in patients with ANL who had a history of prior exposure to radiation, alkylating agents, or pesticides.

E. Future Directions

It is highly desirable to be able to predict, prior to occupational, environmental, or therapeutic exposure (or early in the therapy of primary diseases), those individuals who may exhibit unusual cytogenetic sensitivity to specific cytostatic agents and be at increased risk for development of S-ANLL. Newly diagnosed cancer patients prior to treatment, occupational cohorts, and populations accidentally exposed to clastogenic agents are valuable resources for providing the data required to answer pertinent questions regarding individual susceptibility. A question of primary importance is whether or not specific cytogenetic effects, as observed in PBLs, have any relevance at all to the cytogenetic abnormalities ultimately observed in neoplastic cells, i.e., bone marrow cells in S-ANLL.

Certainly, studies such as those described in the present chapter should be extended in order to discern potential associations between specific cytogenetic parameters. Ideally, chromosome aberration, sister chromatid exchange, and fragile site baselines should be determined prior to occupational or therapeutic exposure; at various times during chronic exposures; and at the time of diagnosis, if a malignancy were to develop. In the case of a developing malignancy, cytogenetic analysis of neoplastic tissue is also essential. Several questions might then be addressed:

1. Following repeated exposure to cytostatic agents, do those individuals who express higher baseline frequencies of specific cytogenetic parameters exhibit enhanced susceptibility to neoplasia?
2. Do specific fragile sites coincide with chromosomal break points observed in neoplastic cells and/or with break points induced by the cytostatic agent in chromosomes in PBLs?
3. Is fragile site expression enhanced following repeated exposure?
4. Are persistent elevations of specific cytogenetic parameters associated with increased risk of neoplasia?

Additional studies are warranted to determine whether or not individual susceptibility may be predicted prior to exposure based on the in vitro response of their PBLs to specific agents. Such cytogenetic studies promise to be of continued value in elucidating potential long-term effects of radiation and cytostatic agents on bone marrow.

REFERENCES

1. Moorehead, P. S., Nowell, P. C., Mellman, W. J., Battips, D. M., Hungerford, D. A. Chromosome preparations of leukocytes cultured from human peripheral blood. *Exp. Cell Res. 20,* 613-616 (1960).
2. Natarajan, A. T., Obe, G. Screening of human populations for mutations induced by environmental pollutants: use of human lymphocyte system. *Ecotoxicol. Environ. Safety 4,* 468-481 (1980).
3. Latt, S. A. Sister chromatid exchanges and indices of human chromosome damage and repair: detection by fluorescence and induction by mitomycin C. *Proc. Natl. Acad. Sci. USA 71,* 3162-3166 (1974).
4. Perry, P., Wolff, S. New Giemsa method for the differential staining of sister chromatids. *Nature 251,* 156-158 (1974).
5. Finnon, P., Lloyd, D. C., Edwards, A. A. An assessment of the metaphase finding capability of the Cytoscan 110. *Mutat. Res. 164,* 101-108 (1986).
6. Otto, F. I., Oldiges, H. Flow cytogenetic studies in chromosomes and whole cells for the detection of clastogenic effects. *Cytometry 1,* 13-17 (1980).
7. Green, D. K., Fantes, J. A., Spowart, G. Radiation dosimetry using the methods of flow cytogenetics. In: *Biological dosimetry.* Eisert, W. G., Mendelsohn, M. L. (Eds.). Springer-Verlag, New York, pp. 67-76 (1984).
8. Heddle, J. A. A rapid in vivo test for chromosomal damage. *Mutat. Res. 18,* 187-190 (1973).
9. Muller, H. J. Artificial transmutation of the gene. *Science 66,* 84-87 (1927).
10. Sax, K. Chromosomal aberrations induced by x-rays. *Genetics 23,* 494-516 (1939).
11. Lea, D. E. *Actions of radiations on living cells.* Cambridge University Press, London (1946).
12. Buckton K. E., Langlands, A. O., Smith, P. G., Woodcock, G. E., Looby, P. C. Further studies on chromosome aberration production after whole-body irradiation in man. *Int. J. Rad. Biol. 19,* 369-378 (1971).
13. Lloyd, D. C. An overview of radiation dosimetry by conventional cytogenetic methods. In: *Biological dosimetry.* Eisert, W. G., Mendelsohn, M. L. (Eds.). Springer-Verlag, New York, pp. 3-14 (1984).
14. Lloyd, D. C., Edwards, A. A., Prosser, J. S., Moquet, J. E., Finnon, P. Doses in radiation accidents investigated by chromosome aberration analysis. XVI: A review of cases investigated, 1985. U.K. National Radiological Protection Board Report, R-192 (1986).
15. Evans, H. J., Buckton, K. E., Hamilton, G. E., Carothers, A. Radiation-induced chromosome aberrations in nuclear-dockyard workers. *Nature 277,* 531-534 (1979).
16. Lloyd, D. C., Purrot, R. J., Reeder, E. J. The incidence of unstable chromosome aberrations in peripheral blood lymphocytes from unirradiated and occupationally exposed people. *Mutat. Res. 72,* 523-532 (1980).
17. Bauchinger, M., Kolin-Gerresheim, J., Schmid, E., Dresp, J. Chromosome analyses of nuclear-power plant workers. *Int. J. Radiat. Biol. 38,* 577-581 (1980).

18. High Background Radiation Research Group, China. Health survey in high background radiation areas in China. *Science 209,* 877-880 (1980).
19. Fliedner, T. M., Andrews, G. A., Cronkite, E. P., Bond, V. P. Early and late cytological effects of whole body irradiation on human marrow. *Blood 23,* 471-487 (1964).
20. Countryman, P. I., Heddle, J. A. The production of micronuclei from chromosome aberrations in irradiated cultures of human lymphocytes. *Mutat. Res. 41,* 321-332 (1976).
21. Krepinsky, A. B., Heddle, J. A. Micronuclei as a rapid and inexpensive measure of radiation-induced chromosomal aberrations. In: *Radiation-induced chromosome damage in man.* Isihara, T., Sasaki, M. S. (Eds.). Alan R. Liss, New York, pp. 93-109 (1983).
22. Perry, P., Evans, H. J. Cytological detection of mutagen-carcinogen exposure by sister chromatid exchange. *Nature 258,* 121-125 (1975).
23. Morgan, W. F., Crossen, P. E. X-irradiation and sister chromatid exchange in cultured human lymphocytes. *Environ. Mutat. 2,* 149-155 (1980).
24. Gundy, S., Vara, L., Bender, M. A. Sister chromatid exchange frequency in human lymphocytes exposed to ionizing radiation in vivo and in vitro. *Radiat. Res. 100,* 47-54 (1984).
25. Musilova, J., Michalova, K., Urban, J. Sister-chromatid exchanges and chromosomal breakage in patients with cytostatic agents. *Mutat. Res. 67,* 289-294 (1979).
26. Abe, T., Tsuda, S., Maekawa, T., Taniwaki, M., Sonoda, Y., Ide, T., Misawa, S., Takino, T., Inoue, K. Sister chromosome exchange induced by cancer chemotherapeutic agents in vitro and in vivo: consideration of the hazard of drugs as possible mutagens and carcinogens causing secondary malignancies. *Cancer Treat. Rep. 69,* 505-514 (1985).
27. Gebhart, E. Chromosomal aberrations in lymphocytes of patients under chemotherapy. In: *Mutations in man.* Obe, G. (Ed.). Springer-Verlag, Berlin, Heidelberg, pp. 198-222 (1984).
28. Raposa, T. SCE induction by cytostatics and its relation to iatrogenic leukemogenesis. In: *Sister chromatid exchanges—25 years of experimental research.* Tice, R. R., Hollaender, A. (Eds.). Basic Life Sciences, Vol. 29B, Plenum, New York, pp. 859-884 (1984).
29. McDonald, M. A., Fitzgerald, P. H. Sister chromatid exchange and cell cycle progression in cultured lymphocytes from patients with chronic lymphatic leukemia. *J. Natl. Cancer Inst. 62,* 1169-1171 (1979).
30. Mourelatos, D., Dozi-Vassiliades, J., Tsigalidou-Balla, V., Granitsas, A. Enhancement by methylxanthines of sister-chromatid exchange frequency induced by cytostatics in normal and leukemic lymphocytes. *Mutat. Res. 121,* 147-152 (1983).
31. Palmer, R. G., Dore, C. J., Denman, A. M. Chlorambucil-induced chromosome damage to human lymphocytes is dose-dependent and cumulative. *Lancet 1* (8371), 246-249 (Feb. 4, 1984).
32. Palmer, R. G., Varonos, S., Dore, C. J., Denman, A. M., Ansell, B. M. Chlorambucil induced chromosome damage in juvenile chronic arthritis. *Arch. Dis. Child. 60,* 1008-1013 (1985).

33. Reeves, B. R., Casey, G., Harris, H., Dinning, W. T. Long-term cytogenetic follow-up study of patients with uveitis treated with chlorambucil. *Carcinogenetics 6,* 1615-1619 (1985).
34. Reeves, B. R., Lawler, S. D., Casey, G., Harris, H. Long-term effects of chemotherapy on lymphocyte chromosomes from patients treated for gestational trophoblastic tumours. *Brit. J. Cancer 52,* 719-724 (1985).
35. Ohtsuru, M., Ishii, Y., Takai, S.-I., Kosaki, G. Sister chromatid exchanges in lymphocytes of a patient treated with cyclophosphamide and vincristine for non-Hodgkin's lymphoma. *Gann 73,* 433-438 (1982).
36. Szollar, J., Fekete, G., Schuler, D. Sister chromatid exchange in childhood malignancies. *Teratogen., Carcinogen., Mutagen. 3,* 527-533 (1983).
37. Bochkov, N. P., Filippova, T. V., Kuzin, S. M., Stukalov, S. V. Cytogenetic effects of cyclophosphamide on human lymphocytes in vivo and in vitro. *Mutat. Res. 159,* 103-107 (1986).
38. Lambert, B., Holmberg, K., Einhorn, N. Persistence of chromosome rearrangements in peripheral lymphocytes from patients treated with melphalan for ovarian carcinoma. *Hum. Genet. 67,* 94-98 (1984).
39. Wulf, H. C., Husum, B., Plesner, A. M., Niebuhr, E. Distribution of SCEs in lymphocytes in persons with normal, slightly increased, and heavily increased SCEs. *Mutat. Res. 125,* 263-268 (1984).
40. Turner, J. H., Conner, M. K., Rockette, H. Studies of SCE induction in human PBLs by L-PAM. *Environ. Mutagen. 8, Suppl. 6,* 87A (1986).
41. Harrod, E. K., Cortner, J. A. Prolonged survival of lymphocytes with chromosomal defects in children treated with 1,3-bis(2-chlorethyl)-1-nitrosourea. *J. Natl. Cancer Inst. 40,* 269-279 (1968).
42. International Agency for Research on Cancer. IARC monographs on the evaluation of the carcinogenic risk of chemicals to humans. *Some antineoplastic and immunosuppressive agents,* Vol. 26. IARC, Lyon (1981).
43. Tominaga, K., Shinkai, T., Saijo, N., Eguchi, K., Shimizu, E., Sasaki, Y., Fujita, J., Nakajima, T. Sister chromatid exchanges induced in human lymphocytes by *cis*-diamminedichloroplatinum(II). *Jap. J. Clin. Oncol. 14,* 659-666 (1984).
44. Sorsa, M., Hemminki, K., Vainio, H. Occupational exposure to anticancer drugs–potential and real hazards. *Mutat. Res. 154,* 135-149 (1985).
45. Lambert, B., Ringborg, U., Harper, E., Lindblad, A. Sister chromatid exchanges in lymphocyte cultures of patients receiving chemotherapy for malignant disorders. *Cancer Treat. Rep. 62,* 1413-1419 (1978).
46. Littlefield, L. G., Colyer, S. P., DuFrain, R. J. Comparison of sister-chromatid exchanges in human lymphocytes after G_0 exposure to mitomycin in vivo vs. in vitro. *Mutat. Res. 69,* 191-197 (1980).
47. Ohtsuru, M., Ishii, Y., Takai, S.-I., Higashi, H., Kosaki, G. Sister chromatid exchanges in lymphocytes of cancer patients receiving mitomycin C treatment. *Cancer Res. 40,* 477-480 (1980).
48. Xu, Z.-D., Yajima, A., Abe, Y., Soh, K., Ozawa, N., Takabayashi, T., Sato, S., Mehara, S., Suzuki, M. Effects of radiotherapy and radiochemistry on sister chromatid exchanges in peripheral lymphocytes of the patients with gynecologic cancer. *Tohoku J. Exp. Med. 141,* 175-181 (1983).

49. Kucerova, M., Kocandrle, V., Matousek, V., Polivkova, Z., Reneltova, I. Chromosomal aberrations and sister-chromatid exchanges (SCEs) in patients undergoing long-term Imuran therapy. *Mutat. Res. 94,* 501-509 (1982).
50. Schuler, D., Dobos, M., Fekete, G., Miltenyi, M., Kolmar, L. Chromosome mutations and chromosome stability in children treated with different regimes of immunosuppressive drugs. *Hum. Hered. 29,* 100-105 (1979).
51. Lindskov, R., Wulf, H. C., Wantzin, G. L., Niebuhr, E. Sister chromatid exchange in patients treated with methotrexate for psoriasis. *J. Invest. Dermatol. 82,* 458-459 (1984).
52. Otter, M., Palmer, C. G., Baehner, R. L. Sister chromatid exchanges in lymphocytes from patient with acute lymphoblastic leukemia. *Hum. Genet. 52,* 185-192 (1979).
53. Grunwald, H. W., Rosner, F. Acute leukemia and immunosuppressive drug use. A review of patients undergoing immunosuppressive therapy for non-neoplastic diseases. *Arch. Intern. Med. 139,* 461-466 (1979).
54. Rieche, K. Carcinogenicity of antineoplastic agents in man. *Cancer Treat. Rep. 11,* 39-67 (1984).
55. International Agency for Research on Cancer, *IARC monographs on the carcinogenic risk of chemicals to humans,* Suppl. 4. IARC, Lyon (1982).
56. van Imhoff, G. W., Sleijfer, D. Th., Breuning, M. H., Anders, G. J. P. A., Mulder, N. H., Halie, M. R. Acute nonlymphocytic leukemia 5 years after treatment with cisplatin, vinblastine, and bleomycin for disseminated testicular cancer. *Cancer 57,* 984-987 (1986).
57. Zwelling, L. A., Kohn, K. W. Mechanisms of action of *cis*-dichlorodiammineplatinum(II). *Cancer Treat. Rep. 63,* 1439-1444 (1979).
58. Friedberg, E. C. *DNA repair.* W.H. Freeman, New York (1985).
59. Collins, A. R. S., Johnson, R. T. *The inhibition of DNA repair* (*Adv. Rad. Biol.,* Vol. 11). Academic Press, New York, pp. 72-129 (1984).
60. Preston, R. J. Radiation damage to DNA and its repair in the formation of chromosome aberrations. In: *Radiation-induced chromosome damage in man.* Ishihara, T., Sasaki, M. S. (Eds.). Alan R. Liss, New York, pp. 111-125 (1983).
61. Natarajan, A. T., Obe, G. Influence of DNA repair on radiation-induced chromosomal aberrations in human peripheral lymphocytes. In: *Radiation-induced chromosome damage in man.* Ishihara, T., Sasaki, M. S. (Eds.). Alan R. Liss, New York, pp. 127-140 (1983).
62. Virsik-Peuckert, R. P., Harder, D. Kinetics of the effect of ara C on chromosome aberration yield in irradiated human lymphocytes. *Int. J. Radiat. Biol. 49,* 103-108 (1986).
63. Natarajan, A. T., Darroudi, F., Mullenders, L. H. F., Meijers, M. The nature and repair of DNA lesions that lead to chromosome aberrations induced by ionizing radiations. *Mutat. Res. 160,* 231-236 (1986).
64. Holmberg, M., Gumauskas, E. The role of short-lived DNA lesions in the production of chromosome-exchange aberrations. *Mutat. Res. 160,* 221-229 (1986).

65. Preston, R. J. The use of inhibitors of DNA repair in the study of the mechanisms of induction of chromosome aberrations. *Cytogenet. Cell Genet. 33,* 20-26 (1982).
66. Evans, H. J. What has been achieved with cytogenetic monitoring? *Prog. Clin. Biol. Res. 207,* 3-24 (1986).
67. Evans, H. J. Effects on chromosomes of carcinogenic rays and chemicals. In: *Chromosome mutation and neoplasia.* German, J. (Ed.). Alan R. Liss, New York, pp. 253-279 (1983).
68. Evans, H. J. Cytogenetic and allied studies in populations exposed to radiations and chemical agents. In: *Assessment of risk from low-level exposure to radiation and chemicals.* Woodhead, A. D., Shellabarger, C. J., Pond, V., Hollaender, A. (Eds.). Plenum, New York, pp. 429-447 (1985).
69. Wolff, S. Chromosome aberrations, sister chromatid exchanges, and the lesions that produce them. In: *Sister chromatid exchange.* Wolff, S. (Ed.). John Wiley, New York, pp. 41-58 (1982).
70. Speit, G., Hochsattel, R., Vogel, W. The contribution of DNA single-strand breaks to the formation of chromosome aberrations and SCEs. In: *Sister chromatid exchange–25 years of experimental research.* Tice, R. R., Hollaender, A. (Eds.). Basic Life Sciences, Vol. 29A, Plenum, New York, pp. 229-244 (1984).
71. Wolff, S., Bodycote, J., Painter, R. B. Sister chromatid exchanges induced in Chinese hamster cells by UV irradiation at different stages of the cell cycle; the necessity of cells to pass through S. *Mutat. Res. 25,* 73-81 (1974).
72. Shafer, D. A. Replication bypass model for sister chromatid exchanges and implications for Bloom's syndrome and Fanconi's anemia. *Hum. Genet. 39,* 177-190 (1977).
73. Painter, R. B. A replication model for sister-chromatid exchange. *Mutat. Res. 70,* 337-341 (1980).
74. Carrano, A. V., Thompson, L. H., Stetka, D. G., Minkler, J. R., Mazrimas, J. A., Fong, S. DNA cross-linking, sister chromatid exchange and specific locus mutations. *Mutat. Res. 63,* 175-188 (1979).
75. Haynes, R. H. Molecular mechanisms in genetic stability and change: the role of deoxyribonucleotide pool balance. In: *Genetic consequences of nucleotide pool imbalance.* de Serres, F. J., Hollaender, A. (Eds.). Basic Life Sciences, Vol. 31, Plenum, New York, pp. 1-24 (1985).
76. Singer, B., Grunberger, D. *Molecular biology of mutagens and carcinogens.* Plenum, New York (1983).
77. Bender, M. A., Gooch, P. C. Persistent chromosome aberrations in irradiated human subjects. *Radiat. Res. 16,* 44-53 (1962).
78. Goh, K. Total-body irradiation and human chromosomes. IV. Cytogenetics follow-up studies eight and ten and one-half years after total-body irradiation. *Radiat. Res. 62,* 364-373 (1975).
79. Littlefield, L. G., Joiner, E. E. Cytogenetics follow-up studies in six radiation accident victims 16 years post-exposure. In: *Late biological effects of ionizing radiation,* Vol. I. International Atomic Energy Agency, Vienna, pp. 297-308 (1978).

80. Pendic, B., Barjaktarovic, N., Kostic, V. Chromosomal aberrations in persons accidentally irradiated in Vinca 19 years ago. *Radiat. Res. 81,* 478-482 (1980).
81. Norman, A., Sasaki, M. S., Ottoman, R. E., Fringerhut, A. G. Lymphocyte lifetime in women. *Science 147,* 745 (1965).
82. Norman, A., Sasaki, M. S., Ottoman, R. E., Fingerhut, A. G. Elimination of chromosome aberrations from human lymphocytes. *Blood 27,* 706-714 (1966).
83. Court Brown, W. M., Buckton, K. E., McLean, A. S. Quantitative studies of chromosome aberrations in man following acute and chronic exposure to x-rays and gamma rays. *Lancet i,* 1239-1241 (1965).
84. Buckton, K. E. Chromosome aberrations in patients treated with x-irradiation for ankylosing spondylitis. In: *Radiation-induced chromosome damage in man.* Ishihara, T., Sasaki, M. S. (Eds.). Alan R. Liss, New York, pp. 491-511 (1983).
85. Ishihara, T., Kumatori, T. Chromosome aberrations in human leukocytes irradiated in vivo and in vitro. *Acta Haematol. Jap. 28,* 291-307 (1965).
86. Awa, A. A., Neriishi, S., Honda, T., Yoshida, M. C., Sofuni, T., Matsui, T. Chromosome aberration frequency in cultured blood cells in relation to radiation dose of A-bomb survivors. *Lancet ii,* 903-905 (1971).
87. Sasaki, M. S., Miyata, H. Biological dosimetry in atomic bomb survivors. *Nature 220,* 1189-1193 (1968).
88. Kamada, N., Kudamot, A., Katsuki, T., Hinuma, Y. Chromosome aberrations in B-lymphocytes of atomic bomb survivors. *Blood 53,* 1140-1147 (1979).
89. Tonaka, K., Kamada, N., Ohkita, T., Kudamoto, A. Chromosome breakpoints in T-lymphocytes from atomic bomb survivors. *Hiroshima Med. J. 35,* 1214-1221 (1982).
90. Kamada, N., Tonaka, K. Cytogenetic studies of hematological disorders in atomic bomb survivors. In: *Radiation-induced chromosome damage in man.* Ishihara, T., Sasaki, M. S. (Eds.). Alan R. Liss, New York, pp. 455-474 (1983).
91. Loewe, W. E., Mendelsohn, E. Revised dose estimates at Hiroshima and Nagasaki. *Health Phys. 41,* 663-666 (1981).
92. Kerr, G. D. Review of dosimetry of the atomic bomb survivors. In: *Fourth symposium on neutron dosimetry.* Gurger, G., Ebert, H. G. (Eds.). EUR7448 EN, Vol. I, pp. 501-514 (1981).
93. Awa, A. A., Sokuni, T., Honda, T., Hamilton, H. B., Fujita, S. Preliminary reanalysis of radiation-induced chromosome aberrations in relation to past and newly revised dose estimates for Hiroshima and Nagasaki A-bomb survivors. In: *Biological dosimetry.* Eisert, W. G., Mendelsohn, M. L. (Eds.). Springer-Verlag, Berlin, pp. 77-82 (1984).
94. Awa, A. A. Chromosome damage in atomic bomb survivors and their offspring—Hiroshima and Nagasaki. In: *Radiation-induced chromosome damage in man.* Ishihara, T., Sasaki, M. S. (Eds.). Alan R. Liss, New York, pp. 433-453 (1983).

95. Lisco, H., Conard, R. A. Chromosome studies on Marshall Islanders exposed to fallout radiation. *Science 157,* 445-447 (1967).
96. Ishihara, T., Kumatori, T. Cytogenetic follow-up studies in Japanese fishermen exposed to fallout radiation. In: *Radiation-induced chromosome damage in man.* Ishihara, T., Sasaki, M. S. (Eds.). Alan R. Liss, New York, pp. 475-490 (1983).
97. Marshall, E. Juarez: an unprecedented radiation accident. *Science 223,* 1152-1154 (1984).
98. Littlefield, G. Personal communication (1986).
99. Littlefield, G., Joiner, E., DuFrain, R. J., Colyer, S., Breitenstein, B. Six-year cytogenetic follow-up study of an individual heavily contaminated with americium-241. Paper E3-05. In: *Dosimetry, radionuclides and technology* (Proceedings 7th Int. Congress Radiation Res.). Broerse, J. J., Barendsen, G. W., Kal, H. B., Van Der Kogel, A. J. (Eds.). Martinus Nijhoff, Amsterdam (1983).
100. Wald, N., Sherer, C. R. Chromosomal alterations after therapeutic use of radionuclides. In: *Therapy in nuclear medicine.* Spencer, R. P. (Ed.). Grune and Stratton, Philadelphia, pp. 45-52 (1978).
101. Conner, M. K., Wald, N. Chromosomal methods and population studies. *Environ. Health Perspec. 42,* 107-113 (1981).
102. Wald, N. The status of cytogenetic screening. In: *New and sensitive indicators of health impacts of environmental agents* (Proceedings 3rd Annual Symp. Environmental Epidemiology, 1982). Underhill, D. W., Radford, E. P. (Eds.). University of Pittsburgh Graduate School of Public Health, Center for Environmental Epidemiology, Pittsburgh, PA, pp. 187-199 (1986).
103. Bloom, A. D. (Ed.). *Guidelines for studies of human population exposed to mutagenic and reproductive hazards.* March of Dimes Birth Defects Foundation, New York (1981).
104. Bauman, A., Horvat, D. The impact of natural radioactivity from a coal-fired power plant. *Sci. Total Environ. 17,* 75-81 (1981).
105. Boyd, J. T., Court Brown, W. M., Vennart, J., Woodcock, G. E. Chromosome studies on women formerly employed as luminous-dial painters. *Brit. Med. J. 1,* 337-382 (1966).
106. Brandom, W. F., Saccaman, A. G., Archer, V. E., Archer, P. G., Bloom, A. D. Chromosome aberrations as a biological dose-response indicator of radiation exposure in uranium miners. *Radiat. Res. 76,* 159-171 (1978).
107. Brandom, W. F., Bloom, A. D. Chromosome aberrations in workers with internal deposits of plutonium. In: *Radiation-induced chromosome damage in man.* Ishihara, T., Sasaki, M. S. (Eds.). Alan R. Liss, New York, pp. 513-526 (1983).
108. Dolphin, G. W. The biological problems in the radiological protection of workers exposed to ^{239}Pu. *Health Phys. 20,* 549-557 (1971).
109. Hempelmann, L. H., Langham, W. H., Richmond, C. R., Voelz, G. L. Manhattan project plutonium workers: a 27-year follow-up study of selected cases. *Health Phys. 25,* 461-479 (1973).

110. Voelz, G. L., Hempelmann, L. H., Lawrence, J. N. P., Moss, W. D. A 32-year follow-up of the Manhattan Project plutonium workers. *Health Phys. 37,* 445-485 (1979).
111. Tawn, E. J., Hall, J. W., Schofield, G. B. Chromosome studies in plutonium workers. *Int. J. Radiat. Biol. 47,* 599-610 (1985).
112. Pohl-Ruling, J., Fischer, P. Chromosome aberrations in inhabitants of areas with elevated natural radioactivity. In: *Radiation-induced chromosome damage in man.* Ishihara, T., Sasaki, M. S. (Eds.). Alan R. Liss, New York, pp. 527-560 (1983).
113. Pohl-Ruling, J., and others. Effect of low-dose acute x-irradiation on the frequencies of chromosomal aberrations in human peripheral lymphocytes in vitro. *Mutat. Res. 110,* 71-82 (1983).
114. Nevstad, N. P. Sister chromatid exchanges and chromosomal aberrations induced in human lymphocytes by the cytostatic drug adriamycin in vivo and in vitro. *Mutat. Res. 57,* 253-258 (1978).
115. Wiencke, J. K., Chervenka, J., Kennedy, B. J., Prlina, J., Gorlin, R., Sister-chromatid exchange induction by cisplatin/adriamycin cancer chemotherapy. *Mutat. Res. 104,* 131-136 (1982).
116. Apelt, F., Kolin-Gerresheim, J., Bauchinger, A. Azathioprine, a clastogen in human somatic cells? Analysis of chromosome damage and SCE in lymphocytes after exposure in vivo and in vitro. *Mutat. Res. 88,* 61-72 (1981).
117. Bornstein, R. S., Hungerford, D. A., Haller, G., Engstrom, P. F., Yabro, J. W. Cytogenetic effects of bleomycin therapy in man. *Cancer Res. 31,* 2004-2007 (1971).
118. Dresp, J., Schmid, E., Bauchinger, M. The cytogenetic effect of bleomycin on human peripheral lymphocytes in vitro and in vivo. *Mutat. Res. 56,* 341-353 (1978).
119. Lambert, B., Ringborg, U., Lindblad, A. Prolonged increase of sister-chromatid exchanges in lymphocytes of melanoma patients after CCNU treatment. *Mutat. Res. 59,* 295-300 (1979).
120. Lambert, B., Ringborg, U., Lindblad, A., Sten, M. The effects of DTIC, melphalan, actinomycin-D, and CCNU on the frequency of sister chromatid exchanges in peripheral lymphocytes of melanoma patients. In: *Adjuvant therapy of cancer,* Vol. 2. Jones, S. E., Salmon, S. E. (Eds.). Grune and Stratton, New York, pp. 55-62 (1979).
121. Gebhart, E., Losing, J., Wopfner, F. Chromosome studies on lymphocytes of patients under cytostatic therapy. I. Conventional chromosome studies in cytostatic interval therapy. *Hum. Genet. 55,* 53-63 (1980).
122. Gebhart, E., Windolph, B., Wopfner, F. Chromosome studies on lymphocytes of patients under cytostatic therapy. II. Studies using the BUDR-labeling technique in cytostatic interval therapy. *Hum. Genet. 56,* 157-167 (1980).
123. Gebhart, E., Losing, J., Mueller, R. L., Windolph, B. Interindividual variation of cytogenetic damage by cytostatic therapy. In: *Mutagens in our environment.* Sorsa, M., Vainio, H. (Eds.). Alan R. Liss, New York, pp. 89-98 (1982).

124. Dobos, M., Shuler, D., Gekete, G. Y. Cyclophosphamide-induced chromosomal aberrations in nontumorous patients. *Humangenetik 22,* 221-227 (1974).
125. Kurvink, K., Bloomfield, C. D., Kennan, K. M., Levitt, S., Cervenka, J. Sister chromatid exchange in lymphocytes from patients with malignant lymphoma. *Hum. Genet. 44,* 137-144 (1978).
126. Duker, D. Investigation into sister chromatid exchange in patients under cytostatic therapy. *Hum. Genet. 58,* 198-203 (1981).
127. Clare, M. G., Taylor, J. H., Blain, E., Jones, W. G. The quantitation of sister chromatid exchanges in lymphocytes of cancer patients at intervals after cytotoxic chemotherapy. *Eur. J. Cancer Clin. Oncol. 19,* 1509-1515 (1983).
128. Van den Akker, J., Gorin, N. C., Laporte, J. P., Donay, L., Lopez, M., Taillemite, J. L., Najman, A., Duhamel, G. Chromosome abnormalities after autologous bone marrow transplantation with marrow treated by cyclophosphamide derivatives. *Lancet 1,* 1211-1212 (1985).
129. Einhorn, N., Eklund, G., Franzen, S., Lambert, B., Lindsten, J., Soderhall, S. Late side effects of chemotherapy in ovarian carcinoma. A cytogenetic, hematologic, and statistical study. *Cancer 49,* 2234-2241 (1982).
130. Inoue, S., Brown, L., Ravindranath, Y., Ottenbreit, M. J. Normal sister chromatid exchange frequency in long-term survivors with acute leukemia. *Cancer Res. 42,* 2906-2908 (1982).
131. Lawler, S. D., Walden, P. A. M. Chromosome studies in patients treated with chemotherapy for trophoblastic tumours. In: *Mutagen-induced chromosome damage in man.* Evans, H. J., Lloyd, D. C. (Eds.). Edinburgh Univ. Press, pp. 239-246 (1978).
132. Aronson, M. M., Miller, R. C., Hill, R. B., Nichols, W. W., Meadows, A. T. Acute and long-term cytogenetic effects of treatment in childhood cancer. Sister-chromatid exchanges and chromosome aberrations. *Mutat. Res. 92,* 291-307 (1982).
133. Haglund, U., Hayden, S., Zech, L. Sister chromatid exchanges and chromosome aberrations in children after treatment for malignant lymphoma. *Cancer Res. 40,* 4786-4790 (1980).
134. Miller, R. C., Hill, R. B., Nichols, W. W., Meadows, A. T. Acute and long-term cytogenetic effects of childhood cancer chemotherapy and radiotherapy. *Cancer Res. 38,* 3241-3246 (1978).
135. Robison, L. L., Arthur, D. C., Ball, D. W., Danze, T. J., Wesbit, M. E. Cytogenetic studies of long-term survivors of childhood acute lymphocytic leukemia. *Cancer Res. 42,* 4289-4292 (1982).
136. Bradley, E. C., Schechter, G. P., Matthews, M. J., Whang-Peng, J., Cohen, M. H., Bunn, P. A., Ihde, D. C., Minna, J. D. Erythroleukemia and other hematologic complications of intensive therapy in long-term survivors of small cell lung cancer. *Cancer 49,* 221-223 (1982).
137. Carrano, A. V., Moore, D. H. The rationale and methodology for quantifying sister chromatid exchange in humans. In: *Mutagenicity: new horizons in genetic toxicology.* Heddle, J. A. (Ed.). Academic Press, New York, pp. 268-305 (1982).

138. Sandberg, A. A., Abe, S., Kowalcyzk, J. R., Zedgenidze, A., Takeuchi, J., Kakati, S. Chromosomes and causation of human cancer and leukemia. V. Cytogenetics of leukemias complicating other diseases. *Cancer Genet. Cytogenet.* *7,* 95-136 (1982).
139. Rowley, J. D., Golomb, H. M., Vardiman, J. Nonrandom chromosomal abnormalities in acute nonlymphocytic leukemia in patients treated for Hodgkin's disease and other non-Hodgkin's lymphomas. *Blood 50,* 759-770 (1977).
140. Rowley, J. D. Chromosome changes in leukemia cells as indicators of mutagenic exposure. In: *Chromosomes and cancer, from molecules to man.* Rowley, J. D., Ultmann, J. E. (Eds.). Bristol Myers Cancer Symposium, Vol. 5. Academic Press, New York, pp. 139-159 (1983).
141. Bernstein, M. L., Vekemans, M. J. J. Chromosomal changes in secondary leukemias of childhood and young adults. *CRC Crit. Rev. Oncol./Hematol.* *5*(4), 325-360 (1986).
142. Wilmoth, D., Feder, M., Finan, J., Nowell, P. Preleukemia and leukemia with 12 p− and 19 q+ chromosome alterations following alkeran therapy. *Cancer Genet. Cytogenet. 15,* 95-98 (1985).
143. Pederson-Bjergaard, J., Preben, P., Pederson, N. T., Hou-Jensen, K., Svejgaard, A., Jensen, G., Nessen, N. I. Acute nonlymphocytic leukemia, preleukemia, and acute myeloproliferative syndrome secondary to treatment of other malignant diseases. II. Bone marrow cytology, cytogenetic results of HLA typing, response to anti-leukemic chemotherapy, and survival in a total series of 55 patients. *Cancer 54,* 452-462 (1984).
144. Group Francais de Cytogenetique Hematologique. Chromosome analysis of 63 cases of secondary nonlymphoid blood disorders: a comparative study. *Cancer Genet. Cytogenet. 12,* 95-104 (1984).
145. Arthur, D. C., Bloomfield, C. D. Banded chromosome analysis in patients with treatment-associated acute nonlymphocytic leukemia. *Cancer Genet. Cytogenet. 12,* 189-199 (1984).
146. Scheres, J. M. J. C., Hustinx, T. W. J., Geraedts, J. P. M., Leeksma, C. H. W., Meltzer, P. S. Translocation 1:7 in hematologic disorders: a brief review of 22 cases. *Cancer Genet. Cytogenet. 18,* 207-213 (1985).
147. Sandberg, A. A., Vuopio, P. Fourth international workshop on chromosomes in leukemias 1982: Secondary leukemias associated with neoplasia, treated and untreated. *Cancer Genet. Cytogenet. 11,* 319-321 (1984).
148. Mitelman, F., Brandt, L., Nilsson, P. G. Relation among occupational exposure to potential mutagenic/carcinogenic agents, clinical findings, and bone marrow chromosomes in acute nonlymphocytic leukemia. *Blood 52,* 1229-1237 (1978).
149. Golomb, H. M., Alimena, G., Rowley, J. D., Vardiman, J. W., Testa, J. R., Sovik, C. Correlation of occupation and karyotype in adults with acute nonlymphocyte leukemia. *Blood 60,* 404-411 (1982).
150. Scheres, J. M. J. C., Hustinx, T. W. J., Holdrinet, R. S. G., Geraldts, J. P. M., Hagemeijer, A., Van der Blij-Philipsen, M. Translocation 1:7 in dyshematopoiesis: possibly induced with a nonrandom geographic distribution. *Cancer Genet. Cytogenet. 12,* 283-294 (1984).

151. Rowley, J. D. Biological implications of consistent chromosome rearrangements in leukemia and lymphoma. *Cancer Res. 44,* 3159-3158 (1984).
152. Yunis, J. J. Comparative analysis of high-resolution chromosome techniques for leukemia bone marrows. *Cancer Genet. Cytogenet. 7,* 43-50 (1982).
153. Testa, J. R., Oguma, N., Misawa, S., Wiernik, P. H. Chromosome abnormalities in acute leukemia: a higher incidence than previously assumed (letter to the editor). *Cancer Genet. Cytogenet. 8,* 305-306 (1983).
154. Carrano, A. V., Gray, J. W., Langlois, R. G., Yu, L. C. Flow cytogenetics: methodology and applications. In: *Chromosomes and cancer, from molecules to man.* Rowley, J. D., Ultmann, J. E. (Eds.). Academic Press, New York, pp. 195-210 (1983).
155. Young, B. D., Jeanpierre, M., Goyns, M. H., Stewart, G. D., Elliot, T., Krumlauf, K. Construction and characterization of chromosomal DNA libraries. In: *Chromosomes and cancer, from molecules to man.* Rowley, J. D., Ultmann, J. E. (Eds.). Academic Press, New York, pp. 211-224 (1983).
156. Tomonaga, M., Tomonaga, Y., Kusano, M., Ichimaru, M. Sequential karyotypic evolutions and bone marrow asplasia preceding acute myelomonocytic transformation from myelodysplastic syndrome. *Brit. J. Haematol. 58,* 53-60 (1984).
157. Nowell, P. C. Cytogenetic clues in some confusing disorders. *Amer. J. Pathol. 89,* 459-476 (1977).
158. Mitelman, F. Restricted number of chromosomal regions implicated in aetiology of human cancer and leukemia. *Nature 310,* 325-327 (1984).
159. Erikson, J., Ar-Rushid, A., Drwinga, H. L., Nowell, P. C., Croce, C. M. Transcriptional activation of translocated c-myc oncogene in Burkitt's lymphoma. *Proc. Natl. Acad. Sci. USA 80,* 820-824 (1983).
160. Sandberg, A. A. A chromosomal basis of oncogenesis. *Cancer Genet. Cytogenet. 8,* 277-285 (1983).
161. Chaganti, R. S. K., Jhanwar, S. C. Chromosomal mechanisms of cancer etiology. In: *Genetics in clinical oncology.* Chaganti, R. S. K., German, J. (Eds.). Oxford Univ. Press, New York, pp. 60-79 (1985).
162. Hecht, F., Sutherland, G. R. Fragile sites and cancer break points. *Cancer Genet. Cytogenet. 12,* 179-181 (1984).
163. LeBeau, M. M., Rowley, J. R. Heritable fragile sites in cancer. *Nature 308,* 607-608 (1984).
164. Yunis, J. J., Soreng, A. L. Constitutive fragile sites and cancer. *Science 226,* 1199-1203 (1984).
165. Leonard, A., Deknudt, G. R., Leonard, E. D., Decat, G. Chromosome aberrations in employees from fossil-fueled and nuclear-power plants. *Mutat. Res. 138,* 205-212 (1984).
166. Kapadia, S. B., Krause, J. R., Ellis, L. D., Pan, S. F., Wald, N. Induced acute non-lymphocytic leukemia following long-term chemotherapy. *Cancer 45,* 1315-1321 (1980).

8

Mutational Effects of Radiotherapy and Chemotherapy

ALEXANDER A. MORLEY
Flinders University and Medical Centre, Adelaide, South Australia, Australia

I. INTRODUCTION

Many of the important late effects of cytotoxic drugs and radiation such as carcinogenesis, leukemogenesis, proliferative stem cell failure, teratogenesis, and inherited defects are likely to be due to direct genetic damage. Development of indices of genetic damage is important in order to understand its mechanism, determine its magnitude, and predict the later development of biological effects. Conventionally, the study of genetic damage has been by way of study of visible chromosome abnormalities, but this end point is relatively insensitive since the frequency of genetic changes is likely to be several orders of magnitude greater than the frequency of visual chromosome abnormalities, and gross visual chromosome changes represent only one of many different types of damage to DNA.

Recently, methods have been developed for study of mutations in human somatic cells in vivo. The method that is best characterized studies mutations at the hypoxanthine phosphoribosyl transferase (HPRT) locus in lymphocytes. It is based on two technical advances: the ability to select the rare HPRT$^-$ mutants by elimination of wild-type cells (1) and the ability to clone lymphocytes at high efficiency (2) so that the mutant lymphocytes can be detected by clonal expansion. The HPRT locus is on the X chromosome, and since there is only one locus active in both male and female cells a single mutation will cause a phenotypic change. HPRT is a purine salvage enzyme and catalyzes formation of purine nucleotides both from the natural bases hypoxanthine and guanine and from analogs such as thioguanine (TG). When wild-type cells are grown in the presence of TG they incorporate it into DNA and are killed, whereas mutant HPRT$^-$ cells are unable to incorporate it and hence survive. Since mutant cells also have an intact pathway for de novo synthesis of purines, they are still able to proliferate if appropriately stimulated, for example by culturing at limiting dilution in microplates in the presence of phytohemagglutinin, irradiated feeder lymphocytes, and interleukin-2. The efficiency of this system is such that nearly all peripheral blood lymphocytes will proliferate and form clones and, when selected by adding TG, the rare mutant $HPRT^-$ lymphocytes can be detected by clone formation and studied further (3,4).

This technique enables the study of both spontaneous and induced mutations in vivo in both man and mouse. In healthy young adults the frequency of mutant $HPRT^-$ lymphocytes in human peripheral blood is approximately 10^{-6}-10^{-5}, and it increases with age (5); the frequency of $HPRT^-$ mutant lymphocytes in the spleen in mice is approximately 2-4 $\times 10^{-6}$ (6,7). The process of mutagenesis can also be studied in vitro by exposing lymphocytes to a physical or chemical mutagen, allowing 7-10 days for expression of the mutation as a phenotypic change, and then selecting with TG to enable detection of mutants. Detailed studies of mutant cells can be performed by expanding the selected clones and, for example, studying the HPRT gene, mRNA for HPRT, and the HPRT enzyme itself.

Another genetic locus that is being used for the study of mutagenesis is the locus for the erythrocyte membrane protein glycophorin, the terminal portion of which carries the epitopes for the M and N blood groups. Erythrocytes from individuals heterozygous for MN are studied, and cells that have lost one allele and may be mutants are enumerated using flow cytometry to detect cells that are $M^+ N^-$ or $N^- M^+$ (8). This system has the advantage that a larger number of cells can be studied, so rare events are more readily detectable, but it has the real disadvantage that further study of the presumptively mutant cells is not possible and, in particular, it is not possible to confirm by gene analysis that they are truly mutant cells. If $M^+ N^-$ or $N^- M^+$ cells are in fact mutants, then they represent mutations that occurred early in hemopoietic maturation, probably even in the stem cell.

II. EXPERIMENTAL STUDIES

A. Radiation

Mutagenesis in vitro produced by x-radiation has been studied (9), and an example of the effect of 100-kV x-rays on human lymphocytes in vitro is shown in Figure 1. The lymphocytes were irradiated immediately after isolation, i.e., in G_0, and were then cultured for 10 days to allow for expression. The effect of ^{60}Co gamma irradiation of lymphocytes in vivo in mice is shown in Figure 2. Mice were irradiated at a high dose rate (15 Gy/hr) and at a low dose rate (2.5 cGy/hr), and the spleens were assayed 30-40 days after irradiation. The dose-

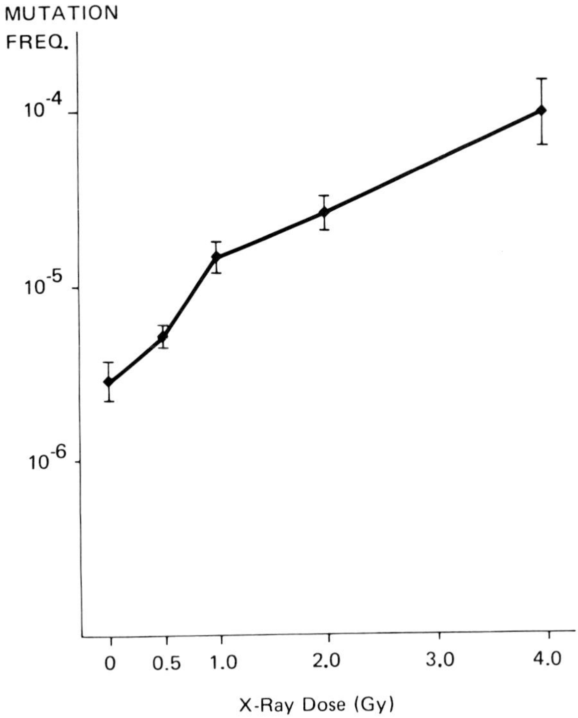

Figure 1 The relationship between dose of x-radiation in vitro and frequency of mutant human lymphocytes. (From Ref. 9.)

response curve for the high dose rate gamma radiation is very similar to the dose-response curve for in vitro irradiation of human lymphocytes, and this suggests that both in vitro data on human lymphocytes and in vivo data on murine lymphocytes are likely to mimic closely the situation for human lymphocytes in vivo.

The dose-response curve for low dose rate irradiation shows that fewer mutations are produced for a given total dose, and a similar observation has been made after irradiation when other end points such as inherited mutations or tumor production have been used. The most likely explanation for this reduced effect of low dose rate radiation is the existence of some type of DNA repair pathway that either minimizes or removes the initial radiochemical lesions produced by radiation or repairs these lesions in an error-free fashion so that the original information content of the DNA is restored.

Several inducible DNA repair lesions are already recognized (reviewed in Ref. 10). The inducible "SOS" repair system can repair damage produced by UV radiation in bacteria, but its activity results in increased mutagenesis and its existence

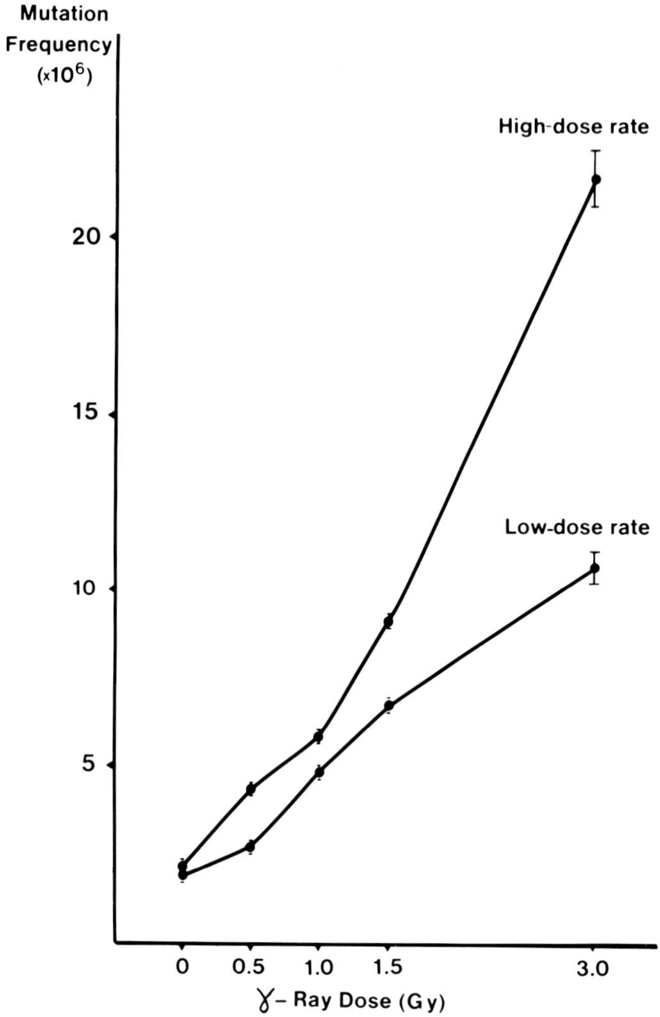

Figure 2 The frequency (mean +1 SE, 13 mice/point) of in vivo mutant splenic lymphocytes in mice irradiated with various doses of x-radiation either at a high dose rate (15 Gy/hr) or a low dose rate (2.5 cGy/hr).

in eukaryotes is unproven. The "adaptive system" in eukaryotes is induced following alkylation of DNA, and it repairs damage to DNA by transferring methyl and ethyl groups to a protein containing glutathione. There is some recent evidence that a third system, which repairs or removes premutational lesions following ionizing radiation, can be detected in human lymphocytes. Mitogenic stimulation of human lymphocytes with phytohemagglutinin results in a marked decrease

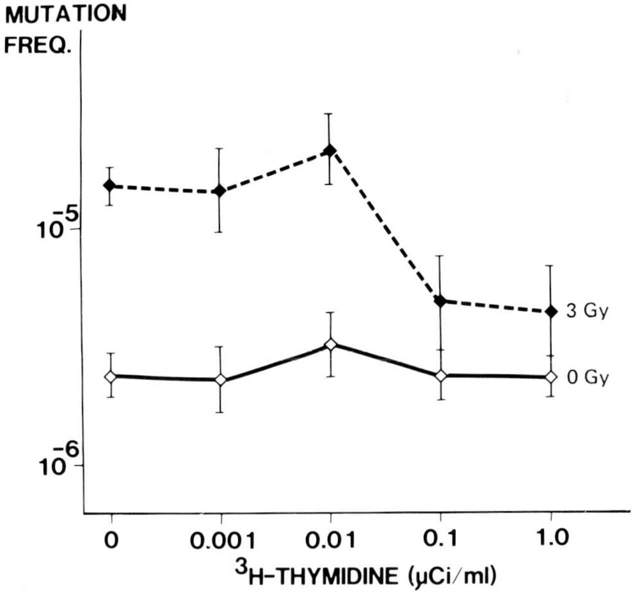

Figure 3 Effect on lymphocytes of exposure to [^{3}H] thymidine for 6 hr at 37°C prior to x-radiation with 3 Gy. (From Ref. 12.)

in the number of mutations produced by a subsequent dose of x-radiation (11). Mitogenic activation is associated with transcription of many new proteins, and it seems likely that certain repair enzymes are among the proteins transcribed. Ionizing radiation itself may induce a similar type of error-free repair system (12). Figure 3 shows data from an experiment in which lymphocytes in G_0 were incubated for 6 hr with various doses of [^{3}H] thymidine and the number of mutations produced by x-radiation was then measured. It can be seen that at high levels of [^{3}H] thymidine the number of induced mutations is much decreased.

These various factors that affect the yield of mutations are of potential importance, since much human exposure, including some types of radiotherapy, occurs at low dose rates and thus is potentially able to be modulated by inducible repair systems. The effect of mitogenic stimulation is of interest because it suggests that the proliferative state of the cell may influence the yield of mutations after DNA damage. Since hemopoietic stem cells and committed progenitor cells differ in their proliferative state, they may have different susceptibilities to mutagenesis.

B. Chemotherapy

Mutagenesis can also be demonstrated following exposure of lymphocytes to cytotoxic drugs either in vitro or in vivo. The effects of various cytotoxic drugs in vivo

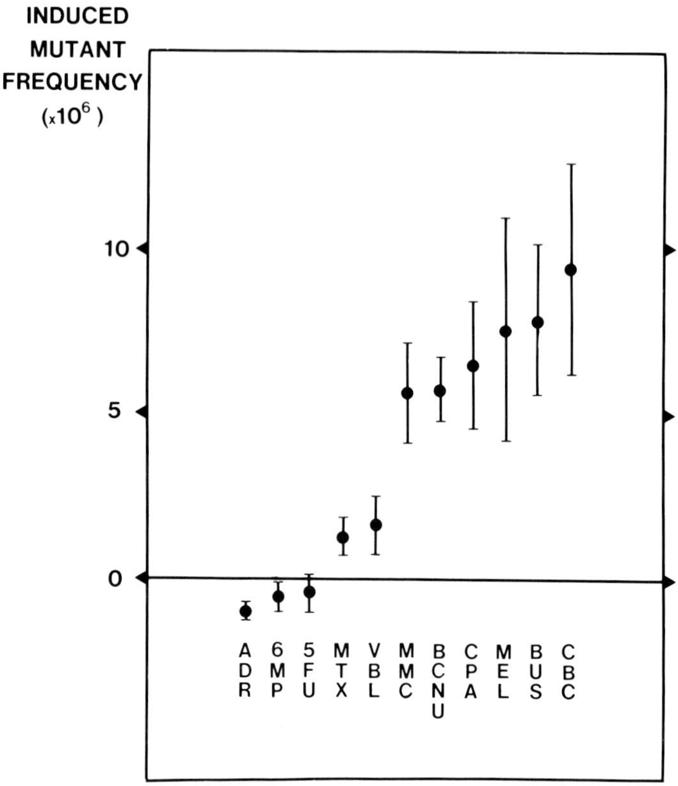

Figure 4 Number of mutations induced in murine splenocytes by a single dose of adriamycin (ADR), 6-mercaptopurine (6MP), 5-fluorouracil (5FU), methotrexate (MTX), vinblastine (VBL), mitomycin C (MMC), bischloronitrosourea (BCNU), cyclophosphamide (CPA), melphalan (MEL), busulfan (BUS), or chlorambucil (CBC). The results are the mean +1 SE for 6 mice/point and are calculated as the mutation frequency in drug-injected mice minus the mutation frequency in control mice.

are illustrated in Figure 4, which shows the results of studies in which mice were treated with a single dose of drug at approximately one-half to two-thirds of the LD_{50} dose and the mutation frequency in splenic lymphocytes was assayed 30-40 days later. The particular agents studied were chosen to cover a broad range of chemical classes and also to reveal any correlations between mutagenesis and the production of residual bone marrow damage. This latter complication occurs particularly following treatment with busulfan, mitomycin, and bischloronitrosourea, but is also seen with other alkylating agents (13,14), and it is of interest that the greatest mutagenic effect follows treatment with the same drugs. Theories on the etiology of residual marrow damage are either selective, postulating that stem cells of high proliferative ability are selectively killed, leaving a stem cell population of low proliferative ability (15), or inductive, postulating that in some way chemotherapy or radiation damages all stem cells so that proliferative ability is impaired (16). Selective theories cannot explain the observation that the more mature progenitor cells in residual damage also show impaired proliferation (17), and the above data, showing a correlation between the drugs that produce residual damage and those that produce mutations, provide direct evidence that residual damage is the result of mutational damage to hemopoietic stem cells.

III. CLINICAL STUDIES

Several studies have shown directly that chemotherapy and/or radiotherapy produce somatic mutations in patients with cancer. In a study of mutations at the HPRT locus in 41 patients with solid tumors or lymphoma, a threefold increase in mutations was seen in patients treated with chemotherapy and a fivefold increase in patients treated with chemotherapy plus radiotherapy (18). Too few patients were treated with radiotherapy alone to determine the effect of this modality by itself. Updated data on patients with solid tumors treated with chemotherapy alone are shown in Figure 5. Studies by other workers on patients with carcinoma of the breast have shown an increase in HPRT mutations following radiotherapy (19) and an increase in glycophorin mutations following chemotherapy (20).

The association between inherited disorders of DNA repair such as xeroderma pigmentosum and Fanconi's anemia and the development of cancer has suggested that genetic susceptibility to DNA damage may be an important predisposing factor in patients with the common forms of cancer. However, mutation frequency in untreated patients does not differ from that in controls of the same age, and this is indirect evidence against this possibility. Direct study of lymphocytes exposed to various doses of x-radiation or the chemical mutagen methyl nitrosourea has also shown no difference between cancer patients and controls in the number of induced mutations (18,21). Thus at present there is no evidence that inherited susceptibility to mutagenesis is a predisposing factor to development of cancer in most patients.

Since mutation assays in treated patients with cancer have been performed some time after the mutagenic exposure, the results obtained have depended both on the initial number of mutations produced and on the biological half-life of mutant $HPRT^-$ cells. This is presently unknown but is under investigation. However, there is some evidence from tissue culture, from preliminary studies on induced mutations in mice, and from study of female heterozygotes with Lesch-Nyhan syndrome (inherited HPRT deficiency) that there is weak in

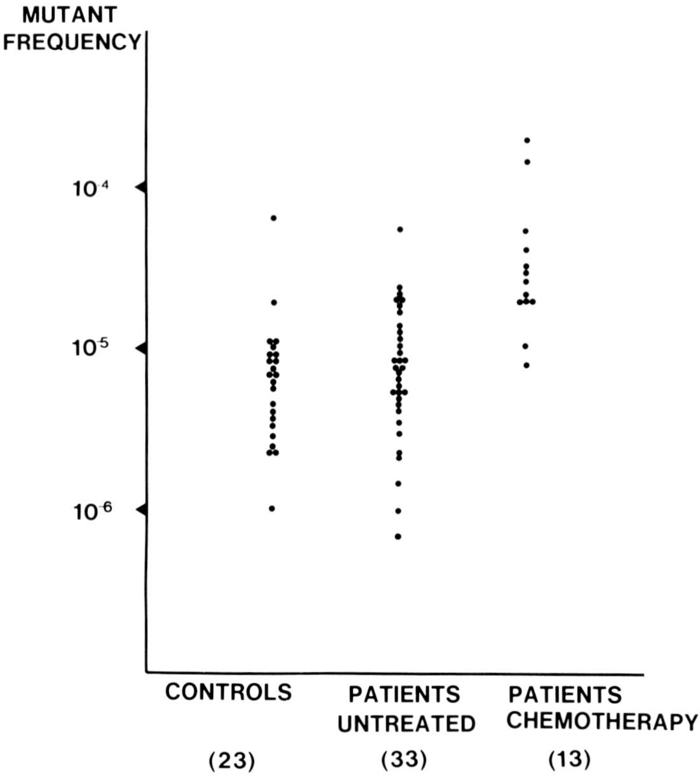

Figure 5 Mutation frequency in untreated patients with solid tumors, patients treated with various forms of chemotherapy, and age-method controls.

vivo selection against HPRT⁻ lymphocytes (22). If so, then measurement of mutation frequency in an individual following exposure to a mutagen may underestimate the mutagenic effect, particularly if the measurement is performed some time after the exposure. This point is relevant to the important question of whether enumeration of mutation frequency in patients who have received chemotherapy or radiotherapy is of any value in predicting future complications.

Pharmacists and nurses who prepare or administer cancer chemotherapy are also potentially exposed to cytotoxic drugs, albeit at lower doses than patients with cancer, and there has been concern about the possible hazard to which these individuals are exposed. In an epidemiological study of Finnish nurses, an increased incidence of fetal loss was observed in those who had been involved with preparing or administering cancer chemotherapy (23). In experimental studies, material showing mutagenic activity in microbial tests has been detected in urine, and in other studies chromosomal abnormalities have been detected in lymphocytes of exposed individuals. However, such findings have been difficult to confirm either by other investigators or by the same investigators in subsequent studies. Nurses and pharmacists handling cytotoxic drugs have also been studied using lymphocyte mutation frequency as the end point. In the initial study, a small but significant difference was found between exposed individuals and age- and sex-matched controls, and there was a suggestion of a relationship between mutation frequency and duration of exposure (24). However, a subsequent and larger study involving monitoring of individuals from hospitals around Australia has failed to show any difference between oncology workers and controls (21).

One difficulty with all the studies on nurses and pharmacists is that they used a biological indicator of genetic damage that is undoubtedly insensitive or is affected by other variables. This factor may explain some of the discrepancies between the various studies, but another factor, possibly of equal importance, is that occupational practices in respect of cytotoxic drugs have changed substantially during the last few years. This has occurred in response to both the perceived theoretical risk of cytotoxic drugs and the results of the studies in which genetic effects were reported. Thus both the positive and negative studies may have given results that were correct at the time they were obtained.

IV. MOLECULAR CHANGES

The molecular basis for HPRT mutations has been studied using Southern analysis with a cDNA probe for HPRT. A surprisingly large number of spontaneous mutations have been found to be due to substantial gene changes, deletions, and/or amplifications of portions of the HPRT gene (25,26), and, given the resolution of Southern analysis, it is likely that the majority of spontaneous mutations represent DNA changes involving a number of bases rather than representing point mutations. Similarly, many of the mutations induced by x-rays are associated with partial or complete deletions of the HPRT gene (27,28), although these deletions are rarely large enough to be visible as chromosomal abnormalities (21). Examples of partial and complete gene deletions following x-irradiation are shown in Figure 6. The molecular basis for mutations produced by cytotoxic drugs is likely to be more variable and depend upon the chemical damage produced to DNA. Thus changes on Southern analysis are rare following mutagenesis by methyl nitrosourea, which produces small alkylations in DNA, whereas deletions are very common following mitomycin, which cross-links the two DNA strands (21). However, the picture that is emerging suggests that the size and nature of the ultimate mutation depends not so much on the nature of the primary chemical lesion in DNA as on the secondary process of repair that results from that lesion.

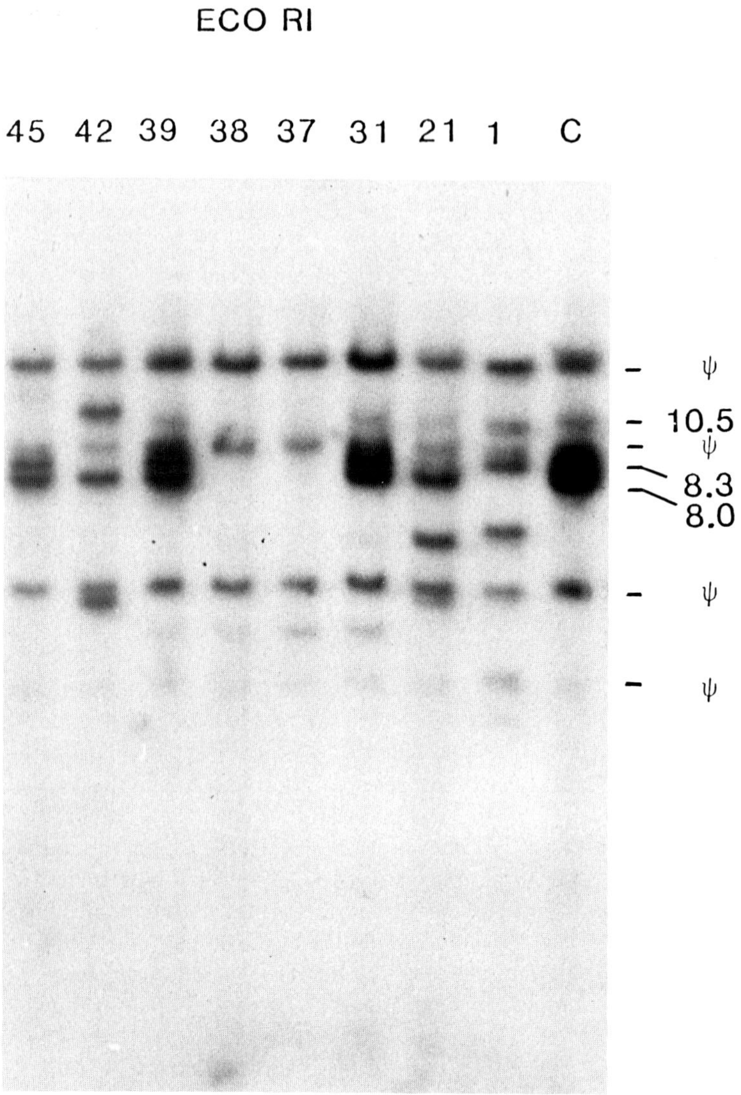

Figure 6 Autoradiagraphs of Southern transfers of DNA from eight mutant clones induced by x-radiation (numbered) and one control clone (C). Clones 45, 42, 21, and 1 show partial deletions, and clones 38 and 37 show complete deletion of the HPRT gene. Note preservation of the pseudogene bands. (From Ref. 27.)

V. CONSEQUENCES OF MUTAGENESIS

In studies of mutagenesis, lymphocytes have been used as nucleated mammalian cells rather than as specific immune cells. Nevertheless there are good data that both chemotherapy and radiation result in long-term effects on the immune system, both in experimental animals and in humans, and produce long-term qualitative and/or quantitative changes in various immune populations (29-32; see also Chapter 9). The peripheral blood lymphocyte, however, may well be quite a good model for the hemopoietic stem cell, since both cells are normally in G_0 and both have very extensive proliferative capacity. Thus individual circulating human T lymphocytes are able to give rise to between 10^8 and 10^{32} descendants (21), and individual murine stem cells are capable of completely restoring hemopoiesis, implying that they are able to give rise to at least 10^{11}-10^{12} descendants (33). If mutations occur in hemopoietic stem cells as they do in T lymphocytes, then one could readily envisage how late effects such as carcinogenesis and proliferative failure might result.

The finding of large deletions in a high proportion of spontaneous and induced mutations is of great interest in view of the evidence that mutations involving both alleles of critical regulatory genes are important in oncogenesis (reviewed in Refs. 34 and 35). In inherited Wilms's tumor and retinoblastoma there is an inherited deletion in all body cells of a portion of one chromosome, 11 or 13, respectively. In the tumor cells the corresponding region of the homologous chromosome is also lost, by mechanisms such as interstitial deletion, recombination, or whole chromosome loss, and this is believed to result in loss of the second allele of a regulatory gene important for control of cell growth. One can readily envisage that if sizable genetic events such as deletions occur widely and randomly throughout the genome, as suggested by the molecular data on mutations, then loss of genes at one or more critical sites could occur and lead to the development of cancer. Chromosomes 5 and 7 are commonly abnormal in the secondary leukemias that follow chemotherapy, which suggests that such regulatory genes may be present on these chromosomes.

REFERENCES

1. Szybalski, W., Szybalski, E. H. Drug sensitivity as a genetic marker for human cell lines. *Univ. Mich. Med. Bull 28,* 277 (1962).
2. Morley, A. A., Trainor, K. J., Seshadri, R. Cloning of human lymphocytes using limiting dilution. *Exp. Hematol. 11,* 418-424 (1983).
3. Albertini, R. J., Castle, K. L., Borcherding, W. R. T-cell cloning to detect the mutant 6-thioguanine-resistant lymphocytes present in human peripheral blood. *Proc. Natl. Acad. Sci. USA 79,* 6617-6621 (1982).
4. Morley, A. A., Trainor, K. J., Seshadri, R. S., Ryall, R. G. Measurement of in vivo mutations in human lymphocytes. *Nature 302,* 155-156 (1983).

5. Trainor, K. J., Wigmore, D. J., Chrysostomou, A., Dempsey, J. L., Seshadri, R. S., Morley, A. A. Mutation frequency in human lymphocytes increases with age. *Mech. Age Develop. 27,* 83-86 (1984).
6. Jones, I. M., Burkhart-Schulz, K., Carrano, A. V. A method to quantify spontaneous and *in vivo* induced thioguanine-resistant mouse lymphocytes. *Mutat. Res. 147,* 97-105 (1985).
7. Dempsey, J. L., Morley, A. A. Measurement of *in vivo* mutant frequency in lymphocytes in the mouse. *Environ. Mutagen. 8,* 385-391 (1986).
8. Jensen, R. H., Bigbee, W., Branscomb, E. W. Somatic mutations detected by immunofluorescence and flow cytometry. In: *Biological dosimetry cytometric approaches to mammalian systems.* Eisert, W. G., Mendelsohn, M. L. (Eds.). Springer-Verlag, Berlin, pp. 161-170 (1984).
9. Sanderson, B. J. S., Dempsey, J. L., Morley, A. A. Mutations in human lymphocytes: effect of X- and UV-irradiation. *Mutat. Res. 140,* 233-227 (1984).
10. Friedberg, E. C. *DNA repair.* Freeman, New York (1985).
11. Sanderson, B. J. S., Morley, A. A. Mitogenic stimulation may induce an antimutagenic repair system in human lymphocytes. *Mutagenesis 1,* 131-133 (1986).
12. Sanderson, B. J. S., Morley, A. A. Exposure of human lymphocytes to ionizing radiation reduces mutagenesis by subsequent ionizing radiation. *Mutat. Res.* (in press).
13. Trainor, K. J., Morley, A. A. Screening of cytotoxic drugs for residual bone marrow damage. *J. Natl. Cancer Inst. 57,* 1237-1239 (1976).
14. Trainor, K. J., Seshadri, R. S., Morley, A. A. Residual marrow injury following cytotoxic drugs. *Leuk. Res. 3,* 205-210 (1979).
15. Botnick, L. E., Hannon, E. C., Hellman, S. Limited proliferation of stem cells surviving alkylating agents. *Nature 262,* 68-70 (1976).
16. Morley, A. Residual marrow damage from cytotoxic drugs. *Aust. N.Z. J. Med. 10,* 569-571 (1980).
17. Trainor, K. J., Morley, A. A., Seshadri, R. S. A proliferative defect of marrow cells in experimental chronic hypoplastic marrow failure (aplastic anaemia). *Exp. Hematol. 8,* 674-682 (1980).
18. Dempsey, J. L., Seshadri, R. S., Morley, A. A. Increased mutation frequency following treatment with cancer chemotherapy. *Cancer Res. 45,* 2873-2877 (1985).
19. Messing, K., Bradley, W. E. C. In vivo mutant frequency rises among breast cancer patients after exposure to high doses of γ-radiation. *Mutat. Res. 152,* 107-112 (1985).
20. Langlois, R. Personal communication.
21. Dempsey, J. L., Morley, A. A., Trainor, K. J., Osborne, Y., McCarron, M., Turner, D. R. Unpublished observations.
22. Dempsey, J. L., Morley, A. A., Seshadri, R. S., Emmerson, B., Gordon, R., Bhagat, C. Detection of the carrier state for an X-linked disorder, the Lesch-Nyhan syndrome, by the use of lymphocyte cloning. *Human Genet. 64,* 288-290 (1983).

23. Selevan, S. G., Lindbohm, M.-L., Hornung, R. W., Hemminki, K. A study of occupational exposure to antineoplastic drugs and fetal loss in nurses. *New Engl. J. Med. 313,* 1173-1178 (1985).
24. Chrysostomou, A., Seshadri, R. S., Morley, A. A. Mutation frequency in nurses and pharmacists exposed to cytotoxic drugs. *Aust. N.Z. J. Med. 14,* 831-834 (1984).
25. Turner, D. R., Morley, A. A., Haliandros, M., Kutlaca, R., Sanderson, B. J. S. *In vivo* somatic mutations in human lymphocytes are frequently due to major gene alterations. *Nature 315,* 343-345 (1985).
26. Albertini, R. J., O'Neill, J. P., Nicklas, J. A., Heintz, N. H., Kelleher, P. C. Alterations of the HPRT gene in human in vivo-derived 6-thioguanine-resistant T lymphocytes. *Nature 316,* 369-371 (1985).
27. Skulimowski, A. W., Turner, D. R., Morley, A. A., Sanderson, B. J. S., Haliandros, M. Molecular basis of X-ray induced mutation at the HPRT locus in human lymphocytes. *Mutat. Res. 162,* 105-112 (1986).
28. Thacker, J. The nature of mutants induced by ionising radiation in cultured hamster cells. *Mutat. Res. 160,* 267-275 (1986).
29. Pugsley, C. A. J., Forbes, I. J., Morley, A. A. Immunological abnormalities in an animal model of chronic hypoplastic marrow failure induced by busulfan. *Blood 51,* 601-610 (1978).
30. Gale, R. J., Morley, A. A. The mononuclear phagocyte system in experimental chronic marrow failure. *Exp. Hematol. 8,* 16-24 (1980).
31. MacKay, I. R., Goodyear, M. D., Riglar, C., Penschow, J., Whittingham, S., Russell, I. S., Kitchen, P. R. B., Collins, J. P. Effect on immunologic and other induces of adjuvant cytotoxic chemotherapy including melphalan in breast cancer. *Cancer 53,* 2619-2627 (1984).
32. Jakobsson, M., Taskinen, P. J., Ryhän, P., Hollmen, A., Herva, E., Kärkölä, P., Saloheimo, M. The effect of surgery, radiation therapy, and combined radiation therapy and chemotherapy on immunocompetence in patients with lung carcinoma. *Acta Radiol. Oncol. 24,* 481-486 (1985).
33. Abramson, S., Miller, R. G., Phillips, R. A. The identification in adult bone marrow of pluripotent and restricted stem cells of the myeloid and lymphoid systems. *J. Exp. Med. 145,* 1567-1579 (1977).
34. Murphree, A. L., Benedict, W. F. Retinoblastoma: clues to human oncogenesis. *Science 223,* 1028-1033 (1984).
35. Solomon, E. Recessive mutation in aetiology of Wilms' tumour. *Nature 309,* 111-112 (1984).

9

Long-Term Damage to the Immune System After Irradiation

ELIZABETH NAPARSTEK and SHIMON SLAVIN
Hadassah University Hospital, Jerusalem, Israel

I. INTRODUCTION

The continuing improvement in survival rates of patients with malignant disorders in the last decade can be attributed to a variety of factors. Among these are an increase in the proportion of cancers diagnosed in a controllable stage, improvement in diagnostic and surgical techniques; and, above all, improvement in therapeutic strategies that involve new chemotherapeutic agents, high-energy megavoltage radiation equipment, and combined therapeutic modalities. Although the aim of both modalities is to attain the greatest effect on the tumor and the least effect on normal tissues, the immediate toxicity of these potential therapeutic modalities is almost inevitable. Improvement in the supportive care of cancer patients is therefore another important contribution to the higher survival in recent years.

The long-term complications and consequences of chemoradiotherapy, which now can be followed for long periods of disease-free survival, are still not fully recognized and far from being controlled. Dose-dependent toxicities to specific organs caused by various chemotherapeutic agents are under constant surveillance. Phase I and phase II studies provide the initial information on various side effects of new drugs, while long-term follow-up and monitoring of patients who received chemo- or radiotherapy provides further information on late secondary complications. Combination of various chemotherapeutic agents is generally considered more effective for tumor eradication, reducing the chance of the emergence of resistant mutations, and in addition it enables the use of smaller doses of each drug that would complement or act in synergy with another. Such an approach may reduce to some extent those side effects that are dose-dependent. It is generally accepted, however, that high-dose chemoradiotherapy or even radiation therapy alone may cause direct and remote immediate and late effects on the immune system and also to a lesser extent on the hemopoietic tissue.

Among the most intriguing complications is the development of a second malignancy, related in particular to radiation and alkylating agents or, much more likely, following a combination of both. It is well accepted that a somatic mutation initiates the development of the secondary malignancy. The extent to which an altered immune surveillance, induced by chemoradiotherapy, causes induction or permits escape of the clonogenic mutation, is still controversial.

In the following section we discuss delayed effects of radiation therapy on the immune system, its components, and its function in experimental animals and humans.

II. THE EFFECT OF IONIZING RADIATION ON TISSUES

A. Cellular Damage Caused by Irradiation

Two types of ionizing radiation, electromagnetic (x or γ rays) and subatomic particle (electrons, protons, neutrons) radiation, are commonly used in clinical practice for both primary and palliative treatment of malignant diseases (1,2). Both types of radiation transfer energy as photons, which upon penetration into the tissue cause ionization, resulting in cellular damage. The cellular DNA is susceptible to damage by either direct ionization caused by a passage of an ionizing particle or indirect ionization through energy transferred from free radicals. Ionization of the DNA results in structural damage to the chromosomes: a single-strand DNA break that can frequently be repaired by proper enzymes or double-strand DNA breaks that result in irreversible lesion and loss of replication potential and eventually in cell death.

Radiation at clinically utilized dose ranges has no effect on the enzymatic and biochemical processes, and therefore the ability of specialized cells to function and synthesize tissue-specific proteins is maintained until the cells attempt to undergo mitosis, where failure results in cell death.

B. Tissue Response to Irradiation

The expression of radiation injury in tissue depends on various factors. The most important is the amount of radiation absorbed by the tissue, which is a function of the energy of irradiation and the physical and biological characteristics of the tissue.

Tissues vary in their susceptibility to irradiation. Radiosensitivity of a specific tissue is best described by a survival curve, obtained by irradiation of cells in vitro (3,4), which shows the relation between the surviving fraction and the radiation dose. For most of its length the curve is linear, indicating that cells are killed in an exponential fashion. The slope of the curve at a point when the dose kills 63% of the cells is termed D_0. Small D_0 thus indicates greater radiosensitivity. At low doses of radiation the curve flattens. The nonlinear portion of the curve, termed the "shoulder," indicates that cells are not being killed exponentially but are accumulating radiation damage that can be subsequently repaired.

Another important factor in tissue response is the proliferative organization of the tissue, i.e., its kinetics of self-renewal (5). Tissues that have a defined clonogenic stem cell compartment and postmitotic mature fractional cells, such as the hemopoietic tissue, epidermis, and alimentary and testicular epithelia, are more vulnerable to radiation and express radiation injury by a steady, dose-dependent depletion of the mature cells as a result of the loss of stem cells; such tissues also respond early by rapid repopulation of surviving cells provided the total dose was insufficient to kill all cells. Other tissues, defined as "flexible," are tissues that ordinarily do not undergo mitosis but may do so upon appropriate stimulus, such as damage or loss of cells. Finally, tissues that consist of fixed postmitotic, highly differentiated cells such as neurons are usually highly radioresistant. Regeneration or repair of sublethal cell damage also depends on the proliferative organization of each tissue, and this forms the basis for dose fractionation or hyperfractionation (5,6). Dose fractionation enables regeneration of surviving clonogenic cells during the course of therapy, thus protecting the tissue from permanent damage.

III. THE IMMUNE SYSTEM

The major cellular components of the immune system are lymphocytes, macrophages, and accessory cells (7). The lymphocytes are located in a variety of lymphoid organs from which they can be delivered by efferent lymphatic channels and the bloodstream to peripheral locations. Two other components of the immune system are (1) the primary lymphoid organs, including the thymus and the bone marrow, and (2) the secondary lymphoid organs, such as spleen, lymph nodes, and the lymphatic tissues associated with the gastrointestinal tract. All cell types of the immune system interact with each other directly and/or through active factors that they secrete in response to different signals, resulting in recognition of antigens, induction and modulation of the specific cell-mediated and humoral responses, and storage of immunological memory.

The main function of the primary lymphoid organs is to produce committed lymphocytes by providing an environment permissive to the maturation of T and B cells from their immunologically incompetent precursors, while the secondary lymphoid organs serve to maximize the function, by controlling the traffic and homing of the cells involved and their targets, leading to efficient interactions of different cell subsets in response to antigen. Recirculation of the lymphocytes among the various lymphoid organs and their interactions with self and foreign antigens through accessory cells is an essential feature of the dynamic and complex function of the immune system.

The stem cells from which lymphocytes derive arise from the yolk sac and the fetal liver. Later in the prenatal development, both T and B lymphocytes are derived from a population of primordial hematolymphoid cells located in the bone marrow. For B cells, the bone marrow is also the site of cellular maturation, through which the cells acquire immunoglobulin gene rearrangement, characteristic cell-surface receptors, and the development of MHC-encoded structures required for interaction with other immune cells. T cells undergo their major maturational stages in the thymus. Thymic maturation involves the induction of specific genes, some of which are expressed only during intrathymic stage, while others are expressed throughout the life span of the cell: expression of antigen-specific receptors; development of MHC restriction required for immune cell interaction; production of regulatory and effector T cells associated with help, suppression, and cytolysis; and the induction of T-cell surface receptors that most likely are responsible for their homing characteristics in the secondary lymphoid tissues.

Neither T nor B lymphocytes constitute a homogeneous population of cells; each group comprises several subsets differentiated by surface markers and specific functions. In addition, there is a heterogeneous group of lymphocytes that are neither T nor B cells that seem to play an essential role in several in vitro systems and therefore most likely have important biological functions in vivo, particularly as part of the natural defense mechanisms against tumors.

IV. THE RESPONSE OF THE IMMUNE SYSTEM TO IRRADIATION

A. Radiosensitivity of the Immune System

The response of the immune system to ionizing radiation has been thoroughly studied in animal models in vivo as well as in vitro. Most of the data have been reviewed in detail by Anderson (8,9). From these studies, some distinct features that characterize the response of the immune system to radiation injury became clear. One is a phenomenon termed "interphase" death, and another is a heterogeneous response of the various cell types that constitute the immune system.

Radiation sensitivity of a particular cell type is described by D_0, the slope of the exponential portion of the survival curve, and by D_q, the projected slope of the "shoulder" part of the curve, which represents the dose that can be accumulated and subsequently repaired. The steeper the slope, the smaller the D_0, indicating greater radiosensitivity. Most proliferating cells die a mitotic death after irradiation and are thus defined as radiosensitive, while resting cells that do not divide often may survive very high doses of radiation and are thus defined as radioresistant (1,5). Of all mammalian tissues, lymphocytes (but not all subsets) and sperm cells are the most sensitive to irradiation and have the lowest D_0 of

25-35 cGy (1,8,9). Moreover, while most cells exposed to irradiation do not die until they attempt to undergo mitosis, most lymphocytes are killed *without* entering the mitotic cycle. The immediate death of lymphocytes after small doses of irradiation is thus nonmitotic or "interphase." The knowledge of this extreme radiosensitivity of lymphocytes to irradiation is based on old observations in animals. Whole body exposure of rats to 1 Gy results in a rapid decrease in the number of circulating lymphocytes to 25% within 4 hr (10). Within 1 hr after exposure to an LD_{50} dose of x-rays, necrosis of various lymphoid tissues is evident, and within a few days the lymphoid tissues are almost devoid of lymphocytes (11). Data obtained from patients treated with radiation for malignant disorders and from persons exposed to accidental irradiation similarly show a significantly faster decrease in the number of circulating lymphocytes than in other blood elements (9).

The second feature that characterizes the response of the immune system to irradiation is the marked variability in the radiosensitivity of various lymphoid organs, various areas of the same organ, and various lymphoid subsets. This contrasts with the rather uniform response of most other tissues to radiation.

Most studies of the differential radiosensitivity of defined B and T lymphocyte subsets were performed in vivo by serial determination of the percentage of T and B lymphocytes obtained by thoracic duct cannulation following whole body irradiation (12) and some by adoptive transfer of cells irradiated in vitro and assayed in vivo (13,14). These studies clearly demonstrated that B cells are more sensitive to irradiation than T cells, yielding D_{37} values of 0.7-1.45 Gy.

As for T cells, however, the results demonstrated distinct differences among the various T cell subsets; generally, T suppressor cells are more radiosensitive than helper T cells. However, two important variables should be considered in evaluating the data; one is the maturational and functional state of a given cell population. Thus, although cytotoxic T cells are radiosensitive, they do express cytotoxic activity after exposure to high-dose radiation when activated 7 days prior to irradiation (15). The other important variable is the method employed to study the regulative responses of T cells, whether totally in vitro, in vivo, or by adoptive transfer experiments (13,14,16-18). Unprimed T helper cells, for example, are radiosensitive regardless of whether irradiation is given in vivo or in vitro or whether the assay system is in vitro or involves adoptive transfer. In contrast, primed T helper cells are radioresistant when assayed in vitro but radiosensitive when assayed by adoptive transfer.

Difficulties in interpreting data employing in vivo studies result in part from the effect of irradiation on cell traffic. Cells of the immune system constantly recirculate through the blood, thoracic duct, small afferent and efferent lymphatic channels, and various lymphoid organs. Irradiation does seem to alter the homing and the recirculation pattern of lymphocytes and thus alters the interaction of certain lymphocyte subsets with their proper microenvironment and with other accessory cells. This may account for radiosensitivity of helper function observed in adoptive transfer experiments in contrast to relative radioresistance of the same cells when assayed in vitro.

Histological appearance and specific assessment of size, weight, and cell number of various lymphoid organs afford yet another method to determine the relative radiosensitivity of lymphocytes located within these organs (13). Since 30-40% of the spleen mass is composed of cells other than lymphocytes that by nature are less radiosensitive, the loss in splenic mass is less pronounced than that in the thymus, in which the microenvironmental cell mass is much smaller in proportion. As shown histologically and by immunofluorescence, non-thymic-dependent areas are extremely radiosensitive, resulting in greater and faster depletion of B cells from B-dependent areas than from T-dependent areas (19).

The response of the thymus to radiation is more complex. It is generally agreed that the thymus is a relatively radiosensitive organ; however, there is a discrepancy in the response of thymic lymphocytes and thymic stroma to radiation therapy. Alteration in the morphology of the thymic lymphocytes can be documented after exposure to 5 cGy (8), while the stromal cells compartment does not show morphological alteration even after 50 Gy (20). The repopulation of the thymus after irradiation is of particular importance, since failure of thymic microenvironment has often been suggested to be responsible for the delayed recovery of several functions of the T-cell-dependent immune system after irradiation.

Following low-dose irradiation (1.5-2 Gy) the thymus regains its initial weight within 12 days. However, following higher doses of irradiation there seems to exist a biphasic pattern of response: initial recovery, presumably due to regeneration of radioresistant subsets of intrathymic precursors, and later a second regenerative phase due to influx of lymphocytes from regenerating bone marrow (21,22). This phenomenon was elegantly shown by preservation of marrow cell supply by selective shielding of the hind limbs, or alternatively by administration of syngeneic bone marrow cells, both of which prevented the second spontaneous decrease in thymic repopulation and loss of weight (22).

B. Alterations in the Immune Functions Following Irradiation

The function of the immune system is altered remarkably following irradiation. As a result of the broad spectrum of radiosensitivities exhibited by various lymphocyte subpopulations, the functional impairment is not uniform. This results from the differential radiosensitivity of the various cells participating in antibody production. As previously mentioned, primed T helper cells and plasma cells are relatively radioresistant, whereas unprimed T helper cells and T suppressor cells are radiosensitive. The immunoglobulins themselves are not affected by irradiation. Therefore, high-dose irradiation given before antigenic stimulation will decrease antibody production as it affects the unprimed T and B lymphocytes. On the other hand, the same dose of irradiation given after antigenic stimulation might enhance antibody production by preferential inhibition of suppressor cells as opposed to the primed T helper and B cells (23). As suppressor cells are even more radiosensitive than unprimed T cells, low-dose irradiation given prior to antigenic challenge will lead to enhanced antibody production (24). Similar mechanisms may explain the radioresistance of the secondary as compared to the primary antibody response.

The cell-mediated responses in general are less affected by irradiation than antibody production, again due to relative radioresistance of T as compared to B cells. This can be demonstrated by the effect of irradiation on delayed-type hypersensitivity (DTH), graft-versus-host reaction (GVH), and allograft rejection.

Delayed-type hypersensitivity appears to be radioresistant. Exposure of guinea pigs to sublethal whole body irradiation of 3 Gy prior to immunization with diphtheria toxoid resulted in reduction of antitoxin antibody, while it did not alter the delayed-type hypersensitivity to the toxin (25). Larger radiation doses (8 Gy), however, totally suppressed both antibody formation and delayed-type hypersensitivity responses (26). Graft-versus-host reactivity, which is mediated by T cells, is also affected by irradiation. Inoculation of parental lymphocytes into F_1 hybrid elicits graft-versus-host response in the recipient. This response is inhibited by irradiation of the donor lymphocytes prior to inoculation (27).

It has been known for many years that irradiation of the recipient prior to transplantation promotes survival of the graft (28). This is mainly true for the first-set allograft, whereas second-set response is more radioresistant. The dose required for sufficient immunosuppression, however, is high and results in bone marrow aplasia. Thus, irradiation cannot be used as the sole mode of conditioning for organ transplantation. When used in lower doses, irradiation may sometimes even lead to acceleration of graft rejection.

Irradiation has been shown also to be useful in aiding tolerance induction (29). This may be due to the fact that the postirradiation recovery phase is characterized by preponderance of immature lymphoid cells, which are particularly susceptible to tolerance induction. This state of tolerance is, however, transient in most situations. Moreover, in certain experimental conditions, irradiation of tolerant animals may result in termination of the unresponsive state, presumably due to removal of suppressor cells or alternatively to depletion of clonally unresponsive cells.

V. DELAYED EFFECTS OF IRRADIATION ON THE IMMUNE FUNCTION IN HUMANS

In the previous section we reviewed the short-term or acute effects of irradiation on the immune system in experimental models. It seems clear that ionizing radiation has a profound effect on all facets of the immune response. Due to their extreme radiosensitivity, irradiation causes an acute decrease in the number of circulating lymphocytes and the size of the primary and secondary lymphoid organs. This, however, does not necessarily lead to a uniform decrease in the various functions of the immune system, due to the marked differential radiosensitivity among lymphocyte subsets.

Ionizing radiation is a common therapeutic modality for various malignant disorders. Its beneficial efficacy on certain tumors outweighs its immediate and expected untoward effects on the immune system. In recent years it has become apparent that radiation may cause late effects on the immune system. The major bulk of information on the delayed outcome of irradiation on the immune system in humans originates from two sources: (1) survivors of atomic bomb explosions and individuals exposed to accidental irradiation at nuclear plants; (2) patients exposed to high cumulative doses of irradiation as a part of therapy for malignant or nonmalignant diseases. Although much information has been gathered during the last decade, conclusions from these data are confusing. The atomic bomb survivors, for example, comprise a previously basically healthy population; however, the immune functions in these survivors have not been monitored, and, moreover, 30-40 years ago, basic knowledge, techniques, and methods for analyzing the immune functions were lacking. As to the second group, the heterogeneity of this patient population, the effects of the underlying disease on the immune system, and the shortened life span frequently do not allow meaningful conclusions and long-term monitoring of the immune responses.

A. Immune Function in Patients Treated with Local Irradiation

Accumulating knowledge and understanding of the biological effect of radiation on normal and malignant tissues in recent years has resulted in significantly improved techniques of irradiation that have increased its therapeutic efficacy while minimizing side effects. Development of new sophisticated equipment with increasing radiation energy permits the delivery of higher doses of radiation at more homogeneous and precise distribution into the tissues, with less scatter and greater sparing of skin. Local and extended-field irradiation has become a treatment of choice for a variety of localized tumors, with or without adjuvant chemotherapy. It appears, though, that even when localized, radiation has a marked delayed effect on the immune system. This can be best documented in patients treated with limited-field irradiation for local malignancy, even if the nonspecific effects of the malignant process per se on the immune function are excluded.

Two factors of major importance should be considered while evaluating the long-term effects of irradiation on the immune system. Derangement in the immune surveillance has been frequently considered permissive for the development of malignancy (30,31). Indeed, many studies have demonstrated various immune dysfunctions in patients with malignant disorders, regardless of therapy (31-38). None of the clinical and experimental studies, however, has demonstrated or characterized a specific immunological failure responsible for tumor development.

Excluding patients with hematological malignancies and lymphomas, in whom the primary organs involved in the disease process are those normally producing and homing the cells associated with the immune defense mechanism, the degree and frequency of immune dysfunction vary greatly between different tumor types, stage of disease, age of the patient, and other co-morbid conditions. These observations make the interpretation of the severity of immune dysfunction in patients treated with irradiation extremely difficult. In one study, it appeared that patients with head and neck cancers seemed to have a greater degree of immune dysfunction than those with other malignancies (37). Controversial data exist in patients with carcinoma of the lung or the gastrointestinal tract. Therefore, when evaluating the long-term effects of radiation therapy on the immune system, one should rely only on those studies in which a group of patients undergoing the immune monitoring were studied before and after exposure to irradiation, or studies carried out in patients who did not show any immune aberrations at diagnosis. Patients treated by combined modalities such as radiation plus cytotoxic agents, or plus biological reagents such as interferon, which may also affect the immune system, should also be excluded.

Thus, when monitoring the immune function in patients receiving local irradiation, it is of major importance to study those individuals with sufficient disease-free survival after radiotherapy to consider them cured, and thus to eliminate nonspecific tumor-related effects and immunological derangements that normally appear immediately after irradiation.

Since the first report by Millard in 1965 (39), many investigators have described significant abnormalities in the immune function following local irradiation. The majority of these data are summarized in Table 1. Persistent and prolonged decrease in the number of lymphocytes (40-52), particularly circulating T lymphocytes, is a most constant finding years after termination of the therapy (36,42,45-47,51-56). Many have reported a functional decrease in PHA response (39,42-46,48,52,57-63). Decreased or absent cell-mediated skin reactivity to T-cell-mediated antigens was documented by some investigators as late as 12 years following radiation therapy (43,55,59,64,65).

Although serum immunoglobulin levels are as a rule normal, attempts were made to find out whether the B-cell compartment is affected as well. Some investigators demonstrated a decrease in the proportion of SmIg-positive cells and EAC-rosetting cells (50-53,59).

Only a few investigators performed the immunological monitoring of the same group of patients prior to and after therapy (50,52,55,59,64). Likewise, most of the studies were performed on heterogeneous groups of patients with various malignancies, some of whom had received prior chemotherapy while others were at the initial stage of disease. Nevertheless, the data are quite uniform: Local radiation results in prolonged and persistent decrease in the number of circulating T cells with concomitant decrease in PHA responsiveness on a cell-per-cell basis and decreased delayed-type skin reactivity.

Table 1 Delayed Abnormalities in Immune Function in Patients Treated with Local Radiation

Reference	Year	Type of tumor	No. of patients	Time after radiotherapy	Immune derangements
Millard (39)	1965	Testicular ca	5	19 mo	dec PHA response
Meyer (40)	1970	Breast ca	103	4-8 yr	dec circulating T cells
Thomas et al. (57)	1971	Lung ca Pelvic ca	11	>11 mo	dec PHA response
McCredie et al. (41)	1972	Breast ca Cervix ca	112 105	1-5 yr 1-5 yr	dec circulating T cells inc PHA response
Stjernsward et al. (42)	1972	Breast ca	34	1 yr	dec T cells dec PHA response
Cosimi et al. (43)	1973	Breast ca	16	22 mo	dec circulating T cells dec PHA response dec skin reactivity
Blomgren et al. (59)	1974	Prostatic and bladder ca	19	2-3 mo	dec PHA response dec response to PPD dec EAC rosetting cells
Chee et al. (60)	1974	Various	12	6-12 mo	dec PHA response
Wood et al. (53)	1974	Breast	14	>2 yr	dec T and EAC rosetting cells
Jenkins et al. (44)	1975	Uterine ca	31	3-6 mo	dec circulating T cells dec PHA and conA response
Stratton et al. (45)	1975	Various ca	21	1 yr	dec T cells dec PHA and PWM response
Ghossein et al. (61)	1975	Various ca	144	3-6 mo	dec PHA response

Trapley et al. (46)	1975	Larynogopharyngeal	35	4-5 yr	dec circulating T cells dec PHA response
Heier et al. (47)	1975	Seminoma testis	7	6 mo	dec circulating T cells
Campbell et al. (54)	1976	Testicular ca	11	1 yr	dec T cells dec PHA response
Stefani et al. (55)	1976	Head and neck ca	29	6 mo	dec DNCB reaction dec circulating T cells
Yamagata and Green (48)	1976	Cervical ca	138	2-10 mo	dec circulating lymphocytes dec PHA response
Stein et al. (62)	1976	Breast ca	63	5-12 yr	dec PHA response
Raben et al. (49)	1976	Breast ca Pelvic ca	11	1-2 mo	dec circulating T and B cells
Blomgren et al. (64)	1976	Breast ca	48	3 mo	dec B cells dec PPD response
Petrini et al. (50)	1977	Breast ca	11	1-2 mo	dec circulating lymphocytes dec SIg and EAC rosetting cells
Rand et al. (51)	1978	Cervical ca	23	5 yr	dec T cells and SIg-post cells
Hancock et al. (52)	1979	Cervical ca	15	1 yr	dec T and SmIg-post cells, dec PHA response and MI
Lichtenstein et al. (36)	1980	Various ca	27	1-5 yr	dec T cells dec PHA response
Onsrud and Thorsby (56)	1981	Endometrial ca	12	3-5 yr	dec T cells dec PHA response inc NK activity
Haim et al. (65)	1981	Gynecological tu	24	3-12 yr	dec skin reactivity and NBT
Hancock et al. (63)	1984	Cervical ca	9	1-9 yr	dec PHA response

None of the studies showed any correlation between the severity of the immunological derangements and the probability of relapse or cure. Meyer (40) and Stjernsward (42) even suggested that, in general, irradiation may fail to improve survival by preventing proper immune responsiveness to metastasis due to the direct radiation-induced modification of the immune response.

A closer look at the data base of most of these studies indicates that they were carried out primarily in patients with breast carcinoma and gynecological tumors (the majority of them carcinoma of the cervix and ovaries), bladder carcinomas, testicular seminoma, and larynogopharyngeal tumors. In most of these cases, a considerable bulk of lymphoid and bone marrow tissue falls into the radiation field. Such is the case with gynecological and testicular cancers in which the pelvic, paraaortic, and iliac lymph nodes, as well as the pelvis and lower vertebral spines, are often included in the radiation field. Similarly, in head and neck as well as breast and lung cancers, the thymic gland as well as cervical and frequently axillary and mediastinal lymph nodes are irradiated, in addition to adjacent bones containing viable marrow, including cervical and upper thoracic vertebrae, sternum, and ribs. It has been suggested that irradiation of the thymus plays a major role in the reduced number and function of T lymphocytes (42) due to reduced capacity to regenerate T cells de novo. McCredie (41) compared immune functions in patients with breast and squamous cell carcinoma of the uterine cervix and demonstrated similar outcomes in both groups, although the number of lymphocytes recovered more rapidly following radiation exposure of the lower abdomen, suggesting the possible role of thymic irradiation. Raben et al. (49) reported that the impaired T-cell functions were even more severe following pelvic irradiation as compared to thoracic irradiation, thus indicating that thymic irradiation may not be an essential prerequisite for reduced number and function of T cells. Similar T-cell-mediated immune dysfunctions were documented by Chee et al. (60) in patients who received pelvic irradiation for ankylosing spondylitis. These observations argue against the commonly accepted explanation that irradiation of lymphatic tissue itself accounts for the depressed number and function of lymphocytes. Many investigators tend to ascribe some of the effects of irradiation to exposure of cells in the major blood vessels flowing through the radiation field as an explanation for the reduced number and function of lymphocytes shortly after irradiation. To what extent such an exposure affects the persistent reduction of T-cell function is not clear. Ilbery et al. (66) suggested that the impaired lymphocyte responsiveness to PHA may reflect the continued presence of cells bearing sublethal radiation damage. Persistence of lymphocytes with radiation-induced chromosomal aberrations has been described in humans (67 and Chapter 7).

An increase in cell-mediated immune functions following exposure to very low doses of irradiation has also been described. McCredie reported increased PHA responses in patients irradiated for breast and cervical carcinoma (41).

Onsrud and Thorsby reported increased NK activity in patients with endometrial cancer treated with local irradiation (56). This paradoxical increase in cell-mediated immune functions following low-dose irradiation is, however, extremely rare. In summary, immune functions in patients with nonlymphoid malignancies, treated with local irradiation to involved fields, show persisting alterations in the immune system for periods as long as 12-15 years in some studies. The most common abnormality observed in all patients, irrespective of the original diagnosis, is reduced number of circulating T cells and decreased responses to PHA. Other lymphoid subsets show less significant severe abnormalities.

B. Effects of Total Lymphoid Irradiation (TLI) on the Immune System

Analysis of the markedly impaired cell-mediated immune response observed in patients treated for malignant lymphomas that could be ascribed to the fractionated, high-dose radiotherapy (68) has revived an old interest in the concept of using ionizing radiation for suppression of immune responses. In order to explore further the potential utilization of fractionated total lymphoid irradiation (TLI) for immunosuppression, basic treatment protocols were designed in experimental animals in consideration of factors related to the radiobiology of lymphocytes, the anatomy of the immune system, and the possible adverse effects of ionizing irradiation. Radiation was administered by selective exposure of all major lymph nodes, thymus, and spleen with lead shielding of nonlymphoid organs (69,70). High and effective total cumulative doses of irradiation were accomplished with few severe side effects by administration of multiple daily fractions of 1-2 Gy/day.

Fractionated TLI resulted in profound and long-lasting reduction of the pool of lymphocytes in the circulation and in the peripheral lymphoid organs, accompanied by impaired humoral and, especially, cell-mediated immune functions, including markedly delayed capacity to reject an allograft (70). It was originally assumed that the effect of TLI was merely due to dose-dependent elimination of the radiosensitive immunocompetent cells. Indeed, the degree of prolongation of skin graft survival across MHC barriers in mice was clearly dose-dependent. At an optimal TLI dose of 34 Gy, the mean survival of skin allograft in mice was prolonged four- to fivefold (70) and the mean survival of perfused heterotopic cardiac allograft in rats was prolonged ninefold, with occasional permanent survival (71).

Interestingly, studies of adult mice given TLI of 34 Gy have shown that injection of heterologous protein antigens following radiotherapy results in a state of permanent antigen-specific tolerance rather than immunity (72). Rodents inoculated with histoincompatible bone marrow (BM) cells developed durable chimerism along with a state of tolerance to donor-type alloantigens without clinical signs of graft-versus-host disease (GVHD), indicating development of unresponsiveness of host versus graft as well as graft versus host (70). The effects of TLI on the recovery of various cell subsets in rodents and humans have been previously described in detail (68,69,73-75).

The most striking effect of TLI seems to be the generation of suppressor cells capable of abrogating both cellular and humoral responses, including in vitro suppression of T-cell-mediated proliferative responses of MLR, PHA, ConA (73-75); suppression of plaque formation of normal B cells to T-independent antigens (76); in vivo suppression of adoptive antibody response to dinitrophenyl-hapten coupled to heterologous proteins such as bovine serum albumin (72); and suppression of GVHD by allogeneic BM cells in lethally irradiated recipients (73,77). TLI-induced suppressor cells of MLR are antigen-nonspecific; they appear to be large, immature, mononuclear cells, cyclophosphamide-insensitive and extremely radioresistant (≥30 Gy) (73-75,77). Phenotypically, MLR suppressor cells are Thy-1$^-$, LyT-1$^-$, LyT-2$^-$, TL$^-$, Ig$^-$, assialo $GM_1{}^-$, and largely nonadherent to plastic, G-10 Sephadex, and nylon-wool surfaces (75). They have receptors to soybean and, to a lesser extent, peanut agglutinin, similar to immature cells present in the normal marrow. Indeed, TLI-induced spleen cells are capable of colony formation in vitro (78).

Thus, TLI may be regarded as a procedure that results in marked depletion of mature T cells by exposing the lymphoid system to fractionated radiation while shielding nonoverlapping bones with active marrow that serve as the source of uncommitted immunohemopoietic progenitor cells that are capable of acquiring tolerance to new protein antigens or neoalloantigens. In this respect, TLI mimics the immature, tolerance-susceptible fetal or neonatal immune system. Indeed, cells with characteristics similar to those described following TLI can be documented in fetal liver, neonatal spleen, and spleen of nude mice, as well as in the marrow of normal mice (74).

The overall effects of TLI on the immune system can be viewed as the result of a combination of at least four interrelated mechanisms: (1) interphase death of the pool of unprimed radiosensitive lymphocytes by direct lymphocytotoxic effects of ionizing irradiation; (2) emergence of large immature stem-cell-derived non-T suppressor cells capable of potent suppression of in vitro and possibly in vivo cell-mediated immune responses during the process of recovery from TLI; (3) altered processing of immunocompetent cells in the microenvironment of peripheral lymphoid organs (thymus, lymph nodes, and spleen) following radiotherapy; and (4) formation of a transient phase in which a stable state of specific unresponsiveness may be induced, similar to the neonatal period, through an unknown mechanism, most likely facilitated by donor BM cells.

The size of the radiation field seems to play a major role. In rodents, exposure of a wide field including the whole abdomen seems to be an important prerequisite (71). Likewise, whereas permanent transplantation tolerance to perfused organ allografts cannot be established in dogs, pigs, primates, and humans exposed to low (6 Gy) or high (up to 40 Gy) total cumulative doses of TLI using the classical "mantle" and "inverted Y" ports (73), permanent survival of renal and hepatic allografts were reported following low-dose TLI (6-8 Gy) using a wide port of radiation including the whole torso and excluding the skull, limbs, and lungs (79).

The feasibility of clinical application of low-dose TLI in combination with other immunosuppressive modalities for transplantation of perfused organ allografts was investigated using small and large outbred animal models (80-83) as well as in patients at high risk for rejection of a renal allograft (84,85).

In comparing the results of this group with those of a similar group of patients treated with conventional immunosuppression at 1, 2, and 3 years after retransplantation, patient survival was slightly better in the TLI-treated group. Graft survival was significantly superior in the TLI-treated group compared with patients treated with conventional immunosuppression.

The use of a combination of TLI and CY-A in clinical renal transplantation is currently being investigated in a number of centers (86-89).

In clinical bone marrow transplantation, TLI was used either as a single fraction to reduce the morbidity associated with total body irradiation or as small multiple daily fractions as originally described in experimental animals (73).

Single-dose TLI is now routinely used for successful prevention of rejection in multiply transfused patients with severe aplastic anemia (90). Although rejection is a major problem in up to 60% of similar patients conditioned by cytoxan (CTX) (200 mg/kg) alone, 39 out of 40 multiply transfused patients with severe aplastic anemia treated by one-dose of TLI of 7.5 Gy showed sustained engraftment. The use of fractionated TLI in clinical bone marrow transplantation was introduced in 1979 by Slavin et al. (91,92). The use of TLI in clinical bone marrow transplantation to prevent rejection of T-lymphocyte-depleted marrow allografts is also currently under investigation (93-96). The available data suggest that the immunosuppressive effects of TLI may be used as part of the conditioning regimen prior to allogeneic bone marrow transplantation to prevent late graft rejection that is enhanced by using T-cell depletion for prevention of GVHD in both malignant and nonmalignant disorders.

Due to the unique effects of TLI on the immune system, it was suggested that fractionated irradiation might be a rational form of therapy for selected patients with drug-resistant severe autoimmune disorders, as was indeed documented in several murine models of spontaneous systemic lupus erythrematosus-like disease (97,98). On the basis of these studies, TLI was administered to several groups of patients with intractable rheumatoid arthritis (99,100), drug-resistant systemic lupus erythematosus (SLE) (101), and multiple sclerosis (102), with some encouraging, although not yet unequivocal, pilot clinical results. Studies of peripheral blood lymphocytes after TLI in rheumatoid arthritis and SLE revealed marked reduction in the absolute number of T cells (Leu-4), to about one-third of the pretreatment number. This decrease was associated with more than fourfold reduction in the number of helper T cells (Leu-3) with only a slight reduction in the number of suppressor/cytotoxic T cells (Leu-2) (99,100). However, as expected from murine studies, the laboratory manifestations of autoimmunity persisted due to resistance of memory cells to TLI (73).

In summary, a vast amount of experimental data in animals and humans suggest that TLI may be used clinically alone or in conjunction with other immunosuppressive modalities, possibly for the treatment of selected drug-resistant autoimmune disorders but more likely to reduce the likelihood of rejection in recipients of marrow and organ allografts. It is very likely that induction of tolerance of host against perfused organ allografts could be improved by combining the effects of TLI with additional antilymphocyte agents such as monoclonal antilymphocyte antibodies, in order to deplete all the mature and committed lymphocyte reservoir in the host, allowing the newly developing immune system to acquire unresponsiveness to the alloantigens of the "new self"—the grafted organ.

C. Immune Functions in Recipients of High-Dose Whole Body Irradiation

1. Immune Functions Among Atomic Bomb Survivors

Data on the acute systemic effects of whole body exposure to ionizing radiation have been drawn primarily from animal experiments. LD_{50} values were determined in many species, while in humans most observations and extrapolations are based on data from Hiroshima and Nagasaki atomic bomb casualties, the accidental exposure of Marshall Islanders to fallout radiation in 1954, a limited number of nuclear plant accidents, and therapeutic exposures of patients with malignant disorders to whole body irradiation. It is generally accepted that the whole body $LD_{50\text{-}60}$ is around 4.5 Gy for acute exposure (103,104).

The immediate effects of whole body irradiation result mainly from cell death in critical organs such as bone marrow, the gastrointestinal tract, and the central nervous system. Long-term or delayed effects are thought to result from irreparable damage to DNA of cells that survive the radiation exposure. Such effects can be produced by lower doses or by lower dose rates than for acute effects.

The A-bomb survivors comprise the largest group of irradiated human beings. The major cause of late death in this population is malignant disorders. Acute leukemia appearing within a few years after irradiation and reaching a peak at 5-7 years was the most common malignancy (105,106). Recent reviews, however, indicate there was also elevated incidence of other malignancies, in lung, breast, and thyroid (107).

As reviewed in the previous section, local irradiation for malignant tumors of various organs results in marked derangements in the immune function. The effect of single-dose whole body irradiation on the immune system is therefore of general interest, and particularly in association with radiation-induced carcinogenesis. Nothing, however, can be inferred about the dose rate effect, since the survivors all received a single prompt exposure. Individuals located within 10,000 m of the hypocenter of the explosion, which includes a wide range of low-dose exposures, are considered A-bomb survivors.

Reports on the immune functions in atomic bomb survivors are rare. Akiyama et al. (108) studied the percentage of T cells and PHA responses in 1047 survivors during 1974-1977 (i.e., 30-33 years after exposure). Of these, 900 were apparently healthy without evidence of malignant tumors or chromosomal abnormalities. These individuals were presumably exposed to doses between 0 and 2 Gy or more. Decreased responsiveness to PHA was demonstrated years later and was more severe in "healthy" individuals with a chromosomal abnormality. Another study was conducted in a group of A-bomb survivors residing in the United States (109). This study probably represents a selected population that was exposed to very low doses (95% were exposed to less than 50 cGy). In this group of 189 survivors, natural cell-mediated cytotoxicity was significantly higher than in normal controls. Likewise, interferon production and responsiveness to PHA also tended to be higher.

This paradoxical increase in cell-mediated immunity following low-dose irradiation is extremely rare. It may be explained by abrogation of the normal negative feedback, mediated by suppressor cells that are extremely radiosensitive, as demonstrated in experimental animal models.

2. Immune Functions in Bone Marrow Transplant Recipients

Another group of patients exposed to lethal doses of whole body irradiation with chemotherapy for therapeutic purposes comprises bone marrow transplant recipients. Bone marrow transplantation is one of the most radical treatment modalities in modern medicine. It involves ablation of the patient's own lymphohemopoietic system to permit the engraftment of a new healthy (allogeneic or autologous) bone marrow that will substitute for the host's diseased or deficient hemopoietic stem cells. The impact of the procedure and the sequence of events that follow the interaction between the host and the recipient tissues on the host's new immune status are complex and can be strategically defined in three stages: (1) host reactivity against the grafted tissue, against which the ablative chemoradiotherapy of the conditioning regimen prior to transplant is directed; (2) graft reactivity against the recipient, resulting in graft-versus-host disease, against which posttransplantation immunosuppression is commonly used; and (3) prolonged immunoincompetence of the treated host, which results from both, with increased susceptibility to infections.

The immune system of the recipient is derived from the marrow cells of donor origin (110-112) either by passive transfer of donor lymphoid cells with the marrow inoculum or by cells of second ontogeny that differentiate from the donor's stem cells now repopulating the host hemopoietic and lymphoid system. Therefore, all the immunological parameters show pronounced impairment (113-116) due predominantly to immaturity in all types of transplants—allogeneic, syngeneic, and autologous (117-119)—for the first few months to a year following transplantation. These observations suggest that differences across minor histocompatibility loci do not seem to play a major role in the immune dysfunction observed in the posttransplantation period.

Although the number of circulating lymphocytes as well as the absolute number of T and B cells reach near-normal levels at about 3 months after transplantation, severely abnormal in vivo and in vitro functions of lymphoid subsets are the rule, accounting for the increased tendency to develop life-threatening infections.

Serum immunoglobin levels reach normal values within 3 months after marrow transplantation, yet the humoral response, both in vivo and in vitro, demonstrates marked impairment (119-126). Patients fail to produce antibodies in response to neoantigens KLH and bacteriophage X174 (122). These findings correlate with the in vitro observation of failure to respond to PWM (124-126) and to produce immunoglobulin in culture as measured by direct PFC assay (119-121,123). Healthy patients regain normal B cell function within a year after bone marrow transplantation, while patients with chronic GVHD continuously show decreased antibody production, although paradoxically they may have significantly higher immunoglobulin levels (121).

The failure of B cells to produce antibodies in vitro results not from a maturational defect within the B cell population, but rather from deficient helper or excessive suppressor function by T cells. The latter was confirmed by coculture experiments in which in vitro antibody production was assessed in the presence of T cell subsets, demonstrating a presence of radioresistant (activated) suppressor T cells (119,123,125,126). Interestingly, the same suppression was demonstrated in autologous transplants, again indicating that the development of activated suppressor cells occurs even in the absence of any histocompatibility differences. Since in allogeneic transplants the immune system in the recipients is of donor origin, one might speculate that the absence of helper activity is caused by failure of proper differentiation in an adult host environment lacking an intact thymus or other environmental factors or milieu required for proper T cell maturation. Under these circumstances, high-dose whole body irradiation (and/or high-dose chemotherapy) may play an essential role in the posttransplant immune dysfunction through damage to the lymphoid stroma, which may be important for maturation of immunocompetent cells or for cell-to-cell interactions. Alternatively, one might speculate that what seems to be an initial defect in the various lymphoid subsets is merely a reflection of the normal developmental stages that occur in the new reconstituting immune system of the host: during its expansion, various normal maturational stages are transiently expressed as they are during normal ontogeny, exhibiting different activational states within a specific subset. Thus suppressor activity may represent a more primitive function, appearing earlier in the ontogeny of the reconstituting immune system than the more mature helper activity, accounting for overall suppressed immune functions.

Impaired T cell functions, the primary cause of the high incidence of life-threatening infections in patients undergoing marrow grafting, can be demonstrated in vivo by absent skin reactivity to recall antigens such as candida, mumps, PPD, or neoantigens such as KLH or DNCB (122). The number of circulating T lymphocytes remains lower than usual for several months. Significant imbalance in the various subsets of T cells was demonstrated with the use of monoclonal antibodies (127-129). During the early posttransplantation period there is a rapid recovery of immature or activated suppressor T cells, while the helper/inducer subset is markedly depleted for a year or more, resulting in an abnormally low helper/suppressor ratio (125,126,130,131). This excess of T suppressors may explain in part the reduced immunoglobulin production in vitro by B cells mentioned earlier (119,120,124).

The in vitro proliferative responses of T cells to various mitogens (PHA, ConA), alloantigens (MLR), and cell-mediated lympholysis (CML) are also impaired (132, 133). The proliferation of T cells in response to antigen-presenting cells (such as macrophages pulsed with *E. coli*) is also decreased (134). Production of interleukin-2 (IL-2) is also severely impaired, and this may be a key defect in explaining T cell dysfunctions (135). Patients who do not develop chronic GVHD regain near-normal T cell subset number and function near the end of the first year after transplantation.

Interestingly, memory T cells are relatively radioresistant even to supralethal doses of whole body irradiation and chemotherapy. Supralethally irradiated recipients (⩾15 Gy) are still capable of rejecting MHC mismatched marrow allografts, or even HLA-matched, T-lymphocyte-depleted marrow allografts. Residual host T lymphocytes can also be documented by cloning residual host T cells, following supralethal conditioning in the presence of IL-2. All the above suggests that certain T cell subsets are extremely radioresistant.

In summary, although most cells of the immune system are radiosensitive and therefore completely ablated during pretransplantation conditioning with radiochemotherapy, certain potentially alloreactive T cells capable of inducing graft rejection are relatively radioresistant. Allogeneic, syngeneic, and autologous bone marrow recipients demonstrate severe derangements in all immunological parameters during the first year after marrow transplantation. These immune dysfunctions, however, do not reflect impairment of the host immune system due to chemoradiotherapy, but rather represent the outcome of regeneration of donor-type immunity in a microenvironment that was exposed to supralethal chemotherapy or radiotherapy. To what extent the lack of an intact thymic microenvironment capable of maturing stem cells into functioning T cells affects the degree and tempo of these maturational processes is not clear.

REFERENCES

1. Hall, E. J. *Radiobiology for the radiologist.* Harper & Row, New York (1973).
2. Evans, R. G., Donaldson, S. S. Principles of radiation biology and radiation therapy. In: *Cancer in the young.* Levine, A. S. (Ed.). Masson, pp. 257-282 (1982).
3. Puck, T. T., Markus, P. I. Action of X rays on mammalian cells. *J. Exp. Med. 103,* 653-666 (1956).
4. Elkind, M. M., Sutton, H. Radiation response of mammalian cells grown in culture. I. Repair of X-ray damage in surviving Chinese hamster cells. *Radiat. Res. 13,* 556-593 (1960).
5. Wheldon, T. E., Michalowski, A. S., Kirk, J. The effect of irradiation on function in self-renewing normal tissues with differing proliferative organisation. *Brit. J. Radiol. 55,* 759-766 (1982).
6. Withers, H. R. Biologic basis for altered fractionation schemes. *Cancer 55,* 2086-2095 (1985).
7. Paul, W. E. (Ed.). *Fundamental immunology.* Raven, New York, pp. 43-109 (1984).
8. Anderson, R. E., Warner, N. L. Ionizing radiation and the immune response. In: *Advances in immunology*, Vol. 24. Dixon, F. J., Kunkel, A. G. (Eds.). Academic, New York, pp. 216-320 (1976).
9. Anderson, R. E., Standefer, J. C., Tokuda, S. The structural and functional assessment of cytotoxic injury of the immune system with particular reference to the effects of ionizing radiation and cyclophosphamide. *Brit. J. Cancer 53* (*Suppl. VII*), 140-160 (1986).
10. Schrek, R. Qualitative and quantitative reactions of lymphocytes to X-rays. *Ann. N.Y. Acad. Sci. 95,* 839-848 (1961).
11. Jordan, S. W. Ultrastructural studies of spleen after whole body irradiation of mice. *Exp. Mol. Pathol. 6,* 156-171 (1967).
12. Anderson, R. E., Williams, W. L. Radiosensitivity of T and B lymphocytes vs effects of whole body irradiation on numbers of recirculating T cells and sensitization to primary skin grafts in mice. *Amer. J. Pathol. 89,* 367-378 (1977).
13. Anderson, R. E., Olson, G. B., Autry, J. R., Howarth, J. L., Troup, G. M., Bartels, P. H. Radiosensitivity of T and B lymphocytes. IV. Effect of whole body irradiation upon various lymphoid tissues and numbers of recirculating lymphocytes. *J. Immunol. 118,* 1191-1200 (1977).
14. Anderson, R. E., Lefkovits, I. Effects of irradiation on the in vitro immune response. *Exp. Cell Biol. 48,* 255-278 (1980).
15. Denham, S., Grant, C. K., Hall, J. G., Alexander, P. The occurrence of two types of cytotoxic lymphoid cells in mice immunised with allogeneic tumour cells. *Transplantation 9,* 366-382 (1970).
16. Janeway, C. A. Cellular cooperation during in vivo antihapten antibody responses. II. The effect of in vivo and in vitro x-irradiation on T and B cells. *J. Immunol. 114,* 1402-1407 (1975).

17. Ito, T., Cudkowicz, G. Sensitivity to radiation and insensitivity to vinblastine of the inducer function of thymus-derived cells. *Cell Immunol. 2,* 595-601 (1972).
18. Sprent, J., Anderson, R. E., Miller, J. F. A. P. Radiosensitivity of T and B lymphocytes; II. Effect of irradiation on response to T cells to alloantigens. *Eur. J. Immunol. 4,* 204-210 (1974).
19. Durkin, H. G., Thorbecke, G. J. Preferential destruction of germinal centers by prednisolone and X-irradiation. *Lab. Invest. 26,* 53-62 (1972).
20. Trowell, O. A. Radiosensitivity of the cortical and medullary lymphocytes in the thymus. *Int. J. Radiol. Biol. 4,* 163-173 (1961).
21. Kataoka, Y., Sato, T. The radiosensitivity of T and B lymphocytes in mice. *Immunology 29,* 121-130 (1975).
22. Tokada, A., Tokada, Y., Huang, C., Ambrus, J. L. Biphasic pattern of thymus regeneration after whole body irradiation. *J. Exp. Med. 129,* 445 (1969).
23. Dixon, F. J., McConahey, P. J. Enhancement of antibody formation by whole body X-radiation. *J. Exp. Med. 117,* 833-847 (1963).
24. Taliaferro, W. H., Taliaferro, L. G. Effects of irradiation on initial and anamnestic hemolysin responses in rabbits; antigen injection before x-rays. *J. Immunol. 104,* 1364-1376 (1970).
25. Salvin, S. B., Smith, R. F. Delayed hypersensitivity in the development of circulating antibody. The effect of X-irradiation. *J. Exp. Med. 109,* 325-338 (1959).
26. Uhr, J. W., Scharff, M. Delayed hypersensitivity. The effect of X-irradiation on the development of delayed hypersensitivity and antibody formation. *J. Exp. Med. 112,* 65-75 (1960).
27. Biggar, W. D., Meuwissen, H. J., Good, R. A. Effect of in vitro irradiation of cells in graft-versus-host reaction. *Proc. Soc. Exp. Biol. Med. 137,* 1274-1277 (1971).
28. Tyan, M. L., Cole, L. J. Differential response to allogeneic and xenogenic skin grafts by sublethally irradiated (670 rad) and non-irradiated mice sensitized by various means. *J. Immunol. 91,* 396-402 (1963).
29. Nossal, G. J. V., Pike, B. L. Evidence for the clonal aberration theory of B-lymphocyte tolerance. *J. Exp. Med. 141,* 904-917 (1975).
30. Klein, G. Immune and non-immune control of neoplastic development: contrasting effects of host and tumor evolution. *Cancer 45,* 2486-2499 (1980).
31. Penn, I., Starzl, T. E. Malignant tumors arising de novo in immunosuppressed organ transplant recipients. *Transplantation 14,* 407-417 (1972).
32. Sharma, B., Terasaki, P. I. Immunization of lymphocytes from cancer patients. *J. Natl. Cancer. Inst. 52,* 1925-1926 (1974).
33. Ducos, J., Migueres, J., Colorabies, P., Kessoos, K., Poujoulet, N. Lymphocyte response to PHA in patients with lung cancer. *Lancet i,* 1111-1112 (1970).
34. Han, T., Takita, H. Immunological impairment in bronchogenic carcinoma: a study of lymphocyte response to phytohemagglutinin. *Cancer 30,* 616-620 (1972).

35. Lauder, I., Bone, G. Lymphocyte transformation in large bowel cancer. *Brit. J. Cancer 27,* 409-414 (1973).
36. Lichtenstein, A., Zighelboim, J., Dorey, F., Brossman, S., Fahey, J. L. Comparison of immune derangements in patients with different malignancies. *Cancer 45,* 2090-2095 (1980).
37. Catalona, W. J., Chretien, P. B. Abnormalities of quantitative dinitrochlorobenzene sensitization in cancer patients: correlation with tumor stage and histology. *Cancer 31,* 353-356 (1973).
38. Chretien, P. B., Twomey, P. L., Trahan, E. G., Catalona, W. J. Quantitative dinitrochlorobenzene contact sensitivity in preoperative and cured cancer patients. *Natl. Cancer. Inst. Mon. 39,* 263-266 (1973).
39. Millard, R. E. Effect of previous irradiation on the transformation of blood lymphocytes. *J. Clin. Pathol. 18,* 783-785 (1965).
40. Meyer, K. K. Radiation-induced lymphocyte-immune deficiency. *Arch. Surg. 101,* 114-121 (1970).
41. McCredie, J. A., Inch, W. R., Sutherland, R. M. Effect of postoperative radiotherapy on peripheral blood lymphocytes in patients with carcinoma of the breast. *Cancer 29,* 349-356 (1972).
42. Stjernsward, J., Jondal, M., Vanky, F., Wigzell, H., Scaly, R. Lymphopenia and change in distribution of human B and T lymphocytes in peripheral blood induced by irradiation for mammary carcinoma. *Lancet i,* 1352-1356 (1972).
43. Cosimi, A. B., Brunstetter, F. H., Kemmerer, W. T., Miller, B. N. Cellular immune competence of breast cancer patients receiving radiotherapy. *Arch. Surg. 107,* 531-535 (1973).
44. Jenkins, V. K., Olson, M. H., Ellis, H. N., Dillard, E. A. In-vitro lymphocyte response of patients with uterine cancer as related to clinical stage and radiotherapy. *Gynecol. Oncol. 3,* 191-200 (1975).
45. Stratton, J. A., Byfield, P. E., Byfield, J. E., Small, R. C., Benfield, J., Pilch, Y. A. Comparison of the acute effects of radiation therapy including or excluding the thymus on the lymphocyte subpopulations of cancer patients. *J. Clin. Invest. 56,* 88-97 (1975).
46. Tarpley, J. L., Potvin, C., Chretien, P. B. Prolonged depression of cellular immunity in cured laryngopharyngeal cancer patients treated with radiation therapy. *Cancer 35,* 638-644 (1975).
47. Heier, H. E., Christensen, I., Froland, S. S., Engeset, A. Early and late effects of irradiation for seminoma testis on the number of blood lymphocytes and their B and T subpopulations. *Lymphology 8,* 69-74 (1975).
48. Yamagata, S., Green, G. H. Radiation-induced immune changes in patients with cancer of the cervix. *Brit. J. Obstet. Gynecol. 83,* 400-408 (1976).
49. Raben, M., Walach, N., Galili, U., Schlesinger, M. The effect of radiation therapy on lymphocyte subpopulation in cancer patients. *Cancer 37,* 1417-1421 (1976).
50. Petrini, B., Wasserman, J., Blomgren, H., Baral, E. Blood lymphocyte subpopulations in breast cancer patients following radiotherapy. *Clin. Exp. Immunol. 29,* 36-42 (1977).

51. Rand, R. J., Jenkins, D. M., Bulmer, R. T- and B-lymphocyte subpopulations following radiotherapy for invasive cell carcinoma of the uterine cervix. *Clin. Exp. Immunol. 33,* 159-165 (1978).
52. Hancock, B. W., Bruce, L., Heath, J., Sugden, P., Ward, A. M. Effects of radiotherapy on immunity in patients with localized carcinoma of the cervix uteri. *Cancer 43,* 118-123 (1979).
53. Wood, S. E., Campbell, J. B., Anderson, J. M., Kelly, F. Lymphocyte response after radiotherapy. *Lancet i,* 863 (1974).
54. Campbell, A. C., Wiernik, G., Wood, J., Hersey, P., Walker, C. A., Maclennan, I. C. M. Characteristics of the lymphopenia induced by radiotherapy. *Clin. Exp. Immunol. 23,* 200-208 (1976).
55. Stefani, S., Kerman, R., Abbate, J. Immune evaluation of lung cancer patients undergoing radiation therapy. *Cancer 37,* 2792-2796 (1976).
56. Onsrud, M., Thorsby, E. Long-term changes in natural killer activity after external pelvic radiotherapy. *Int. J. Radiat. Oncol. Biol. Phys. 7,* 609-614 (1981).
57. Thomas, J. M., Coy, P., Lewis, H. S., Yuen, A. The effect of therapeutic irradiation on lymphocyte transformation in lung cancer. *Cancer 27,* 1046-1050 (1971).
58. Catalona, W. J., Sample, W. F., Chretien, P. B. Lymphocyte reactivity in cancer patients; correlation with tumor histology and clinical stage. *Cancer 31,* 65-71 (1973).
59. Blomgren, H., Wasserman, J., Littbrand, B. Blood lymphocytes after radiation therapy of carcinoma of the prostatic gland or urinary bladder. *Acta Radiol. (Ther.) 13,* 357-367 (1974).
60. Chee, C. A., Ilbery, P. L. T., Rickinson, A. B. Depression of lymphocyte replicating ability in radiotherapy patients. *Brit. J. Radiol. 47,* 37-43 (1974).
61. Ghossein, N. A., Bosworth, J. L., Bases, R. E. The effect of radical radiotherapy on delayed hypersensitivity and the inflammatory response. *Cancer 35,* 1616-1620 (1975).
62. Stein, J. A., Adler, A., Ben Efraim, S., Maor, M. Immunocompetence, immunosuppression, and human breast cancer. I. An analysis of their relationship by known parameters of cell-mediated immunity in well-defined clinical stages of disease. *Cancer 38,* 1171-1187 (1976).
63. Hancock, B. W., Bruce, L., Whitham, M. D., Ward, A. M. The effects of radiotherapy on immunity in patients with cured localized carcinoma of the cervix uteri. *Cancer 53,* 884-887 (1984).
64. Blomgren, H., Berg, R., Wasserman, J., Glas, U. Effect of radiotherapy on blood lymphocyte population in mammary carcinoma. *Int. J. Radiat. Oncol. Biol. Phys. 1,* 177-188 (1976).
65. Haim, N., Rudik, L., Samuelly, B., Mekori, T., Robinson, E. Immune status in patients cured of breast and gynecological cancer. *Clin. Oncol. 7,* 141-147 (1981).
66. Ilbery, P. L. T., Rickinson, A. B., Thrum, C. E. Blood lymphocyte replicating ability as a measurement of radiation dosage. *Brit. J. Radiol. 44,* 834-840 (1971).

67. Court-Brown, W. M., Bucton, K. E., McLean, A. S. Quantitative studies of chromosome aberrations in man following acute and chronic exposure to X-rays and gamma-rays. *Lancet i,* 1239-1241 (1965).
68. Fuks, Z., Strober, S., Bobrove, A. M., Sasazuki, T., McMichael, A., Kaplan, H. S. Longterm effects of radiation of T and B lymphocytes in the peripheral blood of patients with Hodgkin's disease. *J. Clin. Invest. 58,* 803-814 (1976).
69. Slavin, S., Strober, S., Fuks, Z., Kaplan, H. S. Longterm survival of skin allografts in mice treated with fractionated total lymphoid irradiation. *Science 193,* 1252-1254 (1976).
70. Slavin, S., Strober, S., Fuks, Z., Kaplan, H. S. Use of total lymphoid irradiation in tissue transplantation in mice. *Transplant. Proc. 9,* 1001-1004 (1977).
71. Slavin, S., Reitz, B., Bieber, C. P., Kaplan, H. S., Strober, S. Transplantation tolerance in adult rats using total lymphoid irradiation (TLI): Permanent survival of skin, heart and marrow allografts. *J. Exp. Med. 147,* 700-707 (1978).
72. ZanBar, I., Slavin, S., Strober, S. Induction and mechanism of tolerance to bovine serum albumin after total lymphoid irradiation (TLI). *J. Immunol. 121,* 1400-1404 (1978).
73. Slavin, S., Weiss, L., Morecki, S., Weigensberg, M., Fuks, Z. Immunosuppression and induction of transplantation tolerance by fractionated total lymphoid irradiation. In: *Tolerance in bone marrow and organ transplantation.* Slavin, S. (Ed.). Elsevier, Amsterdam, pp. 105-153 (1984).
74. Weigensberg, M., Morecki, S., Weiss, L., Fuks, Z., Slavin, S. Suppression of cell mediated immune responses following total lymphoid irradiation (TLI). 1. Characterization of suppressor cell of the mixed lymphocyte reaction. *J. Immunol. 132,* 971-978 (1984).
75. Morecki, S., Weigensberg, M., Slavin, S. Lectin separation of nonlymphoid suppressor cells induced by total lymphoid irradiation. *Eur. J. Immunol. 15,* 138-148 (1985).
76. May, R. D., Slavin, S., Vitetta, E. S. A partial characterization of suppressor cells in the spleens of mice conditioned with fractionated total lymphoid irradiation (TLI). *J. Immunol. 131,* 1108-1114 (1983).
77. Strober, S., Slavin, S., Gottlieb, M., ZanBar, I., King, D., Hoppe, R. T., Fuks, Z., Grument, F. C., Kaplan, H. S. Allograft tolerance after total lymphoid irradiation (TLI). *Immunol. Rev. 46,* 87-112 (1979).
78. Slavin, S., Seidel, H. J. Hematopoietic activity in bone marrow chimeras prepared with total lymphoid irradiation (TLI). *Exp. Hematol. 10,* 206-216 (1982).
79. Myburgh, J. A., Smit, J. A., Browde, S. Total lymphoid irradiation in vascularized organ allotransplantation in primates. In: *Tolerance in bone marrow and organ transplantation.* Slavin, S. (Ed.). Elsevier, Amsterdam, pp. 153-166 (1984).
80. Rynasiewicz, J. J., Sutherland, D. E. R., Kawahara, K., Najarian, J. S. Total lymphoid irradiation: Critical timing and combination with cyclosporine A for immunosuppression in a rat heart allograft model. *J. Surg. Res. 30,* 365-371 (1981).
81. Koretz, S. H., Gottlieb, M. S., Strober, S., Pennock, J., Bieber, C. P., Hoppe, R. T., Reitz, B. A., Kaplan, H. S. Organ transplantation in mongrel dogs using total lymphoid irradiation (TLI). *Transplant. Proc. 13,* 443-445 (1981).

82. Bieber, C. P., Jamieson, S., Raney, A., Burton, N., Bogarty, S., Hoppe, R., Kaplan, H. S., Strober, S., Stinson, E. B. Cardiac allograft survival in rhesus primates treated with combined total lymphoid irradiation and rabbit antithymocyte globulin. *Transplantation 28,* 347-350 (1979).
83. Pennock, J. L., Reitz, B. A., Bieber, C. P., Aziz, S., Oyer, P. E., Strober, S., Hoppe, R., Kaplan, H. S., Stinson, E. B., Shumway, N. E. Survival of primates following orthotopic cardiac transplantation treated with total lymphoid irradiation and chemical immune suppression. *Transplantation 32,* 467-473 (1981).
84. Najarian, J. S., Sutherland, D. E. R., Ferguson, R. M., Simmons, R. L., Kersey, J., Mauer, S. M., Slavin, S., Kim, T. H. Total lymphoic irradiation and kidney transplantation: A clinical experience. *Transplant. Proc. 13,* 417-424 (1981).
85. Sutherland, D. E. R., Ferguson, R. M., Rynasiewicz, J. J., Kim, T. H., Fryd, D. S., Dhein, B., Slavin, S., Simmons, R. L., Najarian, J. S. Total lymphoid irradiation vs cyclosporin for retransplantation in recipients at high risk to reject renal allografts. *Transplant. Proc. 15,* 460-464 (1983).
86. Cortesini, R. Personal communication.
87. Sampson, D., Levin, B. S., Hoppe, R. T., Bieber, C. P., Miller, E., Waer, M., Kaplan, H. S., Collins, G., Strober, S. Preliminary observations on the use of total lymphoid irradiation, rabbit antithymocyte globulin, and low-dose prednisone in human cadaver renal transplantation. *Transplant. Proc. 17,* 1299-1303 (1985).
88. Strober, S., Collin, G. Personal communication.
89. Waer, M., Vanrenterghem, Y. Personal communication.
90. Ramsay, N. K. C., Kersey, J. H. Conditioning of bone marrow recipients with cyclophosphamide and total lymphoid irradiation. In: *Tolerance in bone marrow and organ transplantation.* Slavin, S. (Ed.). Elsevier, Amsterdam, pp. 167-174 (1984).
91. Slavin, S., Naparstek, E., Weshler, Z., Brautbar, C., Rachmilewitz, E. A., Fuks, Z. Bone marrow transplantation for severe aplastic anemia in HLA-identical siblings using total lymphoid irradication (TLI) and cyclophosphamide. *Transplant. Proc. 15,* 668-670 (1983).
92. Slavin, S., Naparstek, E., Weshler, Z., Fuks, Z. Total lymphoid irradiation (TLI) as part of the conditioning regimen for allogeneic bone marrow transplantation in severe aplastic anemia. In: *Recent advances in bone marrow transplantation,* Vol. 7. Gale, R. P. (Ed.). UCLA Symposia on Molecular and Cellular Biology. Alan R. Liss, New York, pp. 21-27 (1983).
93. Slavin, S., Waldmann, H., Or, R., Cividalli, G., Naparstek, E., SteinerSalz, D., Michaeli, J., Galun, E., Weiss, L., Samuel, S., Morecki, S., Bar, S., Brautbar, C., Weshler, Z., Hale, G., Rachmilewitz, E. A., Reisner, Y. Prevention of graft vs host disease in allogeneic bone marrow transplantation for leukemia by T cell depletion in vitro prior to transplantation. *Transplant. Proc. 17,* 465-467 (1985).
94. Waldmann, H., Polliack, A., Hale, G., Or, R., Cividalli, G., Weiss, L., Weshler, Z., Samuel, S., Manor, D., Brautbar, C., Rachmilewitz, E. A., Slavin, S. Elimination of graft versus host disease by in vitro depletion of alloreactive lymphocytes with a monoclonal rat antihuman lymphocyte antibody (CAMPATH1). *Lancet 2,* 483-485 (1984).

95. Slavin, S., Or, R., Weshler, Z., Fuks, Z., Morecki, S., Weigensberg, M., Bar, S., Weiss, L. The use of total lymphoid irradiation for allogeneic bone marrow transplantation in animals and man. *Survey Immunol. Res. 4,* 283-252 (1985).
96. Slavin, S., Or, R., Naparstek, E., Cividalli, G., Weshler, Z., Weiss, L., Mumcuoglu, M., Engelhard, D., Aker, M., Pollack, A., BenYehuda, A., Brautbar, C., Hale, G., Waldmann, H. New approaches for prevention of rejection and graft vs host disease (GVHD) in clinical bone marrow transplantation (BMT). *Israel J. Med. Sci. 22,* 264-267 (1986).
97. Slavin, S. Successful treatment of autoimmune disease in (NZB/NZW)F1 female mice by using fractionated total lymphoid irradiation. *Proc. Natl. Acad. Sci. USA 76,* 5274-5276 (1979).
98. Kotzin, B. L., Strober, S. Reversal of NZB/NZW disease with total lymphoid irradiation. *J. Exp. Med. 150,* 371-378 (1979).
99. Kotzin, B. L., Strober, S., Engelman, E. G., Calin, A., Hoppe, R. T., Kansas, G. S., Terrel, C. P., Kaplan, H. S. Treatment of intractable rheumatoid arthritis with total lymphoid irradiation. *New Engl. J. Med. 305,* 969-976 (1981).
100. Trentham, D. E., Belli, J. A., Anderson, R. I., Buckley, J. A., Goetzl, E. J., David, J. R., Austen, K. F. Clinical and immunologic effects of fractionated total lymphoid irradiation in refractory rheumatoid arthritis. *New Engl. J. Med. 305,* 976-982 (1981).
101. BenChetrit, E., Gross, D. J., Braverman, A., Weshler, Z., Fuks, Z., Slavin, S., Eliakim, M. Total lymphoid irradiation therapy in refractory systemic lupus erythematosus. *Ann. Intern. Med. 105,* 58-60 (1986).
102. Devereux, C. Personal communication.
103. Leaf, A. New perspectives on the medical consequences of nuclear war. *New Engl. J. Med. 315,* 905-912 (1986).
104. Kohn, H. I., Fry, M. R. J. Medical carcinogenesis. *New Engl. J. Med. 310,* 504-511 (1984).
105. Beebe, G. W., Kato, H., Land, C. E. Mortality experience of atomic bomb survivors 1950-1974. *Radiat. Res. 75,* 138-201 (1978).
106. Kato, H., Schull, W. J. Studies of the mortality of A-bomb survivors. Report 7. Mortality 1950-1978. Part I. Cancer mortality. *Radiat. Res. 90,* 395-432 (1982).
107. Wakabayashi, T., Kato, H., Ikeda, T., Shull, W. J. Studies of the mortality of A-bomb survivors. Report 7. Part III. Incidence of cancer in 1959-1978, based on the Tumor Registry, Nagasaki. *Radiat. Res. 93,* 112-146 (1983).
108. Akiyama, M., Yamakido, M., Kobuke, K., Dock, D. S., Hamilton, H. B., Awa, A. A., Kato, H. Peripheral lymphocyte response to PHA and T cell population among atomic bomb survivors. *Radiat. Res. 93,* 572-580 (1983).
109. Bloom, E. T., Korn, E. L., Tagasugi, M., Toji, D. S., Onari, K., Makinodan, T. Immune function in aging atomic bomb survivors residing in the USA. *Radiat. Res. 96,* 399-410 (1983).
110. Herzenberg, L. A., Cole, L. J. Presence of donor specific gammaglobulins in sera of allogeneic mouse radiation chimeras. *Nature 202,* 352-353 (1964).

111. Witherspoon, R. P., Schanfield, M. S., Storb, R., Thomas, E. D., Giblett, E. R. Immunoglobulin production of donor origin after marrow transplantation for acute leukemia or aplastic anemia. *Transplantation 26,* 407-408 (1978).
112. Lum, L. G., Munn, N. A., Schanfield, M. S., Storb, R. The detection of specific antibody formation to recall antigens after human bone marrow transplantation. *Blood 67,* 582-587 (1986).
113. Elfenbein, G. J., Anderson, P. N., Humphrey, R. L., Mullins, G. M., Sensenbrenner, L. L., Sands, J. R., Santos, G. W. Immune system reconstitution following allogeneic bone marrow transplantation in man: a multiparameter analysis. *Transplant. Proc. 8,* 641-646 (1976).
114. Noel, D. R., Witherspoon, R. P., Storb, R., Atkinson, K., Doney, K., Mickelson, E. M., Ochs, H. D., Warren, R. P., Weiden, P. L., Thomas, E. D. Does graft-versus-host disease influence the tempo of immunologic recovery after allogeneic human marrow transplantation? An observation on 56 long-term survivors. *Blood 51,* 1087-1105 (1978).
115. Gale, R. P., Opelz, G., Mickey, M. R., Graze, P. R., Saxon, A. Immunodeficiency following allogeneic bone marrow transplantation. *Transplant. Proc. 10,* 223-227 (1978).
116. Witherspoon, R. P., Lum, L. G., Storb, R. Immunologic reconstitution after human marrow grafting. *Semin. Hematol. 21,* 2-10 (1984).
117. Shiobara, S., Harada, M., Mori, T., Kodo, H., Ishino, C., Matsue, K., Odaka, K., Kondo, K., Hattori, K. Difference in posttransplant recovery of immune reactivity between allogeneic and autologous bone marrow transplantation. *Transplant. Proc. 14,* 429-433 (1982).
118. Witherspoon, R. P., Kopecky, K., Storb, R. F., Flournoy, N., Sullivan, K. M., Sosa, R., Deeg, H. J., Ochs, H. P., Cheever, M. A., Fefer, A., Thomas, E. D. Immunological recovery in 48 patients following syngeneic marrow transplantation for hematological malignancy. *Transplantation 33,* 143-149 (1982).
119. Korsmeyer, S. J., Elfenbein, G. J., Goldman, C. K., Marshall, S. L., Santos, G. W., Waldmann, T. A. B cell, helper T cell, and suppressor T cell abnormalities contribute to disordered immunoglobulin synthesis in patients following bone marrow transplantation. *Transplanation 33,* 184-190 (1982).
120. Ringden, O., Witherspoon, R., Storb, R., Ekelund, E., Thomas, E. D. B cell function in human marrow transplant recipients assessed by direct and indirect hemolysis-in-gel assays. *J. Immunol. 123,* 2729-2734 (1979).
121. Ringden, O., Witherspoon, R. P., Storb, R., Ekelund, E., Thomas. E. D. Increased in vitro B-cell IgG secretion during acute graft-versus-host disease and infection; observations in 50 human marrow transplant recipients. *Blood 55,* 179-186 (1980).
122. Witherspoon, R. P., Storb, R., Ochs, H. D., Flournoy, N., Kopecky, K. J., Sullivan, K. M., Deeg, H. J., Sosa, R., Noel, D. R., Atkinson, K., Thomas, E. D. Recovery of antibody production in human allogeneic marrow graft recipients: influence of time posttransplantation, the presence or absence of chronic graft-versus-host disease, and antithymocyte globulin treatment. *Blood 58,* 360-368 (1981).

123. Lum, L. G., Seigneuret, M. C., Storb, R. F.,Witherspoon, R. P., Thomas, E. D. In vitro regulation of immunoglobulin synthesis after marrow transplantation. I. T-cell and B-cell deficiencies in patients with and without chronic graft-versus-host disease. *Blood 58,* 431-439 (1981).
124. Witherspoon, R. P., Lum, L. G., Storb, R., Thomas, E. D. In vitro regulation of immunoglobulin synthesis after human marrow transplantation. II. Deficient T and non-T lymphocyte function within 3-4 months of allogeneic, syngeneic or autologous marrow grafting for hematologic malignancy. *Blood 59,* 844-849 (1982).
125. Lum, L. G., Seigneuret, M. C., Orcutt-Thordarson, N., Noges, J. E., Storb, R. The regulation of immunoglobulin synthesis after HLA-identical bone marrow transplantation. VI. Differential rates of maturation of distinct functional groups within lymphoid subpopulations in patients after human marrow grafting. *Blood 65,* 1422-1433 (1985).
126. Witherspoon, R. P., Goehle, S., Kretschmer, M., Storb, R. Regulation of immunoglobulin production after human marrow grafting. *Transplantation 41,* 328-335 (1986).
127. de Bruin, H. G., Astaldi, A., Leupers, T., van de Griend, R. J., Dooren, L. J., Schellekens, P. T. A., Tanke, H. J., Roos, M., Vossen, J. M. T lymphocyte characteristics in bone marrow-transplanted patients. II. Analysis with monoclonal antibodies. *J. Immunol. 127,* 244-251 (1981).
128. Friedrich, W., O'Reilly, R. J., Koziner, B., Gebhard, D. F., Good, R. A., Evans, R. L. T-lymphocyte reconstitution in recipients of bone marrow transplants with and without GVHD: Imbalances of T-cell subpopulations having unique regulatory and cognitive functions. *Blood 59,* 696-701 (1982).
129. Schroff, R. W., Gale, R. P., Fahey, J. L. Regeneration of T cell subpopulations after bone marrow transplantation: cytomegalovirus infection and lymphoid subset imbalance. *J. Immunol. 129,* 1926-1930 (1982).
130. Atkinson, K., Hansen, J. A., Storb, R., Goehle, S., Goldstein, G., Thomas, E. D. T-cell subpopulations identified by monoclonal antibodies after human marrow transplantation. I. Helper-inducer and cytotoxic-suppressor subsets. *Blood 59,* 1292-1298 (1982).
131. Forman, S. J., Noecker, P., Gallagher, M., Zaia, J., Wright, C., Bolen, J., Mills, B., Hecht, T. Pattern of T cell reconstitution following allogeneic bone marrow transplantation for acute hematological malignancy. *Transplantation 34,* 96-98 (1982).
132. Mori, T., Tsoi, M. S., Gillis, S., Santos, E., Thomas, E. D., Storb, R. Cellular interactions in marrow-grafted patients. I. Impairment of cell-mediated lympholysis associated with graft vs host disease and the effect of interleukin 2. *J. Immunol. 130,* 712-715 (1983).
133. Brkic, S., Tsoi, M. S., Mori, T., Lachman, L., Gillis, S., Thomas, E. D., Storb, R. Cellular interactions in marrow-grafted patients. *Transplantation 39,* 30-35 (1985).
134. Tsoi, M. S., Dobbs, S., Brkic, S., Ramberg, R., Thomas, E. D., Storb, R. Cellular interactions in marrow-grafted patients. II. Normal monocyte

antigen-presenting and defective T-cell-proliferative functions early after grafting and during chronic graft-versus-host disease. *Transplantation 37,* 556-561 (1984).

135. Azogui, O., Gluckman, E., Fradelizi, D. Inhibition of IL-2 production after human allogeneic bone marrow transplantation. *J. Immunol. 131,* 1205-1208 (1983).

10
Considerations of Long-Term Radiation Injury in Nonhemopoietic Tissues

JOLYON H. HENDRY
Paterson Institute for Cancer Research, Christie Hospital and Holt Radium Institute, Manchester, England

I. INTRODUCTION

Acute whole body doses resulting in long-term survival are limited to about 4-5 Gy if successful marrow transplantation is not performed, and the critical tissue at risk is the bone marrow. After doses approaching this limit, long-term somatic injury comprises cataracts, persistent but not permanent infertility in man, and temporary or permanent sterility in some women (1). If marrow transplantation is successful, the acute dose can be increased to about 7.5 Gy. The limiting tissue now becomes the lung, and the limiting effect is pneumonitis. Cataracts and infertility become more prevalent, and other long-term effects become apparent (2-4). The main additional nonhemopoietic somatic effects are restrictive and obstructive lung damage, and hormonal imbalances in children that result in retardation of sexual development and growth. There are also a few secondary malignancies and a few cases of leukoencephalopathy. However, the latter are associated with additional prophylactic treatments for CNS disease (5).

In this review the above main long-term effects of total-body irradiation (TBI) will be described, together with their production by other doses of local irradiation given in various radiotherapy treatments. The main emphasis is on dose-response relationships, the effects of changes in the pattern of dose delivery, i.e., dose rate and fractionation, and the interpretation of the effects in terms of target-cell populations using experimental data where needed. The most comprehensive data and knowledge for tissues under discussion concerns the response of the lung, and this is used as an example in methods described for calculating changes in isoeffective dose concomitant with changes in the pattern of dose delivery. In many cases, radiation treatments are combined with chemotherapy, and this confounds the interpretation of effects due to the separate agents. First, an introduction is given to the renewal rates of tissues and the radiobiology of their responses.

II. TISSUE RENEWAL

The time course of expression of injury depends primarily on the mode of cell death and the normal renewal characteristics of the tissue. These can be influenced by secondary effects such as infections or injury in other associated tissues. The rate of renewal is governed by the lifetime of mature cells, which may be short, as in the GI tract, the skin, and the testis (where the mature cells are constantly shed from a surface or into a lumen), or long, as in many internal organs where cells remain until their metabolic life is ended (e.g., the thyroid). In general, tissues with a rapid renewal of mature cells are known to be hierarchical in structure, and they comprise stem cells, proliferative maturing cells, and

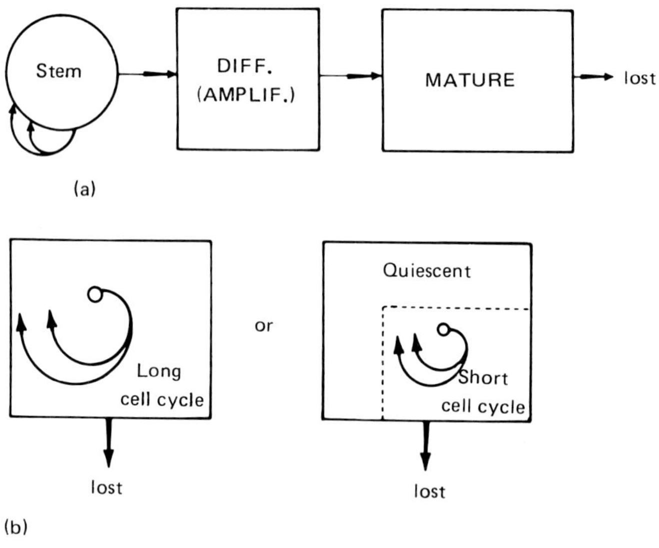

Figure 1 (a) Schematic representation of a hierarchical (type H) cell population, comprising stem cells, differentiating and proliferating transit cells which amplify cell production, and maturing and functionally mature cells. (b) Schematic representation of a flexible (type F) cell population, where either all functional cells are in a long cell cycle and occasionally divide, or the majority are quiescent with others in a short cell cycle. From Michalowski (6). (Reproduced with permission of Springer-Verlag and the author.)

nonproliferative mature cells (see Chapter 1). In contrast, tissues with a very slow renewal of mature cells but with the majority of functional cells capable of proliferation when stimulated are often termed "flexible" (6). Schematic representations of hierarchical and flexible tissues are shown in Figure 1. The ovary is in neither category, as the oocyte population is incapable of renewal and gradually declines from birth.

III. TEMPORAL EXPRESSION OF INJURY

The mode of cell death is another important consideration in the rate of expression of injury. Mitotic failure is the common form of cell death in tissues following radiotherapy or chemotherapy for both early- and late-responding tissues. This is apart from the particular cases of cell death not involving mitosis (interphase death) for lymphocytes, oocytes, salivary glands, and minority cell populations in other tissues. The first division of cells after acute doses up to about 6 Gy is relatively radioresistant, and the ability of cells to undergo further divisions is reduced in a dose-dependent manner. After doses above 6 Gy, it is generally considered (but not proved in vivo) that the ability of cells to divide is either retained or fully destroyed, the ratio depending on the dose.

In hierarchical tissues (e.g., spermatogenesis in this review) the maturing cells are radioresistant because they do not divide, and the sensitivity of the dividing maturing cells after low doses should be progressively greater depending on their proliferative potential. The characteristics of response of hierarchical tissues are shown in Figure 2. Injury is expressed at a rate governed by the lifetime of the mature cells and their lack of replacement by divisions of precursor cells. After high doses all mature cells will be gone after a time equal to the sum of the lifetime of the mature cells and the transit time from the least-differentiated but radioresistant maturing cells. This depletion time may not be the same after radiotherapy as after chemotherapy because of the greater specificity of the latter in some tissues for killing cells in particular stages of differentiation in the cell hierarchy. Recovery after low doses occurs from surviving stem cells, the number of which is dose-dependent. Hence the time to recovery of the mature cell populations will be dose-dependent (Fig. 2).

In flexible-type tissues (e.g., in this review, the thyroid, the Leydig cell population in the testis, and probably the lung), the proportion of mature cells capable of division after irradiation is dependent on the dose. Hence the latency period before the expression of gross tissue injury will be dose-dependent except after very high doses, when virtually all mitotic activity is abolished. This dose-dependent effect is superimposed on the normal slow rate of turnover of the cell population. The latter varies among tissue types, and hence so do latency periods. It should be noted that slowly developing injury in these cell populations may influence injury in associated hierarchical cell populations. The characteristics of response of the flexible tissues are shown diagramatically in Figure 2.

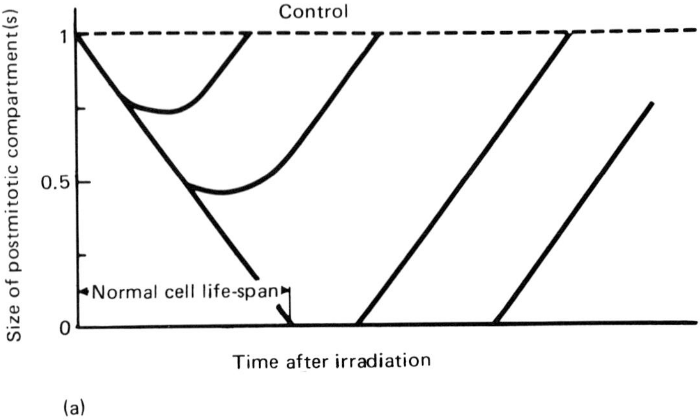

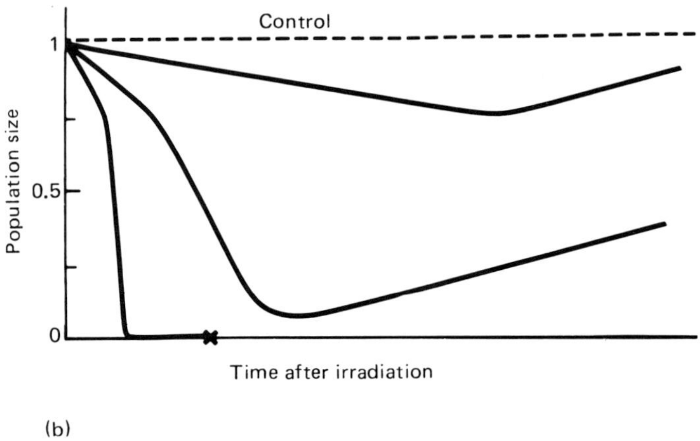

Figure 2 (a) Theoretical response of a type H cell population to a range of single doses of irradiation. During the period of zero input to the mature cell compartment of new mature cells, the total number of these cells declines linearly at a rate equal to that characteristic of steady-state conditions of the tissue concerned. The onset of complete depletion of the mature cells occurs at a time equal to the postmitotic lifetime of cells. Recuperation sets in later the higher the dose (upward-pointing lines moving to the right of the figure), because of the lower number of surviving precursor cells. (b) Theoretical response of a type F cell population to a range of single doses of irradiation. The initial rate of depletion is inversely related to dose (steepening curves) because of the increasing proportion of cells losing mitotic capacity with increasing dose. The latency period to reach a given reduction in the population size is also dose-dependent, with more severe injury appearing earlier. After high doses the steepness of the decline in population size may increase if an avalanche in abortive mitotic activity is induced by homeostatic feedback mechanisms. [From Michalowski (6). Reproduced with permission of Springer-Verlag and the author.]

IV. DOSE-RESPONSE CURVES

The relationship between dose and response can be described by the increasing severity of response with increasing dose, when measured at a particular time after irradiation. This requires that a satisfactory way be found for averaging different responses between individuals, and this is generally not simple. A more useful relationship is obtained when response is defined as the proportion of individuals in whom the injury has exceeded a specified level. A dose-incidence curve is then obtained.

Dose-incidence curves are sigmoid in shape, showing a threshold region, an often-steep increase in incidence with increasing dose, and reaching a plateau at 100% incidence. The sigmoid curve can be linearized for purposes of interpolation or extrapolation by using a probit transformation of the data. The linear plot obtained is characterized by the LD_{50} and the probit width (dose to increase the incidence from 16 to 50%, or from 50 to 84%). This empirical approach is shown in Figure 3 (left panels).

A biologically based transformation is based on the idea that the tissue contains a number K of tissue-rescuing units (7-9). One of these by definition will rescue the tissue from failure, and the units will be depleted exponentially with dose if they are inactivated at random. Within the constraints of applicability of a Poisson model, their surviving fraction (SF) can then be described by SF = $\exp(-D/D_0)$, where D is dose and D_0 is the dose that will inactivate a unit. The mean number that survive a dose D is $K\exp(-D/D_0)$, and the probability of zero units surviving, i.e., of tissue failure (F), is $\exp[-K\exp(-D/D_0)]$. This expression can be transformed by taking logarithms twice to give a function linear with dose, which is

$$\ln(-\ln F) = \ln K - D/D_0$$

The negative slope of this line is $1/D_0$, and the intercept is $\ln K$. Also, when $F = 1/e = 0.37$, $D = D_0 \ln K$. This is the dose giving a 37% incidence of tissue failure, and the dose resulting in the survival on average of one unit. In the commonly measured range of incidences of tissue failure, from 5 to 95%, both probit and double-log transformations (bottom panels, Fig. 3) fit the data equally well.

The biologically based method can be applied to incidences of specified levels of tissue injury as well as tissue failure, but what *is* a tissue-rescuing unit? In hierarchical-type tissues, e.g., in spermatogenesis, a certain number of surviving precursor cells may be required to regenerate the mature cell populations to a given level in time to prevent tissue failure (e.g., infertility). For persistent regeneration and recovery, a given number of stem cells may be required. This minimum number would constitute a rescuing unit. In these cases the number of surviving units would be proportional to the number of surviving regenerative cells. Hence the content of a unit could be calculated, and the sensitivity ($1/D_0$) of the units would equal the sensitivity of the "target" cells. In internal organs where the

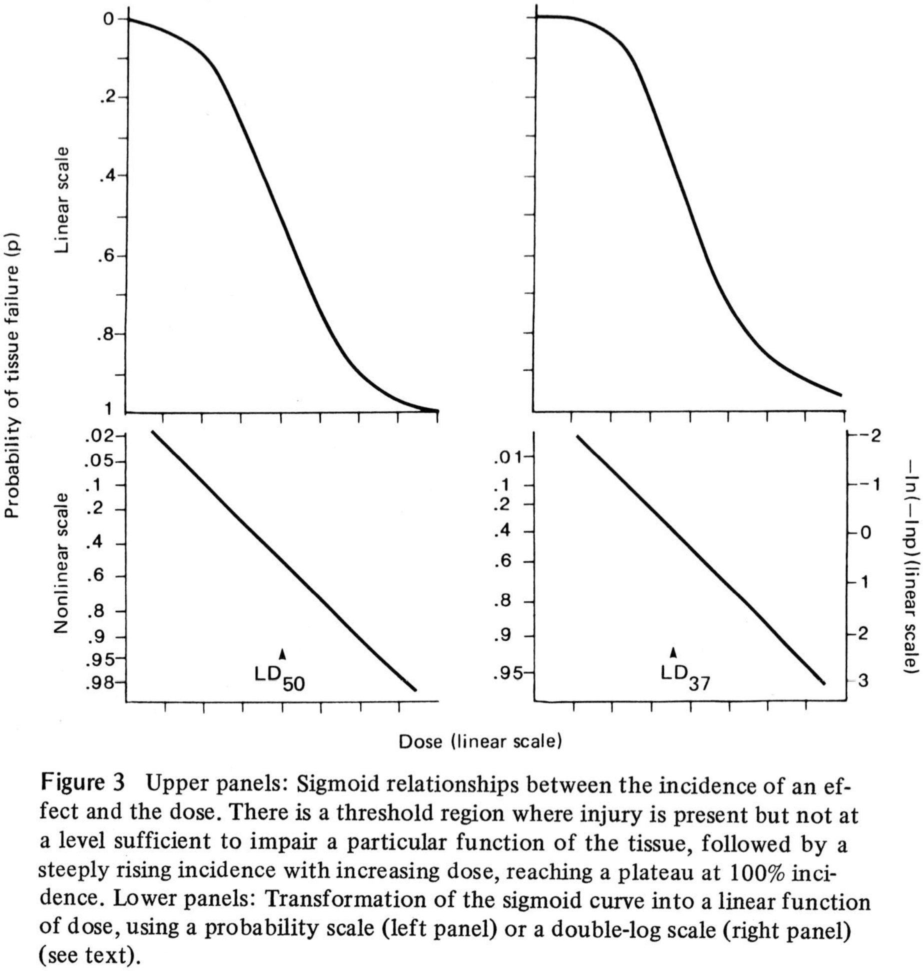

Figure 3 Upper panels: Sigmoid relationships between the incidence of an effect and the dose. There is a threshold region where injury is present but not at a level sufficient to impair a particular function of the tissue, followed by a steeply rising incidence with increasing dose, reaching a plateau at 100% incidence. Lower panels: Transformation of the sigmoid curve into a linear function of dose, using a probability scale (left panel) or a double-log scale (right panel) (see text).

parenchyma is a flexible-type tissue, for example, thyroid and lung, the rescuing unit may be equivalent to a certain number of functional units such as follicles and alveoli. In these cases the steepness of the dose-response curves will depend on whether each independent unit can be regenerated from a single clonogenic cell (cf. hierarchical tissues). If two or even more cells are required, the steepness will increase approximately in proportion to the minimum required number (10,11). This may partly explain the finding that dose-response curves for late-responding tissues such as lung and kidney are indeed steeper, by factors of 2-3, than for many hierarchical-type tissues (12). Another reason for increasing steepness is the failure of tissue due to the inactivation of only one part of a linear series of structures such as exist in the nervous system.

It should be noted that the sensitivity of cells or units deduced from the steepness of dose-response curves may be modified by other factors. There may be variations in cell number or cell sensitivity between the same tissue type in different individuals or the presence of two target-cell populations, e.g., parenchymal and vascular, that fail over dose ranges that overlap. The first possibility would make the dose-response curve shallower; the second would steepen it (13). There is no evidence for the latter effect. The former is likely to be more apparent with human tissues than in well-controlled experimental studies.

V. DOSE FRACTIONATION AND DOSE RATE

Doses are generally less effective when delivered at low dose rates or when fractionated, by amounts that depend on the dose, the tissue, and the overall time. The mechanisms involved are the intracellular repair capacity of the tissue-renewing cells and, in the case of long overall treatment times, repopulation.

One method for calculating changes in isoeffective dose when the schedule of fractionated doses is modified uses the empirical Ellis formula (14):

$$\text{Total dose} = \text{NSD}\, N^{0.24}\, T^{0.11}$$

where NSD is a constant (the nominal standard dose) for a given tissue, N is the number of fractions, and T is the overall time in days. When the overall time is short, of the order of a few days as in high-dose TBI treatments, the number of fractions is by far the most important parameter. Values of the exponents of N, where available for the tissues under discussion, are given in Table 1.

When continuous irradiation is used (i.e., $N = 1$) and the dose rate is varied, the time exponent m can be used to describe the changes in total dose: Total dose = time^m. The time exponent not only varies among tissues, but also depends on the range of dose rate under consideration. This is shown by the varying slope of the lines depicted in Figure 4.

When *fractionated* treatments are given using *low dose rates*, the exponents of N reduce progressively with a decrease in the dose rate.

A more recent and biologically based method of calculating dosage changes is based on the linear-quadratic (LQ) model. This proposes that an effect $E = \alpha D + \beta D^2$, where α and β are parameters and D is the total dose. When the dose is fractionated into N doses, each of size d,

$$E = N(\alpha d + \beta d^2) = D(\alpha + \beta d)$$

When the number of fractions and dose per fraction are changed but are still isoeffective, there is the following equivalence:

$$N_1(\alpha d_1 + \beta d_1^2) = N_2(\alpha d_2 + \beta d_2^2)$$

Table 1 Fractionation and Dose-Rate Parameters Reported for Tissues Discussed in this Review.

Tissue, effect	No. of fractions exponent	Maximum time exponent in continuous irradiation	α/β ratio (Gy) (probable range)
Lung, pneumonitis	0.41, human 0.36 (1-10 fractions), mouse 0.25 (8-30 fractions), mouse	0.37, mouse	3-4, mouse
Testis, stem-cell survival	0.29 (1-4 fractions), mouse 0.07 (10-22 fractions), mouse	–	13.9 (13.4-14.3), mouse
Eye, cataracts	0.22, mouse <0.17, human	–	1.2 (0.6-2.1), mouse

Source: Adapted from Thames and Hendry (15).

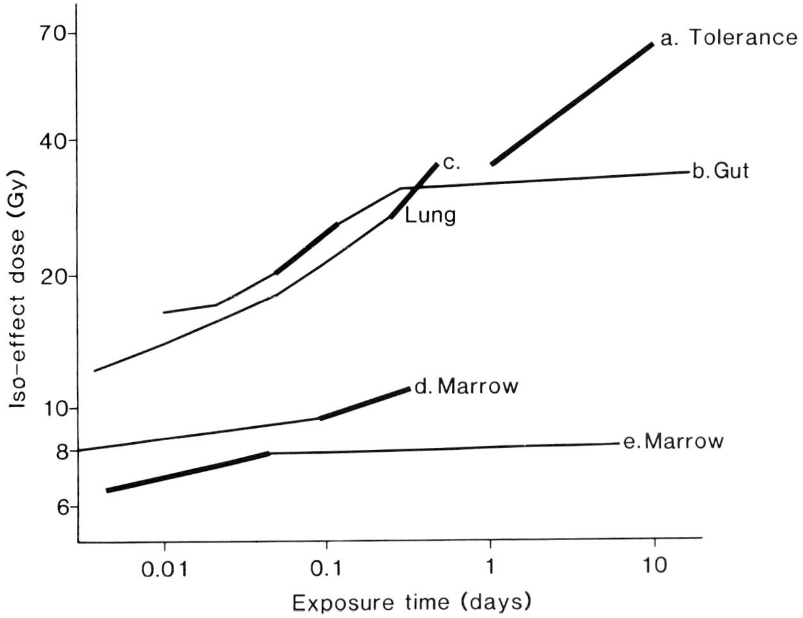

Figure 4 Change in dose for particular effects in various tissues, when a single dose is protracted in time. Maximum slopes are shown by thicker lines. (*a*) $m = 0.29$; (*b*) $m = 0.28$; (*c*) $m = 0.37$; (*d*) $m = 0.11$; (*e*) $m = 0.08$. [From Thames and Hendry (15). Reproduced with permission of Taylor and Francis, Ltd.]

The ratio α/β is tissue-specific and in general terms is high ($\cong$10 Gy) for early-responding tissues and low ($\cong$3 Gy) for late-responding tissues. Values of α/β, where available for the tissues under consideration, are given in Table 1. Values for other tissues can be found elsewhere (16). It should be noted that these values apply specifically to mice, and accurate values for humans are not yet available. However, it is expected that in many cases the differences will be small and that the values for mice can be used to provide initial estimates for humans.

A method has been described for calculating the dosage changes, which incorporates modifications to the dose rate (15). In this method, the quantity $\alpha/\beta + d$ is denoted the fractionation factor, and the quantity D (or $N \times d$) is the dosage factor. The total effect (TE) of a dose D given in fractions of size d is

$$\text{TE} = (\alpha/\beta + d)D = \text{fractionation factor} \times \text{dosage factor}$$

When the treatment schedule includes a change in fraction size from d_1 to d_2, the partial effect (PE) of each part of the treatment may be added to give the total effect:

$$TE = PE_1 + PE_2.$$

If fractions are given close together so that intracellular repair is incomplete, the fractionation factor can be modified to be $\alpha/\beta + d(1 + h_M)$, where h_M is the incomplete repair factor. Furthermore, if a low dose rate is used, the fractionation factor is changed to include a continuous repair factor g and becomes $\alpha/\beta + dg$. Values of these different factors appropriate to different numbers of treatments per day, repair half-times, interfraction intervals, and exposure times can be found elsewhere (Tables 3.1, 3.6, 6.3, and 6.4 in Ref. 15).

The above calculations are designed to estimate isoeffective doses. It is also important to know what increase in effect might occur if the dosage estimations are incorrect. For this purpose one needs to know the steepness of dose-response curves, and this can be characterized by the absolute values of α and β (17). These values can be derived from direct analysis of dose-response curves for fractionated doses. The parameters are related to the probability P of an effect occuring by

$$P = \exp[-\exp(\ln K - \alpha d - \beta dD)]$$

where D is the total dose given in fractions of size d, and K is a constant (12,18). Values of these parameters are available only for tissues in mice, and because of heterogeneity between individuals it is likely that the values applicable to humans will differ more from those for mice than values of the ratio α/β.

VI. LUNG

After the thymus, the lung is the most radiosensitive organ in the thorax. The earliest signs of radiation injury in the lungs are edema and changes in blood circulation, followed by pneumonitis. Although pneumonitis can occur within the first month after irradiation and hence would be called an early effect, it can also occur up to 8 months after irradiation (19) and thus it is also a late effect.

A. Pneumonitis

Pneumonitis is associated with histopathological changes characterized by the collapse of osmotic equilibrium at the alveolocapillary interface, resulting in alveolar instability with atelectasis and passage of blood transudates and hemorrhage into the alveolar lumen. These phenomena can in turn be interpreted as results of the loss of two critical elements of lung function: production of alveolar surfactant and barrier activity.

The most likely candidates for target cells whose depletion results in radiation pneumonitis are the type 2 alveolar cells and the endothelial cells. The latter form a barrier that prevents leakage of water and macromolecules into the interstitium. A constant supply of surfactant is maintained by the renewal of alveolar cells, which disintegrate and liberate surfactant. Radiation reduces the supply of these cells and thus undermines the osmotic balance in the lung.

The histopathological effects are aggravated by immunosuppression and infections (reviewed by Bortin, Ref. 20). Impairment in function and delayed recovery of alveolar macrophages has been found in patients (and dogs) treated with cyclophosphamide, TBI, and methotrexate. Various microorganisms, in particular cytomegalovirus, have been found in some but not all patients with interstitial pneumonitis, and the infection may be associated with immune suppression.

Because lung tissue has a lower density than other soft tissue, a nominal 8 Gy to the lung corresponds to doses 8-15% higher to lung tissue using ^{60}Co γ-rays and 5-8% higher when using 8 MV x-rays (21). Hence 8 Gy becomes 8.6-9.2 Gy (cobalt-60) or 8.4-8.6 Gy (8 MV).

B. Dose Response and Latency Periods

A dose-incidence relationship for pneumonitis using acute irradiation prior to marrow transplantation was described by van Dyk et al. (19). The dose to lung tissue giving pneumonitis in 5% of cases was about 8.3 Gy, and in 50%, about 9.5 Gy (Fig. 5). The dose-incidence data are in agreement with other data for

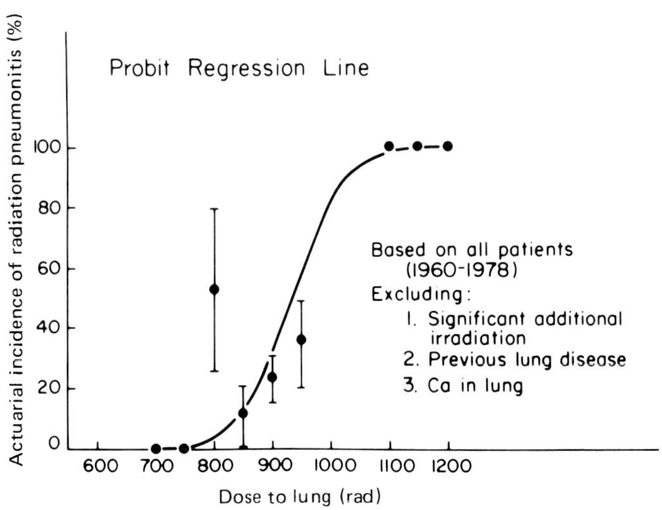

Figure 5 Sigmoidal complications curve for patients irradiated to the lung using single doses, and developing pneumonitis. The point at 8 Gy (800 rad) comprises only 4 patients, and hence the associated error is large. [From van Dyk et al. (19). Reproduced with permission of Pergamon Journals Inc. and the authors.]

upper-half-body irradiation to treat lung metastases (22), where an incidence of pneumonitis of 10-20% was observed after lung doses estimated to be on average 8.8 Gy (19).

The probit width was about 0.75 Gy, and hence the D_0 for the "lung rescuing units" would be about 0.63 Gy. This value is similar to that deduced for mice (8) and smaller than expected considering the depletion rate of single cells, $D_0 \geqslant 1$ Gy.

The frequency distribution of time of onset of pneumonitis was analyzed for 52 patients (19), and in about 90% of these pneumonitis appeared 1-7 months after irradiation. The time of onset was not significantly dose-dependent between 6.5 and 12.5 Gy, but this may reflect the limited sample size. Other data for humans (22), dogs (23), and mice (6,8) indicate a decrease in latency interval with an increase in dose. This is expected in an F type tissue (Fig. 2).

C. Low Dose Rate

The human lung is spared by the use of low-dose-rate irradiation (24,25). The dose for 5% incidence of pneumonitis was increased from 8.2 Gy to 9.5 Gy using 0.05 Gy/min instead of 0.3-0.5 Gy/min (24). Larger increases are indicated from experiments in mice, where the ratio of doses at the two dose rates was about 1.8 (26,27). It was suggested that the difference between mice and humans was due to the addition of cyclophosphamide, which inexplicably reduced the dose-rate effect in mice to a level similar to that observed in humans (28).

D. Fractionation

With fractionated irradiation, the total dose in humans can be increased even further, for example, to 12 Gy given in 6 treatments, or even 15.7 Gy given in 7 treatments. In the Ellis formula, the combined exponents of N and T were estimated to be 0.43, with an NSD of about 9 Gy equivalent (7 Gy with concomitant actinomycin D) (29). This was deduced from a series of 26 patients treated to at least one lung for metastatic lung disease, using ^{60}Co γ-rays or 1-MV x-rays, together with a series of fractionation data using lethality in rats after lung irradiation. The separate exponents of N and T have not been estimated for humans. Values for mice are given in Table 1. Values of α/β in the alternative method for calculating dosage changes associated with changes in fractionation are also given in Table 1.

Various groups of patients have received fractionated doses of irradiation to the lung, for example with prophylactic irradiation in the treatment of osteosarcoma. No pneumonitis was seen in 40 patients given 20-25 Gy to the lung in daily doses of 1.5 Gy (30). This was in contrast to 7 patients in which pneumonitis was observed after 30 Gy given at 3 Gy/day. There was no pneumonitis in a further 14 patients given 24 Gy to the lung in 13 daily doses (31). A recent analysis

Table 2 Incidence of Pneumonitis After Fractionated Irradiation

Total dose (cGy)	Number of fractions	No. of patients	No. of responders	Incidence (%)
3000 3500	15 20	6	2	33
3200 3600	15 20	12	5	42
3000 3800 4500	10 20 30	12	8	67
3100 4200	10 18	10	9	90
4100 5300	16 25	14	12	86

Source: Taken from Mah et al. (32).

of dose-incidence relationships using fractionated doses has been made for 54 patients with various thoracic malignancies treated to various lung volumes (32). No previous treatments had been given. The incidences in five groups of these patients are given in Table 2. The groupings were made on the basis of biologically equivalent doses in different schedules using the NSD formula. A further point is that no significant differences were observed in the incidences of pneumonitis for patients given irradiation to less than one-fourth of the lung volume compared with between one-fourth and one-half. There were only 4 patients in the series with irradiation volumes greater than one-half of the lungs, and hence any effect of volume for large lung volumes was not established.

Clearly, there is insufficient information on the human lung concerning the parameter values necessary for performing accurate calculations of dosage changes resulting from changes in fractionation and/or dose rate. However, rough estimates can be made. First, the increase in dose for 5% incidence of pneumonitis, from 8.2 to 9.5 Gy when the dose rate was decreased from 0.3-0.5 Gy/min to 0.05 Gy/min (24) is commensurate with a repair half-time of about 2 hr or more. Second, taking an acute dose of 9.5 Gy as giving 50% pneumonitis (19), an α/β ratio of 2 Gy would provide doses compatible with the clinical observations concerning fractionation, as follows. For a single exposure,

$$\mathrm{TE} = (2 + 9.5) \times 9.5 = 109$$

With a dose per fraction, d, of 3 Gy, TE = $(2 + 3)D$, and hence the total dose D for an equal TE is 22 Gy.

Similarly, for doses per fraction of 1.5 or 1.85 Gy, the total doses are 31 Gy and 28 Gy, respectively. These total doses are compatible with (1) the lack of pneumonitis after 20-25 Gy given in fractions of 1.5 Gy, or after 24 Gy given in fractions of 1.85 Gy, and (2) its induction by 30 Gy given in fractions of 3 Gy (30-32).

A more detailed example of the method of calculation is as follows. In Manchester, TBI is given to a total dose of 12 Gy, giving two fractions each of 2 Gy/day (6-hr intervals) for 3 days using a dose rate of 10 cGy/min. Knowing that lung is the tissue at risk, what dosage change would be necessary if the dose rate were decreased to 5 cGy/min?

Two sets of parameter values can be tried: (1) values determined in mice, which are accurate but not necessarily applicable to humans, and (2) values compatible with the few observations in humans, which are inaccurate. For mice, the following values are used: $\alpha/\beta = 4$ Gy, repair half-time = 0.72 hr, $h_M = 0.0039$ for two fractions/day, $g \sim 0.9$ for 10 cGy/min. Hence

$$\mathrm{TE} = [4 + 2(1 + 0.0039) \times 0.9] \times 12 = 69.7$$

At 5 cGy/min, each treatment time is 1.3 hr and g is about 0.7. Thus

$$\mathrm{TE} = 69.7 = [4 + (d \times 1.0039 \times 0.7)] \times 6d$$

or

$$4.216d^2 + 24d - 69.7 = 0$$

This is a quadratic equation in d (dose per fraction) with solution $d = 2.12$ Gy. Hence the dose per fraction can be increased by 12 cGy, or 6%.

For humans, the following estimates are used, taken from the above discussion: $\alpha/\beta = 2$ Gy, repair half-time = 2 hr, $h_M = 0.125$, $g \sim 0.95$.

Hence TE = $[2 + 2(1 + 0.125) \times 0.95] \times 12 = 49.7$. At 5 cGy/min, g is about 0.86, and a calculation similar to that given above produces $d = 2.07$ Gy. Hence the dose per fraction can be increased by 7 cGy, or 3%, about half the amount estimated from the mouse data.

E. Residual Effects

There is a second phase of injury in the lung that results in persistent restrictive or obstructive lung disease after irradiation (33,34). Marrow-transplanted patients who suffered but recovered from interstitial pneumonitis had greater restrictive changes than patients without pneumonitis, who nevertheless in many cases showed the long-term changes (34). Restrictive changes improved with time, in contrast to obstructive changes, which became more prominent (Table 3).

The changes were not significantly associated with chronic graft-versus-host disease nor with TBI—comparing patients with hematological malignancies receiving only chemotherapy. It was considered that chemotherapy, in particular

Table 3 Sequential Pulmonary Function in Marrow Transplantation Recipients

	Percent of Patients with Ventilatory Defect at Time of Study					
Total lung capacity	Pretransplant ($N = 340$)	Day 100 ($N = 226$)	1 yr ($N = 136$)	2 yr ($N = 56$)	3 yr ($N = 24$)	4 yr ($N = 35$)
65-79% predicted	11	11	14	11	13	14
50-64% predicted	2	5	6	2	0	0
<50% predicted	0	0	1	0	0	0
Forced Expiratory Volume in 1 s/ Vital Capacity	($N = 358$)	($N = 241$)	($N = 139$)	($N = 60$)	($N = 24$)	($N = 39$)
60-69%	11	9	10	5	16	0
50-59%	3	2	1	0	5	3
<50%	0	0	3	3	8	10

Source: From Sullivan et al. (4). Reproduced with permission of Grune and Stratton Inc. and the authors.

with cyclophosphamide and methotrexate, was likely to be largely responsible for the restrictive changes, in conjunction with the presence of infectious agents (34). The obstructive changes were not found to be associated with previous pneumonitis, TBI, or underlying disease. The abnormalities resembled those found in nontransplant patients with autoimmune diseases and obliterative bronchiolitis, but the cause remains unknown.

Residual lung injury after irradiation has been studied in dogs and in mice with a view to obtaining dose-rate and fractionation parameters. In mice, the late effects are characterized by fibrosis, elevated breathing rate, pleural effusions (uncommon in humans), and, in severe cases, death. The effect of fractionation is slightly greater for late (>6 months) lethality than for early (2-6 months) lethality (8,35), but in contrast the dose-rate effect was less (27).

VII. TESTIS

A. Fertility

Infertility occurs when the sperm count is markedly reduced. In humans, for doses up to 3 Gy, the reduction begins after a latency period of 46 days, which is the maturation time for the radioresistant second and third phases of spermatogenesis (from preleptotene spermatocytes through meiosis and including the spermatids). Azoospermia is reached at about 10 weeks after doses greater than 1 Gy. The drop in the sperm count begins earlier after higher doses, when the spermatids also become affected.

Acute doses of up to 4 Gy cause temporary or prolonged sterility in some men (1). After 6 Gy local irradiation, long-term histological recovery in otherwise normal individuals was reported at 7.5 months, with sperm appearing in seminal fluid at 24 months (36; Table 4).

Table 4 Histological Recovery and Increase in Sperm Counts Following Irradiation in Humans

Single dose (Gy)	Histological recovery (months)	First increase in sperm count (months)	Fractionated dose (Gy)	Recovery from aspermia
0.2	6	6	0.5-1	8-26 mo
1	7	7	1-1.6	13-38 mo
2	7	11	1.2-2.3	11-20 mo
6	7.5	24	2-3	12-14 yr

Source: Adapted from Rowley et al. (36) and Ash (39).

Higher single doses of about 9 Gy were given to the testes of leukemic patients during whole body irradiation prior to marrow transplantation (37). Others had fractionated doses of 11-16 Gy given to the testes in six or seven daily fractions. All men had gonadal failure for up to 5 years after TBI, and 2 of 7 patients receiving single doses and followed for more than 5 years showed eventual recovery of spermatogenesis. Fractionated doses can be equally or even more damaging to spermatogenesis than single doses of the same amount (38,39). The observations following pelvic irradiation for Hodgkin's disease are compatible with this. Most patients remained infertile to 5 years following fractionated doses to the testis totaling 2 Gy, but fertility returned after 2 years following lower doses (40).

In mice, fractionated doses given within a 4-day period are equally or in some cases more effective than single doses, with respect to early testis weight loss and later fertility (41-43). Nonetheless, sparing effects of fractionation are indeed observed (44,45), as they are for most other cell types. However, the responses to fractionated doses given over extended periods of time are complicated by increases in cell sensitivity due to progression of cells into sensitive stages (46), together with loss of cells due to differentiation (44).

The mean time to regain fertility is dependent on dose in mice (Fig. 6; 43), and in humans (Table 4; 36,39,47), as expected for a hierarchial-type tissue (Fig. 2).

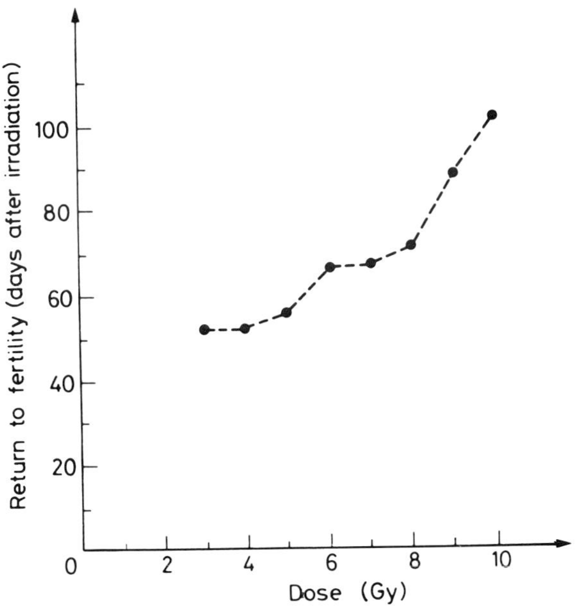

Figure 6 Mean time to regain fertility in mice versus dose. [Redrawn from Cattanach (43)].

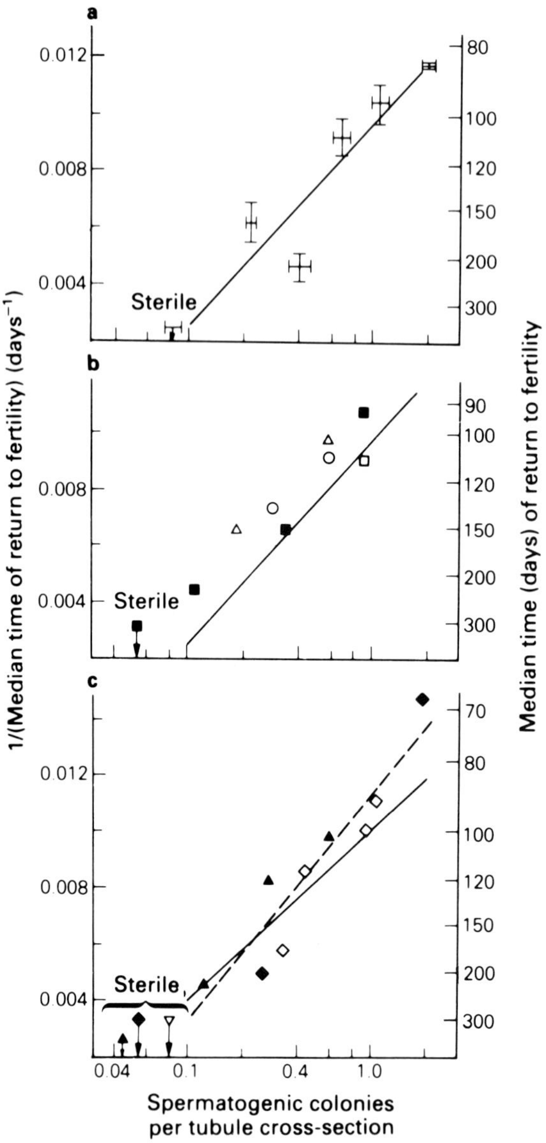

Figure 7 Relationship between time of recovery of fertility and testicular stem-cell survival. From Meistrich (49). The time to recovery of fertility is plotted as the median time after treatment at which fertility was regained (left ordinate); the corresponding number of days are also indicated (right ordinate). Each point represents one dose of radiation or drug. (*a*) 6-10 Gy single dose γ irradiation; (*b*) fractionated doses, doses of neutrons, or a radioprotective drug + γ rays; (*c*) various doses of adriamycin, thiotepa, busulfan, hydroxyurea, or procarbazine. The solid and dashed regression lines are calculated from all the radiation data and all the chemotherapy data, respectively. (Reproduced with permission of Macmillan Ltd. and the author.)

This time period can be prolonged by fractionation (43,48), a feature that would be consistent with greater stem cell killing. Recently it has been shown that the time to regain fertility, and the long-term plateau level of sperm production, are directly related to the level of stem cell killing after irradiation or treatment with a variety of chemotherapeutic agents (Fig. 7; 49). It was suggested that there was little influence of injury in the associated hormonal cell populations, which are required for maintaining spermatogenesis.

In the transplant patients described above, levels of serum testosterone were unchanged. Levels of luteinizing hormone (LH) were elevated in some, and levels of follicle-stimulating hormone (FSH) were elevated in most. These observations are qualitatively in agreement with those in normal individuals receiving lower doses of 6 Gy (36). The transplant patients also received high-dose cyclophosphamide. However, in patients with aplastic anemia, also transplanted but receiving only high-dose cyclophosphamide, the majority recovered spermatogenesis (37). Nonetheless, high-dose chemotherapy can produce permanent azoospermia in the majority of patients, probably as a result of stem cell ablation—e.g., after six courses of MOPP therapy (50), high total doses of chlorambucil (51), and >10 g/m^2 of cyclophosphamide (52).

B. Sexual Development

Sexual development is mediated by testosterone produced in the Leydig cells in the testis and by LH secreted by the anterior pituitary. Radiation injury, in particular to the Leydig cell population, can affect sexual development.

A comprehensive series of studies in rats showed that the threshold for hormonal abnormalities is about 5 Gy to the testes, in both prepubertal (53,54) and pubertal (55,56) animals. The long-term changes after doses higher than 5 Gy were characterized by dose-dependent increases in LH and FSH and decreases in androgen-binding protein (ABP), number of Leydig cells, and LH receptor number. The effects were seen earlier after the higher doses, and the injury was progressive to at least 36 weeks. Spermatogenesis and Sertoli cell function were less radioresponsive in prepubertal and pubertal rats than in adult rats, but in contrast Leydig cells were more affected and there was less recovery (57).

Fractionation of the dose (5, 20, or 30 Gy) into 20 daily fractions produced less reduction in the androgen-dependent weights of the prostate and the seminal vesicles in adult rats (58). However, there was no significant sparing of the Leydig cell population, nor of ^{131}I-hcG (human chorionic gonadotropin) binding, and the increase in serum LH was even greater than after a single dose of the same total amount.

Delayed onset of puberty was shown by 11 out of 16 boys given TBI and marrow transplantation according to the Seattle protocols (4), recently updated to 21 out of 31 (59). Many of these had elevated LH and FSH levels. Shalet et al. (60) studied testicular function in 10 men aged between 17 and 36 who had received irradiation for a nephroblastoma during childhood. The dose of scattered irradiation to the testes ranged from 2.7 to 9.8 Gy, given in 20 fractions over 4 weeks. Eight had oligo- or azoospermia, and seven of these had an elevated FSH level. Further, testicular function was studied in 11 boys who required testicular irradiation (24 Gy in 12-16 fractions over 16-22 days) for a testicular relapse of ALL. Abnormalities in gonadotropin secretion consistent with testicular damage were noted in 9 out of the 11. Evidence of Leydig cell failure through puberty was associated with the increase in total dose from 2.7-9.8 Gy to 24 Gy (61).

VIII. OVARY

A. Fertility

The germ cell population in the ovary is nonrenewing from birth, and it declines with age. Hence any cell death is recorded as a permanent decrease in the oocyte population.

Oocytes die in interphase within a few hours of irradiation. They become pyknotic and are removed by phagocytosis within a few days. Primordial human oocytes are more resistant than oocytes in growing follicles. This is also found in guinea pigs and monkeys, but the reverse is found in mice (reviewed by Bianchi, Ref. 62). An explanation for this may be the inexplicable marked variation in radiosensitivity of oocytes during development and division and the arrest of the oocytes in different stages of their meiotic prophase in various species. Human oocytes are relatively radioresistant, the LD_{50} being between 6 and 18 Gy (63, 64). There are other marked variations between species, which make difficult any quantitative interpretation of human responses on the basis of data in other species. For example, the effect of dose fractionation, not known very precisely in women, is to spare the ovary in mice, but the reverse is found in monkeys (62). Acute doses of up to 4 Gy to the ovaries cause temporary sterility in some women, and doses of 3-10 Gy cause permanent sterility in an increasing proportion of women (1). Older women are more susceptible, due mainly to the decreasing number of follicles with age. The number declines by atresia, from 400,000 at ages 12-16 years to 8000 at 40-44 years.

The total doses of fractionated irradiation required to induce temporary or permanent sterility are higher in some studies than in others using single doses (1), but an accurate assessment of the increase in the total dose is difficult to make. Most of the information comes from the irradiation of women for abdominal tumors or prior to marrow transplantation in the treatment of aplastic anemia and leukemia. Artificial menopause is induced by fractionated doses to the ovaries of the order of 12-15 Gy in young patients and 4-7 Gy in older women (39). Estimates of the total fractionated doses resulting in sterility for 5 years in 50% of women range from 5 Gy for young women (39) to 20 Gy for women aged 40 or more (65). Examples are as follows. Of 38 women treated for leukemia using chemotherapy and 9.2-10 Gy single-dose TBI, 35 had primary ovarian failure for at least 5 years, with amenorrhea and elevated levels of luteinizing and follicle-stimulating hormone (37). Ovarian recovery occurred in 1 out of 6 followed for more than 6 years. Only 1 of 13 who received 12 Gy fractionated TBI instead of a single dose had ovarian recovery after 3 years. Using chemotherapy alone before transplantation in cases of aplastic anemia, all 15 women less than age 26 and 3 of 9 older than age 26 recovered normal gonadotropin levels and menstruation after 200 mg/kg cyclophosphamide. Hence, as with men, irradiation is the main sterilizing agent in these treatments. Ovarian failure is associated with increased serum levels of FSH and LH and low levels of estradiol.

B. Sexual Development

Although younger women are more resistant to sterilization by irradiation, irradiation of girls can delay sexual development (4,59,60). Out of 35 prepubertal girls treated with TBI and marrow transplantation for leukemia according to the Seattle protocols, 10 had delayed development of secondary sexual characteristics (59). All 18 women studied who were treated for abdominal tumors in childhood (20-30 Gy in 25-44 days) had ovarian failure, with very high levels of FSH and low levels of estradiol (66). Other data for children can be found in the review by Shalet (61).

IX. EYE

The lens epithelium is a hierarchical-type tissue, and the dividing cells are limited to the anterior equatorial region. The progeny of the dividing cells migrate posteriorly and then centrally to form the lens fibers. If the lens is irradiated, the maturation of the fiber-forming cells may be abnormal, resulting in opaque fibers. These opacities constitute the beginning of a cataract, which is a focus of opaque fibers.

The incidence and latency period for cataract formation are dose-dependent above a threshold dose of about 2 Gy in humans (67). A single dose of 7.5 Gy causes some degree of cataract formation in 100% of individuals. There is a sparing effect of dose fractionation on cataract formation. An analysis of the difference in incidence following single-dose or fractionated TBI was presented by Deeg et al. (68). The incidence following 10 Gy single dose and chemotherapy rose to 80% after 6 years, in contrast to only 18% using 6 × 2 Gy or 7 × 2.25 Gy instead of a single dose (Fig. 8). The latter incidence was similar to the value of 19% for patients given chemotherapy but no TBI.

Steroids given to control graft-versus-host disease contributed to the incidences in all groups, and for those who received fractionated TBI but no steroids the incidence was only 9%. Further data concerning fractionation were reported by Merriam et al. (69), who showed that 10 Gy given over 3-12 weeks gave 75%

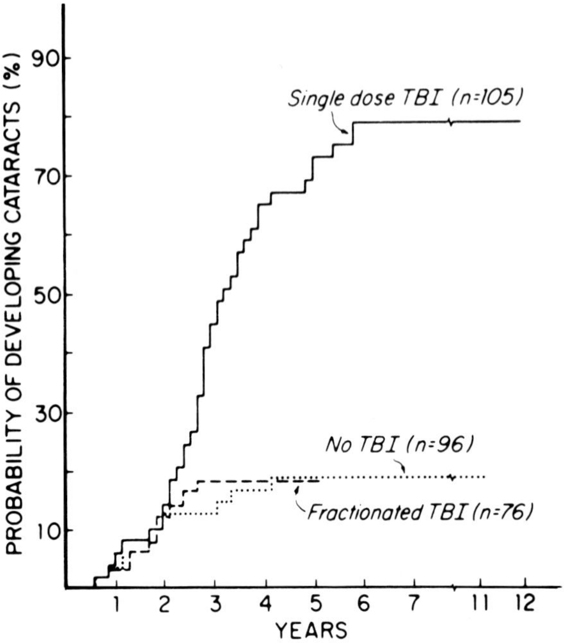

Figure 8 Incidence of cataract following single-dose TBI (10 Gy) or fractionated TBI (6 X 2 Gy or 7 X 2.25 Gy). [From Deeg et al. (68). Reproduced with permission of Pergamon Journals Inc. and the authors.]

incidence of cataracts and 14 Gy over the same period led to 100% incidence. Higher doses of 40-60 Gy given to the eye in the treatment of rhabdomyosarcoma produced cataracts in 90% of the subjects between 1 and 4 years after irradiation (70).

For humans and rats, the time exponent (number of fractions and overall time combined) was estimated as 0.17 (71). In mice, it was higher at about 0.30 (72), and the separate exponents for number of fractions and overall time were, respectively, about 0.22 and 0.11.

X. THYROID

Glandular epithelia are generally considered to be type F tissues because of the capacity of the functional cells to divide following hormonal stimulation. The thyroid is unresponsive because of the radioresistance of most thyroid cell functions and the low rate of division of the follicular cells, but latent injury can be expressed by stimulating cell division (reviewed by Malone et al., Ref. 73). The natural low rate of cell turnover means that hypothyroidism associated with cell (reproductive) death is generally a long-term phenomenon.

TBI induces thyroid dysfunction. Of 23 patients who received single-dose TBI or total lymphoid irradiation using 7.5 Gy, 10 developed thyroid dysfunction within a median time of 13 months. Two had low thyroxine levels as well as raised TSH levels (74). Similar dysfunction was also seen in 45 of 116 children in the Seattle protocols (59). No significant correlation was found with single or fractionated doses or previous cranial irradiation. However, a sparing effect of fractionation is likely, because with localized treatments to the head and neck in adults, thyroid dysfunction is usually characteristic of conventional fractionated doses of more than 20 Gy. Sklar et al. (74) also pointed out that radiation-induced hypothyroidism may be transient rather than permanent.

XI. GROWTH RETARDATION

Stunting after high doses may be due to cell sterilization in the growing bones, for example if the spine receives more than 24 Gy (fractionated) (75). However, if the hypothalamic/pituitary axis is irradiated, growth hormone (GH) is the first pituitary hormone to be affected, and its lack is considered to be the major contributing cause of stunting in unirradiated bones.

Growth retardation occurs in children after TBI used prior to marrow transplantation in treatment of leukemia (59,76). With the Seattle protocols, the effects in boys were less following fractionated than single-dose TBI, but greater when previous cranial irradiation (18-29 Gy fractionated) had been given (59). The effects were also greater in cases of chronic graft-versus-host disease, probably due in part to its treatment using steroids. Even with TBI doses as low as 7.5 Gy, two-thirds of children showed subnormal growth velocities, with mean yearly growth rates 4.6 cm/year below controls (76).

Growth retardation is also seen after localized high-dose treatment for tumors in the head and neck and acute lymphoblastic leukemia (ALL) (61,70,75,77). The doses in these treatments are generally greater than 24 Gy fractionated over at least 3 weeks. Although a fractionation effect is indicated from the above data, this is difficult to quantitate because growth retardation is dose-dependent and isoeffective doses in different schedules are not readily deducible from the literature.

In the marrow-transplant children, partial GH deficiency was present in 6 of 18 who had not received additional cranial irradiation. In children who had, marked GH deficiency was present in 17 out of 25, and there was partial deficiency in 4 others (59). Growth retardation is not due solely to GH deficiency, because treatment with GH does not fully correct the deficiency (reviewed by Shalet, Ref. 77). Experiments with head irradiation in rats by Mosier et al. (e.g., 78) largely concerning the pituitary–size, GH concentration, serum somatomedin activity, GH treatments, pituitary irradiation–have not yet elucidated the mechanisms of growth impairment.

Table 5 Summary of Effects, Doses, and Causes in the Tissues Under Consideration

Tissue, effect	Latency period	Threshold dose	Dose for high incidence	Effect of dose fractionation	Cause	Target-cell population
Lung, pneumonitis	Mean 3 mo (1-7 in 90% of patients)	8.2 Gy single dose	>10 Gy single dose	$N^{0.41}$ or ? $\alpha/\beta \cong 2$ Gy, ? $T_{1/2} \cong 2$ hr [$\alpha/\beta \cong 4$ Gy, mouse] [$T_{1/2} = 0.7$ hr, mouse]	Lack of alveolar surfactant and barrier activity	Type 2 alveolar cells ? endothelial cells
Testis, infertility	≅10 wk, recovery time dose-dependent	⩽4 Gy	>6 Gy single dose. ⩽11-16 Gy, 6-7 fractions	[$\alpha/\beta = 12$ Gy, mouse] Protracted doses often more effective than single doses	Aspermia	Spermatogenic stem cells
Testis, sexual development	Age-dependent	≅10 Gy single dose >(2.7-9.8 Gy), 20 fractions, 4 wk	24 Gy, 12-16 fractions, 16-21 days	Positive sparing	Gonadotropin deficiency	Leydig cells
					Testosterone deficiency	Pituitary

Ovary, infertility	<1 mo	≤4 Gy single dose Higher in younger women	≅10 Gy single dose	Positive sparing	Ovarian failure	Oocytes
Ovary, sexual development	Age-dependent	~10 Gy single dose	20-30 Gy, 25-44 days	Positive sparing	↱Gonadotropin deficiency └ Estrogen deficiency	Ovary Pituitary
Eye, cataract	>1 yr	2 Gy single dose	10 Gy single dose, 40-60 Gy fractionated	$N^{<0.17}$ [$N^{0.22}$ $T^{0.11}$, mouse]	Cell maturation abnormality	Fiber-forming lens epithelial cells
Thyroid, growth and metabolism deficiencies	<1 yr	≤7.5 Gy single dose ≅20 Gy fractionated	–	Positive sparing	Hypothyroidism	Follicular cells
Growth, retardation	Age-dependent	≤7.5 Gy single dose	>24 Gy, 3 wk	Positive sparing	Higher doses: GH deficiency Lower doses: cartilage/bone	In hypothalamic pituitary axis Chondrocytes

Arrows indicate abscopal influence.

XII. CONCLUSIONS

The increasing success of marrow transplantation in leukemia using TBI has put lung second to skin in terms of knowledge of the response of normal human tissues to changes in dose, dose rate, and fractionation. Of the various tissues in which long-term injury appears after high-dose TBI treatments, an accurate estimate of the steepness of the dose-response curve has been obtained only for pneumonitis. This is steeper than expected from considerations of conventional sensitivities of single cells, but it is in agreement with the steep dose-response curves observed for pneumonitis in mice. One possible explanation for the marked steepness is a multicellular origin as a prerequisite for renewal of functional lung subunits. The knowledge has accrued by attempts, largely empirical, to maximize the dose tolerable to the lung and effectively increase the ablative effect on the leukemic marrow, which shows less of a dose-rate and fractionation effect.

The human evidence for lung toxicity is backed up by a large radiobiological data base using mice, which has validated the LQ method for calculating isoeffective dosage changes consequent upon changes in the pattern of dose delivery.

All the tissues discussed in this review (except spermatogenic epithelium with protracted irradiation) show a sparing effect with dose fractionation. However, because of the limited amount of data for tissues, apart from lung, accurate estimates of the dose-response and fractionation parameters are not available.

A summary of information collated for the tissues under discussion is shown in Table 5. In the future we may see (1) further attempts to increase the total dose and hence the therapeutic ratio, perhaps by decreasing the dose rates even further; (2) further detailed analyses of certain effects in TBI patients, similar to those reported in recent years by the Seattle group concerning gonadal function (37), cataracts (68), growth and development (59), and leukoencephalopathy (5) in particular with a view to minimizing late sequelae by variations in fractionation schedule and dose rate; (3) better treatment of the radiation-induced damage based on increasing knowledge of the pathogenesis of the injury in humans and in experimental systems.

ACKNOWLEDGMENTS

I am very grateful to Dr. Godfrey Morgenstern, Dr. Stephen Shalet, and Dr. Joachim Deeg for constructive comments on this article. The work of the author is supported by the Cancer Research Campaign (U.K.).

REFERENCES

1. Annex, J. Non-stochastic effects of irradiation. United Nations Committee on the Effects of Atomic Radiation. Report to the General Assembly, New York, pp. 571-654 (1982).

2. Deeg, H. J. Acute and delayed toxicities of total body irradiation. *Int. J. Radiat. Oncol. Biol. Phys. 9,* 1933-1939 (1983).
3. Deeg, H. J., Storb, R., Thomas, E. D. Bone marrow transplantation: a review of delayed complications. *Brit. J. Haematol. 57,* 185-208 (1984).
4. Sullivan, K. M., Deeg, H. J., Sanders, J. E., et al. Late complications after marrow transplantation. *Semin. Hematol. 21* (1), 53-63 (1984).
5. Thompson, C. B., Sanders, J. E., Flournoy, N., Buckner, C. D., Thomas, E. D. The risks of central nervous system relapse and leukoencephalopathy in patients receiving marrow transplants for acute leukaemia. *Blood 67,* 195-199 (1986).
6. Michalowski, A. Effects of radiation on normal tissues: hypothetical mechanisms and limitations of in situ assays of clonogenicity. *Radiat. Environ. Biophys. 19,* 157-172 (1981).
7. Hendry, J. H., Potten, C. S., Roberts, N. P. The gastrointestinal syndrome and mucosal clonogenic cells: relationships between target cell sensitivities, LD_{50} and cell survival, and their modification by antibiotics. *Radiat. Res. 96,* 100-112 (1983).
8. Travis, E. L., Tucker, S. L. The relationship between functional assays of radiation response in the lung and target cell depletion. *Brit. J. Cancer 53 (Suppl. VII),* 304-319 (1986).
9. Hendry, J. H., Thames, H. D. The tissue-rescuing unit. *Brit. J. Radiol. 59,* 629-630 (1986).
10. Hendry, J. H. Mathematical aspects of colony growth, transplantation kinetics, and cell survival. In: *Cell clones: manual of mammalian cell techniques.* Potten, C. S., Hendry, J. H. (Eds.). Churchill-Livingstone, Edinburgh, pp. 1-12 (1985).
11. Withers, H. R., Mason, K. A., Thames, H. D. Late radiation response of kidney assayed by tubule cell survival. *Brit. J. Radiol. 59,* 587-595 (1986).
12. Thames, H. D., Hendry, J. H., Moore, J. V., Ang, K. K., Travis, E. L. The greater steepness of dose-response curves for late than for early responding normal tissues. (In preparation).
13. Hendry, J. H., Moore, J. V. Is the steepness of dose incidence curves for tumour control or complications due to variation before, or as a result of, irradiation? *Brit. J. Radiol. 57,* 1045-1046 (1985).
14. Ellis, F. Fractionation in radiotherapy. In: *Modern trends in radiotherapy,* Vol. 1. Deeley, T. J., Wood, C. A. P. (Eds.). Butterworths, London, pp. 34-51 (1967).
15. Thames, H. D., Hendry, J. H. *Fractionation in radiotherapy.* Taylor and Francis, London (1987).
16. Fowler, J. F. What next in fractionated radiotherapy? *Brit. J. Cancer 49* (Suppl. VI), 285-300 (1984).
17. Hendry, J. H., Moore, J. V. Deriving absolute values of α and β for dose fractionation, using dose-incidence data. *Brit. J. Radiol. 58,* 885-890 (1985).
18. Thames, H. D., Rozell, M. E., Tucker, S. L., Ang, K. K., Fisher, D. R., Travis, E. L. Direct analysis of quantal radiation response data. *Int. J. Radiat. Biol. 49,* 999-1009 (1986).

19. van Dyk, J., Deane, T. J., Kan, S., et al. Radiation pneumonitis following large single dose irradiation. A re-evaluation based on absolute dose to lung. *Int. J. Radiat. Oncol. Biol. Phys. 7,* 461-467 (1981).
20. Bortin, M. M. Pathogenesis of interstitial pneumonitis following allogeneic bone marrow transplantation for acute leukaemia. In: *Recent advances in bone marrow transplantation,* Vol. 7. Gale, R. P. (Ed.). Liss, New York, pp. 445-460 (1983).
21. McDonald, S. C., Keller, B. E., Rubin, P. Method for calculating dose where lung tumour lies in the treatment field. *Med. Phys. 2,* 210-216 (1976).
22. Salazar, O. M., Rubin, P., Keller, B., et al. Systematic (half-body) radiation therapy: response and toxicity. *Int. J. Radiat. Oncol. Biol. Phys. 4,* 937-950 (1978).
23. Michaelson, J. M., Schreiner, B., Hansen, C. L., et al. Cardiovascular changes in the dog following exposure to X-rays. University of Rochester report UR-596, August 28, 1961.
24. Keane, T. J., van Dyk, J., Rider, W. D., et al. Idiopathic interstitial pneumonia following bone marrow transplantation: the relationship with total body irradiation. *Int. J. Radiat. Oncol. Biol. Phys. 7,* 1365-1370 (1981).
25. Barrett, A., Depledge, M. H., Powles, R. L. Interstitial pneumonitis following bone marrow transplantation after low dose rate total body irradiation. *Int. J. Radiat. Oncol. Biol. Phys. 9,* 1029-1033 (1983).
26. Hill, R. P. Response of mouse lung to irradiation at different dose-rates. *Int. J. Radiat. Oncol. Biol. Phys. 9,* 1043-1047 (1983).
27. Down, J. D., Easton, D. F., Steel, G. G. Repair in mouse lung during low dose-rate irradiation. *Radiother. Oncol. 5,* 1-14 (1986).
28. Lockhart, S. P., Down, J. D., Steel, G. G. The effect of low dose-rate and cyclophosphamide on the radiation tolerance of the mouse lung. *Int. J. Radiat. Oncol. Biol. Phys. 12,* 1437-1440 (1986).
29. Phillips, T. L., Margolis, L. Radiation pathology and the clinical response of lung and oesophagus. *Front. Radiat. Ther. Oncol. 6,* 254-273 (1972).
30. Newton, K. A., Spittle, M. F. Whole lung irradiation. *Clin. Radiol. 20,* 19-22 (1969).
31. Newton, K. A., Barrett, A. Prophylactic lung irradiation in the treatment of osteosarcoma. *Clin. Radiol. 29,* 493-496 (1978).
32. Mah, K., van Dyk, J., Keane, T., Poon, P. Y. Acute radiation induced pulmonary damage: a clinical study on the response to fractionated radiation therapy. *Int. J. Radiat. Oncol. Biol. Phys. 13,* 179-188 (1987).
33. Depledge, M. H., Barrett, A., Powles, R. L. Lung function after bone marrow grafting. *Int. J. Radiat. Oncol. Biol. Phys. 9,* 145-151 (1983).
34. Springmeyer, S. C., Flournoy, N., Sullivan, K. M., Storb, R., Thomas, E. D. Pulmonary function changes in long-term survivors of allogeneic marrow transplantation. In: *Recent advances in bone marrow transplantation,* Vol. 7. Gale, R. P. (Ed.). Liss, New York, pp. 343-353 (1983).
35. Parkins, C. S., Fowler, J. F., Maughan, R. L., Roper, M. J. Repair in mouse lung for up to 20 fractions of X-rays or neutrons. *Brit. J. Radiol. 58,* 225-241 (1985).

36. Rowley, M. J., Leach, D. R., Warner, G. A., et al. Effect of graded doses of ionising radiation on the human testis. *Radiat. Res. 59,* 665-678 (1974).
37. Sanders, J. E., Buckner, C. D., Leonard, J. M., Sullivan, K. M., Witherspoon, R. P., Deeg, H. J., Storb, R., Thomas, E. D. Late effects on gonadal function of cyclophosphamide, total-body irradiation, and marrow transplantation. *Transplantation 36,* 252-255 (1983).
38. Lushbaugh, C. C., Ricks, R. C. Some cytokinetic and histopathologic considerations of irradiated male and female gonadal tissues. *Front. Radiat. Ther. Oncol. 6,* 228-248 (1972).
39. Ash, P. The influence of radiation on fertility in man. *Brit. J. Radiol. 53,* 271-278 (1980).
40. Pedrick, T. J., Hoppe, R. T. Recovery of spermatogenesis following pelvic irradiation for Hodgkin's disease. *Int. J. Radiat. Oncol. Biol. Phys. 12,* 117-121 (1986).
41. Kohn, H. I., Kallman, R. F. The effect of fractionated X-ray dosage upon the mouse testis. I. Maximum weight loss following 80 to 240 rad given in 2 to 5 fractions during 1 to 4 days. *J. Natl. Cancer Inst. 15,* 891-899 (1955).
42. Silini, G., Hornsey, S., Bewley, D. K. Effects of X-ray and neutron dose fractionation on the mouse testis. *Radiat. Res. 19,* 50-63 (1963).
43. Cattanach, B. M. Spermatogonial stem cell killing in the mouse following single and fractionated X-ray dose as assessed by length of sterile period. *Mutat. Res. 25,* 53-62 (1974).
44. Withers, H. R., Hunter, N., Barkley, H. T., Reid, B. O. Radiation survival and regeneration characteristics of spermatogenic stem cells of mouse testis. *Radiat. Res. 57,* 88-103 (1974).
45. Lu, C. C., Meistrich, M. L., Thames, H. D. Survival of mouse testicular stem cells after γ or neutron irradiation. *Radiat. Res. 81,* 402-415 (1980).
46. de Ruiter-Bootsma, A. L., Kramer, M. F., de Rooij, D. G. Survival of spermatogonial stem cells in the mouse after split-dose irradiation with fission neutrons of 1 MeV mean energy or 300 kV X-rays. *Radiat. Res. 71,* 579-592 (1977).
47. Sandeman, T. F. The effects of X-irradiation on male human fertility. *Brit. J. Radiol. 39,* 901-907 (1966).
48. Sheridan, W. The effects of the time interval in fractionated X-ray treatment of mouse-spermatogonia. *Mutat. Res. 13,* 163-169 (1971).
49. Meistrich, M. L. Relationship between spermatogonial cell survival and testis function after cytotoxic therapy. *Brit. J. Cancer 53 (Suppl. VII)*, 89-101 (1986).
50. da Cunha, M. F., Meistrich, M. L., Fuller, L. M., et al. Recovery of spermatogenesis after treatment for Hodgkin's disease: limiting dose of MOPP chemotherapy. *J. Clin. Oncol. 2,* 571-577 (1984).
51. Guesry, P., Lenoir, M., Broyer, M. Gonadal effects of chlorambucil given to prepubertal and pubertal boys for nephrotic syndrome. *J. Pediatrics 92,* 299-303 (1978).
52. Hsu, A. C., Folami, A. O., Bain, J., Rance, C. D. Gonadal function in males treated with cyclophosphamide for nephrotic syndrome. *Fertil. Steril. 31,* 173-177 (1979).

53. Delic, J. I., Hendry, J. H., Morris, I. D., Shalet, S. M. Dose and time related responses of the irradiated prepubertal rat testis. I. Leydig cell function. *Int. J. Androl. 8,* 459-471 (1985).
54. Delic, J. I., Hendry, J. H., Morris, I. D., Shalet, S. M. Dose and time related responses of the irradiated prepubertal rat testis. II. Seminiferous epithelial function. *Int. J. Androl. 8,* 484-496 (1985).
55. Delic, J. I., Hendry, J. H., Morris, I. D., Shalet, S. M. Leydig cell function in the pubertal rat following local testicular irradiation. *Radiother. Oncol. 5,* 29-37 (1986).
56. Delic, J. I., Hendry, J. H., Morris, I. D., Shalet, S. M. Seminiferous epithelial function in the pubertal rat following local testicular irradiation. *Radiother. Oncol. 5,* 39-45 (1986).
57. Delic, J. I., Hendry, J. H., Morris, I. D., Shalet, S. M. Dose and time relationships in the endocrine response of the irradiated adult rat testis. *J. Androl. 7,* 32-41 (1986).
58. Delic, J. I. Studies on testicular function in the rat after cytotoxic injury. Ph.D Thesis, University of Manchester, U.K. (1983).
59. Sanders, J. E., Pritchard, S., Mahoney, P., et al. Growth and development following marrow transplantation for leukaemia. *Blood 68,* 1129-1135 (1986).
60. Shalet, S. M., Beardwell, C. G., Jacobs, H. G., Pearson, D. Testicular function following irradiation of the human prepubertal testis. *Clin. Endocrinol. 9,* 483-490 (1978).
61. Shalet, S. M. The effects of cancer treatment on growth and sexual development. *Clin. Oncol. 4* (2), 223-238 (1985).
62. Bianchi, M. Cytotoxic insult to germinal tissue. In: *Cytotoxic insult to tissue: effects on cell lineages.* Potten, C. S., Hendry, J. H. (Eds.). Churchill-Livingstone, Edinburgh, pp. 258-328 (1983).
63. Lindop, P. J. The effects of radiation on rodent and human ovaries. *Proc. Roy. Soc. Med. 62,* 144-148 (1969).
64. Baker, T. G. Radiosensitivity of mammalian oocytes with particular reference to the human female. *Amer. J. Obst. Gynecol. 110,* 746-761 (1971).
65. Lushbaugh, C. C., Casarett, G. W. The effects of gonadal irradiation in clinical radiation therapy: a review. *Cancer 37,* 1111-1120 (1976).
66. Shalet, S. M., Beardwell, C. G., Morris-Jones, P. H., Pearson, D., Orrell, D. H. Ovarian failure following abdominal irradiation in childhood. *Brit. J. Cancer 33,* 655-658 (1976).
67. Merriam, G. R., Focht, E. F. A clinical study of radiation cataracts and the relationship to dose. *Amer. J. Roent. 77,* 759-785 (1957).
68. Deeg, H. J., Flournoy, N., Sullivan, K. M., et al. Cataracts after total body irradiation and marrow transplantation: a sparing effect of dose fractionation. *Int. J. Radiat. Oncol. Biol. Phys. 10,* 957-964 (1984).
69. Merriam, G. R., Szechter, A., Focht, A. F. The effects of ionising radiations in the eye. *Front. Radiat. Ther. Oncol. 6,* 346-385 (1972).
70. Heyn, R. M. Late effects of therapy in rhabdomyosarcoma. *Clin. Oncol. 4* (2), 287-297 (1985).

71. Merriam, G. R., Focht, E. F. A clinical and experimental study of the effect of single and divided doses of radiation on cataract production. *Trans. Am. Ophthalmol. Soc. 60,* 35-52 (1962).
72. Schenken, L. L., Hagemann, R. F. Time/dose relationships in experimental radiation cataractogenesis. *Radiology 117,* 193-198 (1975).
73. Malone, J. F., O'Connor, M. K., Hendry, J. H. The cellular basis of radiation effects in thyroid, salivary and adrenal epithelia. In: *Cytotoxic insult to tissue: effects on cell lineages.* Potten, C. S., Hendry, J. H. (Eds.). Churchill-Livingstone, Edinburgh, pp. 186-227 (1983).
74. Sklar, C. A., Kim, T. H., Ramsay, N. K. C. Thyroid dysfunction among long-term survivors of bone marrow transplantation. *Amer. J. Med. 73,* 688-694 (1982).
75. Robison, L. L. Delayed consequences of therapy in childhood acute lymphoblastic leukaemia. *Clin. Oncol. 4* (2), 321-332 (1985).
76. Sklar, C. A., Ramsay, N. K. C. Endocrine dysfunction after successful bone marrow transplantation. *Clin. Oncol. 4* (2), 345-352 (1985).
77. Shalet, S. M. Irradiation-induced growth failure. *Clin. Endocrinol. Metab. 15* (3), 591-606 (1986).
78. Mosier, H. D., Jansons, R. A., Swingle, K. F., et al. Growth hormone secretion in the stunted head-irradiated rat. *Pediat. Res. 19,* 543-548 (1985).

11

Long-Term Bone Marrow Damage After Treatment for Acute Lymhoblastic Leukemia

NYDIA G. TESTA
Paterson Institute for Cancer Research, Christie Hospital and Holt Radium Institute, Manchester, England

MANJU BHAVNANI,* ANDREW WILL, and PATRICIA H. MORRIS JONES
Royal Manchester Children's Hospital, Manchester, England

I. INTRODUCTION

Present therapy for acute lymphoblastic leukemia (ALL) in childhood achieves disease-free, long-term survival for about half of the patients. It is therefore important to examine the long-term effects of therapy in these patients, especially because this disease affects mainly children at a tender age. Damage to pulmonary tissue, the heart, the central nervous system, and endocrine and gonadal tissues is well recognized (Chapter 6). Although the bone marrow is one of the limiting tissues for cytotoxic therapy, the acute damage is quickly corrected due to the vast proliferative capacity of the surviving stem and progenitor cells. However, long-term bone marrow damage, which is sometimes hidden and not manifested in lower production of mature functional cells, is known to occur in experimental systems. There are reports in the literature, reviewed elsewhere in this book, of abnormal hemopoiesis following cytotoxic treatment to patients with other types of malignancies. Although the clinical implications of these observations are not clear, the bone marrow damage may in theory be the cause of inadequate response to hemopoietic stress, may predispose to a secondary (hemopoietic) malignancy, or may compromise the reserve capacity of the tissue much later in life.

In this chapter, we analyze available data on long-term bone marrow damage in children treated for ALL and discuss the possible implications for the function of this tissue in the light of our knowledge of the regulation of the production of hemopoietic cells.

**Present affiliation*: Department of Haematology, Royal Albert Edward Infirmary, Lancaster, England.

II. STUDIES OF PROGENITOR CELLS

Studies that have examined the progenitors of granulocytes and macrophages (GM-CFCs) in the bone marrow in patients with ALL in remission and off treatment have in general reported a normal incidence (1-4). In one study, however, a group of children who had received extra chemotherapy for testicular or CNS infiltration or for hematological relapse showed markedly decreased incidence (2). One point worthy of notice is that in the latter study, all patients, even those with low incidences of GM-CFCs, had cellular marrow aspirates, normal numbers of white and red cells in the peripheral blood, and, with one exception, normal numbers of platelets. They could, therefore, be considered hematologically normal by those parameters. However, another study (1) found that platelets were often low. One important observation is that low incidence of GM-CFCs is not predictive of relapse (2,4).

It has to be considered whether the observed low incidence of GM-CFCs (2) is a true reflection of their numbers in vivo. It is possible, as has been described following bone marrow transplantation (5), that an apparently low incidence may be the result of an imbalance in subpopulations of lymphoid cells. However, direct studies on the influence of T cell subpopulations on the GM-CFCs have not yet been performed in these patients.

Studies of erythroid progenitor cells, BFU-E, have shown normal incidence in the bone marrow in adult patients in remission but low incidence in peripheral blood (6). Also, studies of multipotential progenitors, Mix-CFCs, have shown normal incidence in the marrow of adults treated for ALL (7).

III. STUDIES OF STROMAL CELLS

Hemopoiesis, both in vivo and in vitro, takes place within a complex regulatory microenvironment composed by several stromal (and other) cell types and their products (see Chapters 1 and 2). It is known from experimental systems that long-term bone marrow damage may result from the effects of chemotherapy on the stem cells and/or be the result of an altered regulatory microenvironment (Chapter 4). It is reasonable to expect that after intense combined chemotherapy both factors are likely to play a role. As discussed elsewhere in this book (Chapters 2 and 4), the analytical study of the stromal cells in the bone marrow is difficult both because of the several distinct populations involved and because some of the assays are quantitative, but not functional, measurements. In the latter category is the CFU-F assay, which relies on the capacity of a progenitor of reticular-fibroblastoid cells to proliferate and form colonies in culture. Patients with ALL who were off treatment and in remission, studied for periods up to 3 years after cessation of treatment, showed normal incidence of CFU-F in the bone marrow, even those who had low incidence of GM-CFCs (2,3,8). However, this assay measures only one type of the cell populations that compose the hemopoietic microenvironment, and such a cell type may have a more extensive proliferation capacity than other stromal cell populations to recover after cytotoxic injury.

As discussed in Chapters 1, 2, and 4, normal microenvironmental regulation depends on the balance of several cell populations and their products and on the integrity of complex cellular networks. One approach to the study of the functional integrity of the hemopoietic microenvironment is the use of long-term bone marrow cultures; in these cultures active hemopoiesis, which is dependent on the formation of an adherent layer (composed mainly of endothelioid and reticular fibroblastoid cells, adipocytes, and macrophages), is maintained for several weeks.

Long-term bone marrow cultures from 20 patients treated with the protocol UK ALL VIII detailed in Table 1 showed levels of mature granulocytes and macrophages similar to those of control cultures (Fig. 1). This agrees with the clinical picture in those patients who were in full hematological remission, with cellular marrows and normal numbers of granulocytes, red cells, and platelets in peripheral blood. However, the numbers of GM-CFCs measured in the same cultures showed levels 5-10 times lower than in controls in the cells released into the

Table 1 UK ALL VIII Protocol

1. Induction

Vincristine	Asparginase	Prednisolone
1.5 mg/m^2	6000 IU/m^2	40 mg/m^2
Days 1, 8, 15, 22	9 doses in 28 days	Days 1-28

Randomization: Group A: No daunorubicin
Group B: Daunorubicin 45 mg/m^2 on days 1 and 2

2. CNS Prophylaxis

Intrathecal Methotrexate	CNS Irradiation
Dose dependent on age	18 Gy
6 doses in first 7 weeks	Weeks 5-7

3. Maintenance[a]: 28-day cycles

Vincristine	Prednisolone	Methotrexate	Mercaptopurine
1.5 mg/m^2	40 mg/m^2	20 mg/m^2	75 mg/m^2
Day 1	Days 1-5	Days 1, 8, 15, 22	Days 1-28

Randomization: Patients received either 24 or 36 cycles.

[a]Quoted doses may be reduced in the presence of cytopenia.

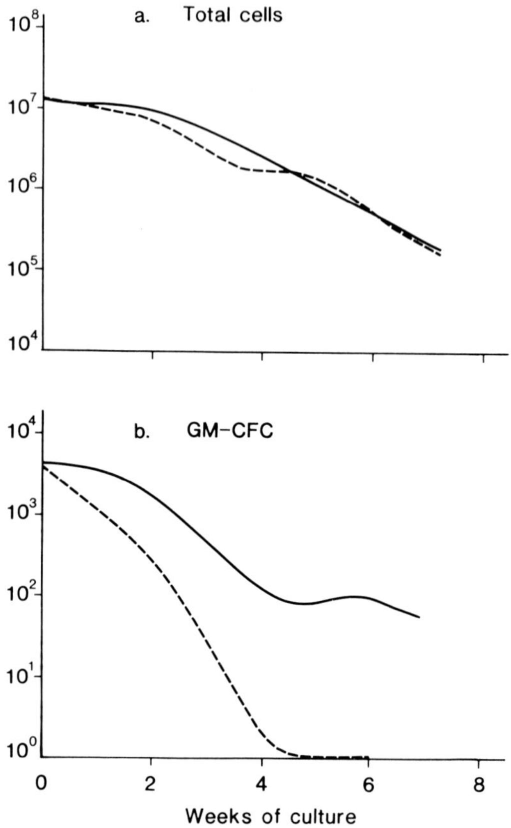

Figure 1 Production of nucleated cells and of GM-CFCs in long-term bone marrow cultures from 20 children in hematological remission after treatment for ALL (dashed line) compared to 9 matched controls (full line). Ordinate shows the numbers measured in suspension at the times indicated.

growth medium harvested every week. The numbers of GM-CFCs that remained within the adherent layer were also lower than in the control cultures; this observation has particular significance since it is within the adherent layer that active hemopoiesis takes place (9,10). The results in Figure 1 indicate that normal production of mature cells in these cultures is achieved from a reduced progenitor (and probably stem cell) population, a situation similar to that seen experimentally in vivo as well as in vitro after varied cytotoxic treatments to mice (Chapter 4). Compensatory mechanisms appear to act in the long-term cultures as effectively as they do in vivo to maintain a normal level of mature cell production, making these cultures a valid means for the study of regulatory mechanisms.

It is, however, not possible to state from these results whether the subnormal numbers of progenitor cells are the result of injury to hemopoietic or to regulatory cell populations. To address this question, two-step cultures were performed: adherent layers from bone marrow of controls or patients were allowed to form and were then irradiated with 16 Gy to stop hemopoiesis. The irradiated but functionally normal adherent layers were then seeded with either normal bone marrow cells or cells from patients. The results indicated that normal adherent layers were able to induce similar numbers of GM-CFCs and mature cells, regardless of whether the second marrow inoculum was from patients or from controls. On the other hand, adherent layers derived from patients' marrow supported only about half as many GM-CFCs as adherent layers derived from normal marrow, and only about 80% of the numbers of mature cells, regardless of the source of the marrow used for the second inoculum (Fig. 2). These observations establish that the marrow stroma of patients treated for ALL is damaged. However, in the one-step cultures shown in Figure 1, the difference in the numbers of GM-CFCs is of greater magnitude than in the two-step cultures, which indicates, as may be expected, that stem and progenitor cells may also be damaged directly.

However, the two-step cultures indicate that the limiting factor in determining the level of hemopoiesis, at least in vitro, is the regulatory microenvironment

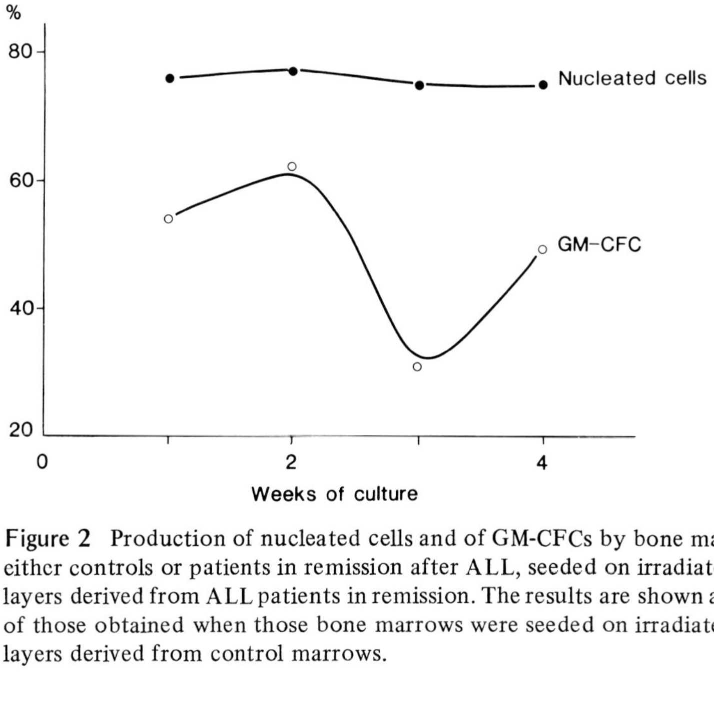

Figure 2 Production of nucleated cells and of GM-CFCs by bone marrow of either controls or patients in remission after ALL, seeded on irradiated adherent layers derived from ALL patients in remission. The results are shown as percentage of those obtained when those bone marrows were seeded on irradiated adherent layers derived from control marrows.

(1) because of the subnormal level of hemopoiesis shown by the normal marrow inoculum on ALL stroma and (2) because the hemopoietic cells from ALL patients generated GM-CFC and mature cell numbers comparable to controls when inoculated on normal stroma.

IV. EVALUATION OF RESIDUAL DEFECTS

The evaluation of the effects of cytotoxic therapy on the hemopoietic system of patients with ALL is complicated by the fact that the leukemic cells infiltrate the bone marrow; it is therefore not possible to separate events that may be due to the development of the leukemia from those that may be the result of therapy. There are indications that the bone marrow environment is abnormal in patients with ALL at presentation: the incidence of CFU-F (a cell population that is not part of the leukemic clone) is markedly subnormal in ALL patients studied at presentation. This has been attributed to inhibitory action of the leukemic cells (8). There is a quick return to normal following treatment, and normal values are maintained during remission (2,3,8).

In acute nonlymphocytic leukemia (ANLL), a high proportion of patients in remission will eventually relapse, and therefore signs of abnormal granulopoiesis seen during remission may be attributed to persistence of leukemic cells. Indeed, metabolic abnormalities and alterations in the production of or response to regulatory molecules as well as the persistence of marker chromosomes in myeloid cells studied in remission suggest that they may belong to the leukemic clone (11-13; Chapter 12). Recently, this view has received support from the observation that 3 of 13 patients of ANLL in remission studied using X-chromosome-linked DNA polymorphisms in bone marrow DNA showed the persistence of clonal (leukemic) hemopoiesis (13). In ALL, however, the myeloid cells are not part of the leukemic process, and therefore any alterations found in this compartment may be the result of therapy.

There are arguments that support the concept that abnormal hemopoiesis in patients treated for ALL may be the result of therapy rather than of the original disease:

1. Sequential determinations of GM-CFCs in patients who eventually relapsed showed that the values obtained were fairly constant (2) and there was not a progressive decline preceding relapse (2,4). However, when bone marrow infiltration becomes apparent during relapse, low values are observed (1). These results are in contrast with the progressive decline seen over several months preceding the diagnosis of secondary ANLL after therapy for non-Hodgkin's lymphoma (14).
2. There appears to be a dose effect with children who have received extra treatment for testicular or CNS infiltration or hematological relapse, showing low incidence of GM-CFCs, while a group of patients treated only with the standard protocol showed no difference from the controls (2). This dose effect

tends to favor the interpretation of therapy-related bone marrow damage. The observation that there is a microenvironmental component causing the subnormal hemopoiesis seen in long-term bone marrow culture may help to clarify further whether the damage is related to the treatment rather than to the leukemic process. Experiments similar to those shown in Figure 2, measuring the capacity to induce hemopoiesis of stromal layers from untreated ALL patients at presentation and during remission, will indicate whether the marrow stroma is further damaged by therapy.

Two facts are important when bone marrow damage in children is assessed. The first is the long prospective life span. It is known that in experimental mice, stem cells are not exhausted with age and have a reserve capacity that far exceeds the needs of a normal life span, even after being subjected to intense induced proliferative stress (15,16). However, it is not yet known whether the first children

Table 2 Hematological Parameters in Children in Remission After Treatment for ALL

Parameter	Status	Ref.
White blood cells	Normal	1,2
Red blood cells	Normal	1,2
Platelets	Normal or low	2 1
Numbers of GM-CFCs in peripheral blood	Low[a]	6
Incidence of GM-CFCs in bone marrow	Normal or low[b]	1-4 2
Cycling status of GM-CFCs	High	Tejero et al., unpublished
Production of mature cells in LTBMC[c]	Normal	Figure 1
Production of GM-CFCs in LTBMC	Low	Figure 1
Capacity of the marrow stroma to support hemopoiesis in LTBMC	Low	Figure 2
Incidence of CFU-F in the bone marrow	Normal	2,3,8

[a]In adults.
[b]Related to dose of cytotoxic drugs.
[c]LTBMC = long-term bone marrow culture.

cured of ALL, who are now in young adulthood, may be at risk of hemopoietic failure later in their lives. The normal level of mature cell production in these children coexists with several abnormalities (summarized in Table 2) all of which suggest stressed hemopoiesis, reaching normal cell production by calling into action compensatory mechanisms. One of those is the increased cell cycling in the GM-CFC compartment (Tejero, Will, and Testa, unpublished), which we are currently investigating. In this context, it is worrying that neither the low incidence of GM-CFCs nor their increased cycling shows a tendency to return to normal values in the 3 years following cessation of treatment (the longest period we have studied to date).

The second factor to consider is the risk of developing a second malignancy, not only therapy-related ANLL, but others later in life. In those cases, a careful assessment of the reserve capacity of the hemopoietic tissue and of its potential capacity to recover after further cytotoxic treatment may have to be considered when deciding the type and extent of therapy.

ACKNOWLEDGMENTS

The authors thank the Cancer Research Campaign (U.K.) for supporting this research.

REFERENCES

1. Inoue, S., Ravindranath, Y., Lusher, J. M., Ito, T. Hematological parameters and marrow in vitro colony forming cells in acute lymphoblastic leukemia after cessation of treatment. *Acta Haematol. Jap. 43,* 61-70 (1980).
2. Haworth, C., Morris Jones, P. H., Testa, N. G. Long-term bone marrow damage in children treated for ALL: evidence from in vitro colony assays (GM-CFC and CFU-F). *Brit. J. Cancer 46,* 918-923 (1982).
3. Katsuno, H., Hirata, J., Kaneko, S., Nishimura, J., Motomura, S., Ibayashi, H. Serial studies of bone marrow derived fibroblastoid colony-forming cells and granulocyte-macrophage precursor cells in patients with acute leukemia. *Acta Haematol. 76,* 185-191 (1986).
4. Shi, L. Y., Chiu, W. F. In vitro granulopoiesis in adult acute lymphoblastic leukemia at various phases of the disease. *Leuk. Res. 11,* 415-420 (1987).
5. Li, S., Champlin, R., Fitchen, J. H., Gale, R. P. Abnormalities of myeloid progenitor cells after "successful" bone marrow transplantation. *J. Clin. Invest. 75,* 234-241 (1985).
6. Peschel, C., Kowalinka, G., Geissler, D., Braunsteiner, H. In vitro growth of erythropoietic progenitor cells in long-term remission of acute leukemia. *Int. J. Cell Cloning 4,* 186-191 (1986).
7. Ganser, A., Hoelzer, D. Effect of intensified chemotherapy on the pluripotent haematopoietic progenitor cells CFU-GEMM in adult acute lymphoblastic leukaemia. *Brit. J. Haematol. 64,* 169-178 (1986).

8. Nagao, T., Yamauchi, K., Komatsuda, M., Noguchi, K., Shimizu, M., Yonekura, S., Nogaki, H. Inhibition of human bone marrow fibroblast colony formation by leukemic cells. *Blood 62,* 1261-1265 (1983).
9. Dexter, T. M., Spooncer, E., Simmons, P., Allen, T. D. Long-term marrow cultures—an overview of techniques and experience. In: *Long-term bone marrow cultures.* Wright, D. G., Greenberger, J. S. (Eds.). Alan R. Liss, New York, pp. 57-96 (1984).
10. Coulombel, L., Eaves, A. C., Eaves, C. J. Enzymatic treatment of long-term human marrow cultures reveals the preferential location of primitive hemopoietic progenitors in the adherent layer. *Blood 62,* 291-297 (1983).
11. Miller, A. M., Gross, M. A., Weiner, R. S. Alteration in the requirement for leukotriene (LT) synthesis in leukemia marrow. *Proc. AACR 27,* 40 (abstr. 156) (1986).
12. Broxmeyer, H. E., Grossbard, E., Jacobsen, N., Moore, M. A. S. Persistence of inhibitory activity against normal bone marrow cells during remission of acute leukemia. *New Engl. J. Med. 301,* 346-351 (1979).
13. Fearon, E. R., Burke, P. J., Schiffer, C. A., Zehnbauer, B. A., Vogelstein, B. Differentiation of leukemia cells to polymorphonuclear leukocytes in patients with acute nonlymphocytic leukemia. *New Engl. J. Med. 315,* 15-24 (1986).
14. Haworth, C., Stevens, R. F., Testa, N. G. Serial incidence of bone marrow GM-CFC prior to the development of acute non-lymphoblastic leukaemia in a child treated for non-Hodgkin lymphoma. *Brit. J. Haematol. 59,* 79-84 (1985).
15. Ross, E. A. M., Anderson, N., Micklem, H. S. Serial depletion and regeneration of the hematopoietic system. *J. Exp. Med. 155,* 432-444 (1982).
16. Valeriote, F., Tolen, S. Extensive proliferative capacity of haemopoietic stem cells. *Cell Tissue Kinet. 16,* 1-6 (1983).

12

Long-Term Bone Marrow Damage After Acute Nonlymphocytic Leukemia

ALAN M. MILLER and ROY SAMUEL WEINER
University of Florida, College of Medicine, Gainesville, Florida

I. CURRENT TRENDS IN THERAPY

Modern therapy for acute nonlymphocytic leukemia (ANLL) has resulted in prolonged disease-free survival for increasing numbers of patients. The improvement in therapeutic results can be attributed to many factors: better drugs, more intensive dosage, better supportive care, and increased utilization of comprehensive leukemia treatment centers by more patients. As the number of long-term survivors increases, it becomes important to examine the long-term effects of both leukemia and its therapy. There have been relatively few reports of hemopoietic function in remission patients and only a few reports of progenitor cell growth and differentiation in patients who are apparently free of disease and who are not receiving chemotherapy. We and others, however, have observed abnormal progenitor cell function in such patients and have raised the question of whether the abnormal growth results from chemotherapy or from the leukemic process. While the clinical consequences of these abnormalities are not known, they may represent a threat to survival by providing inadequate host responses or by predisposing to new or recurrent hemopoietic malignancies. In this chapter we will discuss what is known about hemopoietic function during remission and formulate a framework for future study.

Prolonged remissions, with unmaintained durations of 2 years, were first reported in the early 1980s. Intensification of cytotoxic chemotherapy was the common factor among the more successful regimens. The more successful induction regimens included at least 3 days of anthracycline therapy combined with 7 days of cytosine arabinoside, given by continuous infusion or by twice daily bolus injections (1-4). Consolidation and maintenance chemotherapy usually consisted of anthracyclines, a few of the antimetabolites, and, in some studies, aklylating agents.

We have reported a complete remission rate of 75% with 67% disease-free survival at 2 years and a protracted disease-free survival rate of 38% at 4 years, using four courses of intensive chemotherapy. The first course consisted of 3 days of daunorubicin combined with 10 days of continuous cytosine arabinoside. Subsequent courses included 6-thioguanine and 5-azactidine (5). A larger study evaluated alternatives for postinduction therapy. All patients in that study were induced with 10 days of continuous infusion of Ara-C and three daily injections of daunorubicin, with 65% of 213 patients achieving complete remission. The design of that study includes both intensive and nonintensive consolidation regimens. Although it is still too early for the assessment of long-term effects, there will be patients with durable remission in both arms for evaluation. The questions that may be addressed in studying these patients include those of whether there are more treatment-induced defects in the cells of the patients treated intensively and whether those treated with nonintensive combinations are more likely to have defects associated with residual leukemia. Of the patients in this study who are now more than 2 years past achieving complete remission, approximately half remain in complete remission (6), thus making it likely that long-term hemopoietic effects can be studied.

II. EFFECTS OF COMMONLY USED AGENTS ON HEMOPOIETIC CELLS

Studies of the effects on hemopoietic precursors of the agents commonly used in intensive regimens generally indicate a detrimental effect on the target populations. In a series of papers, Marsh has examined the effects of chemotherapeutic agents on human and experimental animal marrow cells grown in agar contained in diffusion chambers placed intraperitoneally in mice (7-10). The residual drug effect in those studies was assessed by injecting host animals with the particular agent and, after a defined period, transplanting the chambers into untreated mice and following growth within the chambers. Agents that are used in current intensive regimens that have been tested in this system are 5-azacytadine, cytosine arabinoside (Ara-C), m-AMSA, and adriamycin. All four drugs caused significant inhibition of subsequent growth in the diffusion chambers. With Ara-C, a survival plateau of approximately 50% was seen in the dose-response curve supporting a cycle-phase-specific phenomenon. Similarly, a plateau was seen with 5-azacytadine. Adriamycin and m-AMSA, on the other hand, caused exponential dose-related decreases in precursor survival, indicating an ability of the drug to kill cells in all phases of the cell cycle as well as noncycling cells.

Botnick and co-workers have described an exquisite system for determination of the long-term effects on the pluripotent hemopoietic precursors, CFU-S, in mice (11,12). In their studies these authors assess damage to stem cells by measuring self-renewal capacity following single exposure to a chemotherapeutic agent. This self-renewal is measured by the ability of these precursors to repopulate serially lethally irradiated mice. The cytotoxic agents were studied in this system, and treated cells routinely demonstrated a decreased ability to repopulate and therefore a decreased self-renewal capacity. The implications of these results are that long-term survivors of therapy may be at a higher risk for failure or abnormality of one or all hemopoietic lines at a time point remote from their therapy.

The long-term damage from chemotherapy might be subtle and manifested only when marrow is stressed. Using sensitivity to a subsequent exposure to radiation, Kovacs et al. demonstrated that prior in vivo exposure to adriamycin caused increased sensitivity of all hemopoietic precursors to subsequent radiation injury (13). The increased sensitivity to irradiation increased with the post-treatment interval, suggesting that the chemotherapy injury may be abnormally accelerated depletion of the self-renewing population of stem cells.

In another study, Braunschweiger et al. assessed the ability of mice previously treated with adriamycin or daunorubicin to respond to acute anemic stress (14). Four months after therapy animals were bled, and 48 hr later they were sacrificed. Spleen weight and the percentage of nucleated erythroid cells in the spleen and marrow were assessed. In unbled animals there was little difference in these parameters between previously treated and control animals; however, in animals treated with either of the anthracyclines the ability to respond to the acute insult with brisk expansion of the erythroid compartment was markedly decreased.

In addition to affecting bone marrow stem cells directly, chemotherapy has also been shown to affect the bone-marrow-supporting stroma in experimental animals. Ben-Ishay et al. treated normal and leukemic mice with Ara-C and adriamycin. Bone marrow hemopoietic progenitors (GM-CFCs and CFU-D) as well as bone marrow stromal precursors (CFU-F) were assessed serially (15). In nonleukemic mice an initial posttherapy increase was noted in the hemopoietic progenitors, as had previously been described for mice as well as human patients (16,17). Subsequently a period of marked fluctuation was noted both in hemopoietic progenitors and in CFU-F, but eventually levels returned to baseline. There were no studies performed on the long-term effect.

The long-term effects of therapy on stroma may be best studied in the allogeneic bone marrow transplant setting where the host microenvironment but not the donor hemopoietic precursors is exposed to the ablative cytotoxic therapy. Gale et al. studied myeloid progenitors (GM-CFCs) in 41 patients 2-7 years after transplant and found them to be significantly decreased despite normal peripheral blood levels of granulocytes (18). The decrease in apparent number of GM-CFCs was thought to be due to abnormal regulation by T lymphocytes. The CFU-F were not studied nor was the ability of the host fibroblast to produce colony-stimulating factors in response to IL-1 produced by donor monocytes (19). As the methods by which regulating cell populations communicate with each other become known, more definitive assessments of cell injury will be possible.

III. PROGENITOR CELL ASSAYS IN LEUKEMIC PATIENTS

In vitro assays for committed progenitor cells have been studied as potentially useful tools for diagnosis and monitoring of acute leukemia. Moore et al. (20) studied the myeloid-committed progenitor cells from a large series of patients, including 33 with AML, and reported abnormal patterns of in vitro growth, characterized either by complete lack of growth or by production of large numbers of small aggregates of poorly differentiated cells. Further studies demonstrated that although these cells grew abnormally, they still maintained dependence on and sensitivity to normal growth factors (21).

Several studies have examined bone marrow progenitor cells in patients with ANLL in remission (22-26). However, most of these have involved patients continuing to receive maintenance therapy. Galbraith reported abnormal growth patterns in 3 patients in remission, one of whom remained in continuous remission for 18 months, with only cluster formation manifested in vitro (22) He concluded that remission status was not necessarily associated with repopulation of the bone marrow by normal hemopoietic cells. Mertelsman et al. assayed myeloid colony-forming units (GM-CFCs) in bone marrow cells from patients in complete remission from ANLL. They studied 354 samples on 48 patients prior to their next scheduled maintenance treatment and noted marked fluctuations in the number of aggregates and in the growth pattern (23). They divided growth patterns into three groups: no growth, normal growth (<50 colonies and <30-fold excess of clusters), and "AML type" (>30-fold excess of clusters). They noted fluctuations of individual patients changing from normal to abnormal growth patterns and back again, apparently without relationship to chemotherapy cycles and not predictive of eventual relapse. Similar findings were reported by Vincent et al., who showed marked fluctuation and variation in growth of bone marrow of patients with remissions ranging from 100 to 1112 days (24).

Peschel et al. studied 7 patients with ANLL in first stable remission for at least 4 years (6 had been off all therapy for at least 8 months) and concluded that even in patients in long-term remission, certain in vitro abnormalities exist in myelopoietic proliferation and regulation (25). Specifically, the incidence of bone marrow GM-CFC colonies tended to be extremely variable in the patients, particularly after 7 days of culture. Also noted was a significant increase in the presence of microclusters (4-13 cells) during the first 3 days of culture. However, by 7 days the cluster-to-colony ratio was similar to normal controls. No differences were noted between patients and normal individuals in either the number of eosinophil colonies formed or the ability to produce colony-stimulating activity. Although no correlation was seen between number of GM-CFCs in the bone marrow and the number in peripheral blood, the increase in early (3-7 days) clusters and colonies in the marrow and the decreased number of precursors in peripheral blood may represent a compartment shift after therapy for acute leukemia. These authors concluded that although abnormalities in progenitor cells were detectable in patients in long-term remission, they could not clearly be attributed to the effects of therapy rather than to the persistence of an occult leukemic subpopulation.

Eridani et al. studied both GM-CFC and CFU-E in 8 patients in complete remission of AML, two of whom had received no therapy for at least 2 years (26). These patients were treated with a regimen including daunorubicin, Ara-C, and 6-thioguanine. Remission duration at the time of assay was between 3 weeks and 6 years. For the entire group at initial presentation, the number of colony-forming cells was 10% of normal and the number of cluster-forming cells was 33% of normal. The patients in remission, however, had normal numbers of colony- and cluster-forming cells. They did note, however, that in patients with the longest duration of remission, more variability is seen, with marked disparity in colony efficiency. Of their 2 patients with unmaintained remission of 2 years, one had GM-CFC values above normal and the other well below normal. In this group of patients, CFU-E counts at initial presentation were lower than in normal controls when suboptimal concentrations of erythropoietin were used but were indistinguishable from normal at higher erythropoietin concentrations. At remission, CFU-E counts equaled or exceeded normal values, and they remained normal throughout the duration of follow-up during remission.

If any trend can be detected from these studies, it is the great variability in GM-CFC growth and growth patterns during the course of long-term complete remission. There has been no particular pattern or change associated with poor prognosis or durability of remission.

Table 1 Treatment Protocol

	Drug			
Course[a]	Daunorubicin,[b] 40 mg/(m^2-day)	Cytosine arabinoside,[c] 200 mg/(m^2-day)	6-Thioguanine, 100 mg/(m^2-BID)	5-Azacitidine, 150 mg/(m^2-day)
1	X3	X10	–	–
2	X3	X7	X5	–
3	X3	–	X5	X7
4	X3	X7	X5	–

[a]Inverval between courses determined by the return of the peripheral counts to granulocytes $\geqslant$2500/mm^3 and platelets $\geqslant$100,000/mm^3 for at least 1 week.
[b]Number in column represents number of successive days administered.
[c]Cytosine arabinoside administered by continuous infusion.

Table 2 Hemograms of Patients with Complete Remission >24 Months After Therapy[a]

Patient	Months posttherapy[b] 6	12	24	36	Current/ most recent	Comment[d]
CA	7.0/41.1/215	7.3/40.9/210	7.6/42.7/–	7.7/40.7/250	8.3/40.2/208(79M)[c]	CR at 85 mo
WB	7.4/33/133	9.0/45.1/250	8.7/44.2/260	9.2/46.6/274	9.4/46.279(58M)	CR at 62 mo with normal differential, normal marrow at 24 mo
TH	4.8/32.5/156	6.2/40.9/–	6.8/39.8/211	6.5/37/188	7.9/40.0/–(45M)	CR at 45 mo with normal differential, mildly hypocellular marrow at 17 mo
SM	–	9.9/44.4/–	12.6/46.2/–	11.7/47.5/310	12.4/47.7/325(60M)	CR at 83 mo with normal differential, normal marrow at 24 mo
BH	15.8/35.6/–	10.1/39.2/–	7.6/36.8/274	3.5/35.3/250	–––	Relapsed at 41 mo, deceased

[a]All patients treated with protocol described in Table 1.
[b]WBCx10^{-3} per mm^3/hematocrit%/platelet countx10^{-3} per mm^3.
[c]Number of months after treatment of most recent counts.
[d]CR = complete remission.

Our own experience is no different. We studied 12 patients (ages 16-58) with ANLL who were treated with four courses of intensive chemotherapy and followed during unmaintained remission. The treatment protocol used is outlined in Table 1. Of the 12 patients, 9 achieved complete remission; four of those 9 currently remain in complete remission between 43 and 86 months since their last course of therapy. Hemopoietic assessments were done between 6 and 86 months after complete remission on 5 patients from this study who had unmaintained remissions of >24 months. Peripheral hemograms were within normal limits except for mildly decreased leukocytes at 6 months (Table 2). All bone marrows were morphologically normal except for mild megaloblastic changes.

Bone marrow progenitor cells, including GM-CFCs, CFU-E, and BFU-E, from all of these patients showed marked variability compared to those of normal controls (Table 3). All but one patient manifested decreases in one or more marrow progenitor populations regardless of the duration of unmaintained remission. The reason for depressed progenitor cell growth in these patients is unknown, but this severe and durable defect in bone marrow stem cells might be due to (1) inhibition by occult leukemia cells; (2) stem cell injury or depletion due to the cytotoxic therapy; (3) perturbation of other regulatory cells by the cytotoxic therapy; or (4) an inherent defect in the bone marrow stem cells.

Table 3 Progenitor Cell Assays in ANLL Patients with Unmaintained Remission

Patient	Months since last chemotherapy	Percent of normal controls		
		GM-CFC	CFU-E	BFU-E
CA	19	7	9	4
	36	122	141	93
	42	185	81	88
SM	7	61	28	30
	36	74	44	43
	42	97	60	69
	81	57	NT	27
WB	21	155	13.6	25
TH	5	35	49	55
WG	18	7.5	62	59
JG	31	21	95	43

NT = Not tested.

Table 4 Summary of Progenitor Cell Status in Three Groups of ANLL Patients with Unmaintained Remission

Reference	No. of long-term remissions	Range of remission duration (months)	Range of unmaintained remission (months)	Observations
Peschel et al. (25)[a]	6	41-122	7-67	Normal numbers of marrow GM-CFC, increased early marrow clusters, decreased PB GM-CFC, variable CSF levels
Eridani et al. (26)[b]	2	48-72	⩾24	Extreme variability in the two patients, one having GM-CFC values above normal and the other well below normal. However, both had normal CFU-E.
Our patients[c]	6	7-47	5-42	Decreased bone marrow progenitors (at least one line) in most patients.

[a]Rx: All with Ara-C + anthracycline as well as other agents.
[b]Rx: Ara-C, daunorubicin, vincristine, 6-TG, and prednisone.
[c]Rx: As in Table 1.

The reported experiences with patients in protracted unmaintained remission are summarized in Table 4. The major conclusions that can be reached from these 14 patients are that variability exists in marrow precursor numbers and that residual deficiencies may persist. The measurable abnormalities do not appear to have significance. Our patients are not infection-prone.

The effect of ANLL therapy on other cell lineages, particularly megakaryocytes and lymphoid cells, has not been the subject of extensive study. Kovacs et al. looked at T cell function in adriamycin-treated mice. They found significant abnormalities in the ability of cells to produce IL-2 and IL-3 as well as in blastogenesis at 32 weeks posttreatment (27). The effects on these and other cells that produce necessary hemopoietic growth factors may play an important role in the hemopoietic defects manifested following chemotherapy. In the work by Kovacs, IL-3 was decreased by 67% at 32 weeks. This factor is known to be an in vitro multipoietin stimulating erythroid, myeloid, and megakaryocytic lineages (28), and therefore deficiency of this and other factors may affect precursor cells.

IV. ETIOLOGY OF RESIDUAL DEFECTS

Complicating the evaluation of the effects of therapy on the bone marrow is the fact that ANLL is a bone marrow disease. Presumably, patients with certain epithelial malignancies without bone marrow involvement would provide a better model for studying the toxic effects of chemotherapy on hemopoiesis (see Chapter 14). In patients with leukemia, there may be defects as a result of occult residual disease or as a result of genetic events that may have occurred early in the leukemogenic process and that may persist in the absence of overt leukemia. Currently there is no way to separate the relative contributions of therapy and the disease process in evaluating changes in residual marrow.

There are examples of abnormalities in residual marrow that may be attributable to the initial disease process. Broxmeyer et al. have examined peripheral blood and bone marrow cells from acute leukemia patients in remission (29). Bone marrow and blood granulocytes of patients with acute myelogenous leukemia in remission show a defective production of lactoferrin, an inhibitor of colony-stimulating activity. Furthermore, separable populations of cells retain the ability to produce a leukemia-associated inhibitory activity (LIA). This substance is inhibitory to normal but not leukemic CFCs. Residual populations of CFCs resistant to LIA are found in some patients in morphologic complete remission. At the present time, it is unknown whether the resistant populations are clonal or whether their presence portends relapse.

We have previously reported an abnormality in the arachidonic acid metabolism of a subgroup of patients with ANLL (30). While normal GM-CFCs are inhibited in a dose-dependent fashion by inhibitors of the enzyme lipooxygenase, the CFCs from these individuals continue to proliferate despite high concentrations of these inhibitors. This altered sensitivity to lipooxygenase inhibitors persists in bone marrow cells from those individuals through long-term (>2 years) remission.

These leukemia-associated abnormalities appear to persist in remission and are not perturbed by therapy. Mature myeloid cells in remission patients have been shown to bear the clonal molecular markers expressed in the leukemic cells (31). These results suggest that at least some functional mature cells are derived from leukemic progenitors that have differentiated, rather than from residual normal GM-CFCs. Alternatively, chemotherapy may ablate populations of cells that are responsible for the overt manifestations of leukemia but abnormal clones bearing defects characteristic of early events in leukemogenesis persist and may be detectable by new cellular and molecular techniques. The prognostic significance remains unresolved.

It is clear that defective hemopoietic cells are present during complete remission in patients with ANLL. While the chemotherapeutic agents commonly used in ANLL have been shown to cause quantitative and qualitative defects in experimental systems, their contribution to the abnormalities so far described in leukemic patients remain unclear. The data emerging concerning the structured and functional defects associated with leukemogenesis are certainly more intriguing and perhaps more compelling in implicating persisting abnormal clones in the perturbations that have been observed. New techniques of cell separation and the availability of pure growth factors will facilitate more definitive studies of remission cells. As more patients achieve long-term remission status, the prognostic significance of these abnormalities may be defined as well.

REFERENCES

1. Mayer, R. J., Weinstein, J. H., Coral, F. S., Rosenthal, D. S., Frie, E., III. The role of intensive postinduction chemotherapy in the management of patients with acute myelogenous leukemia. *Cancer Treat. Rep. 66,* 1455-1462 (1982).
2. Peterson, B. A., Bloomfield, D. C. Prolonged maintained remissions of adult acute non-lymphocytic leukemia. *Lancet 2,* 158-160 (1977).
3. Priesler, H. D., Rustum, Y., Henderson, E. S., et al. Treatment of acute non-lymphocytic leukemia: use of anthracycline-cytosine arabinoside induction therapy and comparison of the maintenance regimens. *Blood 53,* 455-464 (1979).
4. Gale, R. P., Cline, M. J., UCLA Acute Leukemia Study Group. High remission-induction rate in acute myeloid leukemia. *Lancet 1,* 487-489 (1977).
5. Oblon, D. J., Weiner, R. S., Kramer, B. S., Ross, W., Noyes, W. D., Boyett, J., Kitchens, C. S. Intensive short term chemotherapy for patients with acute myelogenous leukemia: long term follow-up. *Cancer Treat. Rep. 69,* 1425-1427 (1985).

6. Weiner, R. S., Raney, M., Elfenbein, G. J., Kramer, B. S., Vogler, W. R., Winton, E. F., Shina, D. C. Treatment of residual disease in AML: interim analysis of a southeastern cancer study group prospective randomized clinical trial. In: *Minimal residual disease in acute leukemia.* Hagenbeek, A., Lowenberg, B. (Eds.). Martinus Nijhoff, Boston, pp. 167-179 (1985).
7. Marsh, J. C. The effects of cancer chemotherapeutic agents on normal hematopoietic precursor cells: a review. *Cancer Res. 36,* 1853-1882 (1976).
8. Marsh, J. C. Comparison of the sensitivities of human, canine, and murine hematopoietic precursor cells to adriamycin and *N*-trifluoroacetyladriamycin-14-valerate. *Cancer Res. 39,* 360-364 (1979).
9. Marsh, J. C. Comparative effects of methotrexate, two nonclassic folic acid antagonists, and cytarabine on hematopoietic precursor cells. *Cancer Treat. Rep. 66,* 499-504 (1982).
10. Marsh, J. C. Correlation of hematologic toxicity of antineoplastic agents with their effects on bone marrow stem cells: interspecies studies using an in vivo assay. *Exp. Hematol. 13* (*Suppl. 16*), 16-22 (1985).
11. Botnick, L. E., Hannon, E. C., Hellman, S. Late effects of cytotoxic agents on the normal tissue of mice. *Front. Radiat. Therap. Oncol. 13,* 36-47 (1979).
12. Botnick, L. E., Hannon, E. C., Vigneulle, R., Hellman, S. Differential effects of cytotoxic agents on hematopoietic progenitors. *Cancer Res. 41,* 2338-2342 (1981).
13. Kovacs, C. J., Johnke, R. M., Evan, M. J., Emma, D. A., Hoosier, J. L. Development of latent residual drug damage to marrow during the subsequent growth of tumors. *Exp. Hematol. 14,* 165-172 (1986).
14. Braunschweiger, P. G., Kovacs, C. J., Schenken, L. L. Renal and hemopoietic proliferative defects as a delayed consequence of cisplatin, adriamycin and daunomycin treatments. *Brit. J. Cancer 45,* 421-428 (1982).
15. Ben-Ishay, A., Prindull, G., Sharon, S., Borenstein, A. Effects of chemotherapy on bone marrow stroma in mice with acute myelogenous leukemia. Correlation with CFU-C and CFU-D. *Leuk. Res. 9,* 1059-1067 (1985).
16. DeWys, W., Goldin, A., Mantel, M. Hematopoietic recovery after large doses of cyclophosphamide, correlation of proliferative state with sensitivity. *Cancer Res. 30,* 1692-1697 (1970).
17. Richman, C. M., Weiner, R. S., Yankee, R. S. Increase in circulating stem cells following chemotherapy in man. *Blood 47,* 1031-1039 (1976).
18. Gale, R. P., Li, S., Fitchen, J. H., Champlin, R. E. Abnormal CRU-C following bone marrow transplantation in man. *Exp. Hematol. 11* (*Suppl. 14*), 89 (abstr. 162) (1983).
19. Zucali, J. R., Dinarello, C. A., Oblon, D. J., Gross, M. A. G., Anderson, L., and Weiner, R. S. Interleukin 1 stimulates fibroblasts to produce granulocyte-macrophage colony stimulating activity and prostaglandin E2. *J. Clin. Invest. 77,* 1857-1863 (1986).
20. Moore, M. A. S., Williams, N., Metcalf, D. In vitro colony formation by normal and leukemic human hematopoietic cells: characterization of the colony-forming cells. *J. Natl. Cancer Inst. 50,* 630-623 (1972).

21. Metcalf, D., Moore, M. A. S. Growth and responsiveness of human granulocytic leukemic cells in vitro. *Comp. Leuk. Res. 40,* 235-241 (1975).
22. Galbraith, P. R. Remission of acute myeloid leukemia: studies of in vitro colony formation by bone marrow cells. *CMA J. 110,* 1147-1150 (1974).
23. Mertelsmann, R., Moore, M. A. S., Broxmeyer, H. E., Cirrincoine, C., Clarkson, B. Diagnostic and prognostic significance of the CFU-C assay in acute nonlymphoblastic leukemia. *Cancer Res. 41,* 4844-4848 (1981).
24. Vincent, P. C., Sutherland, R., Bradley, M., Lind, D., Gunz, F. W. Marrow culture studies in adult acute leukemia at presentation and during remission. *Blood 49,* 903-912 (1977).
25. Peschel, C., Konwalinka, G., Geissler, D., et al. Studies of myelopoiesis in vitro on blood and bone marrow cells of patients with acute leukemia in long-term remission. *Leuk. Res. 7,* 397-406 (1983).
26. Eridani, S., Sawyer, B., Batten, E. Haemopoietic patterns of acute leukemia in remission: CFU-E and CFU-GM colony formation. *Acta Haematol. 70,* 11-18 (1983).
27. Kovacs, C. J., Evans, M. J., Hooker, J. H., Abernathy, R. S. A permanent defect in T-cell function resulting from adriamycin. *Exp. Hematol. 14,* 505 (abstr. 555) (1986).
28. Quesenberry, P. J., Ihle, J. N., McGrath, E. The effect of interleukin 3 and GM-CSA-2 on megakaryocyte and myeloid clonal colony formation. *Blood 65,* 214-217 (1985).
29. Broxmeyer, H. E., Grossbard, E., Jacobsen, N., Moore, M. A. S. Persistence of inhibitory activity against normal bone marrow cells during remission of acute leukemia. *New Engl. J. Med. 301,* 346-351 (1979).
30. Miller, A. M., Gross, M. A., Weiner, R. S. Alteration in the requirement for leukotriene (LT) synthesis in leukemia marrow. *Proc. AACR 27,* 40 (abstr. 156) (1986).
31. Fearon, E. R., Burke, P. J., Schiffer, C. A., Zehnbauer, B. A., Vogelstein, B. Differentiation of leukemia cells to polymorphonuclear leukocytes in patients with acute nonlymphocytic leukemia. *New Engl. J. Med. 315,* 15-24 (1986).

13

Long-Term Bone Marrow Damage After Treatment for Lymphomas

CLAUDE PARMENTIER, N. MORARDET, and MAURICE TUBIANA
Institut Gustave Roussy and INSERM, Villejuif, France

I. LONG-TERM BONE MARROW DAMAGE INDUCED BY RADIOTHERAPY

A. Introduction

Large-field radiotherapy remains the main modality in the treatment of early-stage malignant lymphomas (1,2). As their survival rate is high, study of these patients provides a unique opportunity for studying the long-term effects of irradiation on the hemopoietic tissues in human beings. Several methods have been used for the investigation of this effect such as peripheral blood count, ferrokinetics, bone marrow scanning, bone marrow biopsy or aspiration, and culture of the bone marrow. The data that have been collected by several groups concern essentially erythropoiesis and are to a large extent consistent. However, several points require further investigation.

B. Methods

1. Radiotherapy

Extended-field irradiation or total nodal irradiation are usually used. Large bone marrow volumes are irradiated by these techniques (3-6). *Mantle-field irradiation* comprises mediastinal, axillary, supraclavicular, and cervical lymph node areas. In adults, approximately 20-30% of the hemopoietic bone marrow is located in the irradiated volume. *Inverted-Y-field irradiation* comprises paraaortic, iliac, and inguinal lymph nodes plus the spleen in nonlaparotomized patients. This includes 30-40% of the hemopoietic bone marrow.

A frequently used technique is subtotal nodal irradiation, which combines a mantle field plus paraaortic and spleen irradiations. Approximately 50% of the bone marrow is irradiated. In *total nodal* irradiation, which associates mantle and inverted Y fields, approximately 60-70% of the hemopoietic bone marrow is irradiated.

The dose received by the bone marrow included in the target volume is generally 40 Gy in fractions of 2 Gy (5 sessions per week). When the irradiation is performed with telecobalt units, the side-scattered irradiation is greater than with megavoltage accelerators. Nevertheless, the different series of patients are approximately comparable with regard to the dose to the irradiated and nonirradiated areas.

2. Investigation Techniques

The erythropoietic regeneration and compensatory mechanisms have been studied mostly by ferrokinetics and whole body scans using ^{59}Fe (7-9), ^{52}Fe (10,11), ^{99m}Tc-sulfur colloid (12), or ^{111}In (13).

All of these techniques have their problems. Their main limitation is that radioisotope uptake is not necessarily a reliable index of hemopoiesis. Ferrokinetic studies appear to be the most specific methods (14-16). For example, the lack of radioiron uptake clearly indicates the absence of erythropoiesis. However, a small uptake may be due to ineffective erythropoiesis or to a metabolic process other than erythropoiesis (17). The results of comparisons between uptake of radioiron and of colloid or ^{111}In render legitimate the clinical use of the latter (18-20). However, the lack of specificity of ^{99m}Tc colloid and of ^{111}In can introduce artifacts in the scintigrams. Therefore, the data obtained with colloids and ^{111}In should be analyzed with great caution (21).

C. Results

1. Blood Cell Count (2)

During the course of radiotherapy a rapid fall is observed both in the blood granulocytes and in the platelet count. In some patients the fall is so severe that the radiotherapy course has to be temporarily interrupted, particularly in elderly patients and patients who have been submitted to chemotherapy prior to the initiation of radiotherapy. When a total nodal irradiation is carried out, a 2-week rest is inserted between the completion of the mantle field and the initiation of the inverted Y field in order to increase hematological tolerance. Similar to what is observed during the radiotherapy course for other types of cancers (22,23), the fall in the number of granulocytes is greater than that which may be ascribed to the proportion of irradiated bone marrow. In most of the patients the rise in the peripheral granulocyte count occurs a few weeks after the completion of radiotherapy and the blood count is back to normal within a few months. In some patients this rise occurs later and is slower, and for several months or even years the lymphocyte and granulocyte blood counts remain lower than normal. The peripheral blood count, however, is not a good indicator of bone marrow damage.

2. Bone Marrow Regeneration

The main result that emerges from the studies is that an irradiation dose greater than 25-30 Gy delivered with the conventional fractionated regimen rapidly induces a profound aplasia. Studies performed as late as 13 years after irradiation showed the persistence of a hypoplasia, indicating that even after long periods complete regeneration does not occur (see Chapter 5).

However, the relationship between the dose and the extent of regeneration remains controversial, as illustrated by the contradictory reports found in the literature. Sykes et al. (24), Slanina et al. (25), and Bajsogolov et al. (26) found persistent aplasia or hypoplasia at doses over 30 Gy and bone marrow restoration below 30 Gy in patients with breast cancer, Hodgkin's disease, and malignant lymphoma, respectively. However, it should be noted that the method they used—sternal marrow aspiration—was only semiquantitative and that the irradiated volumes were relatively small. Parmentier et al. (9), using a ferrokinetic assay and ^{59}Fe scanning, showed that after doses as low as 20 Gy the regeneration remained below normal for several years after irradiation in some patients, but not in all. In contrast, Rubin et al. (12,27), using ^{99m}Tc colloid as a tracer, observed a marked regeneration in most patients a few years after irradiation; however, the specificity of this technique has been questioned.

These apparent inconsistencies are partially explained by the influence of several factors on bone marrow regeneration:

The Irradiated Volume. Morardet et al. (7), using ferrokinetics, and Sacks et al. (13), using ^{111}In as a bone-scanning agent, have shown that there is general correlation between the volume of the central marrow irradiated and the subsequent regeneration of that marrow. They compared patients irradiated on a mantle field or an inverted Y field to patients receiving total or subtotal nodal irradiation and found very little evidence of regeneration in the patients receiving limited irradiation, whereas some regeneration was observed in the vast majority of patients following large-field irradiation. Kaplan has presented autopsy evidence of regeneration to normal cellular levels in patients receiving total nodal irradiation (2). These observations were confirmed and extended by Parmentier et al. (8), who up to 13 years after irradiation demonstrated a more pronounced hypoactivity in the irradiated sites after a mantle-field irradiation than after a more extended irradiation. They are also consistent with the data of Steere et al. (11), although these authors did not mention this volume effect. Thus it can be concluded that only minimal regeneration occurred at dose levels over 30 Gy when major portions of bone marrow were spared irradiation. The influence of the size of the irradiated volume on the regeneration pattern of the irradiated bone marrow suggests the role of stimulating factors different from erythropoietin (11,28), which are discussed later. This is in keeping with the observation that those regions that were treated first regenerated better than those treated during the second half of treatment (10).

Influence of Age. Sacks et al. (13) reported a marked superiority in the capacity for regeneration in patients under 20 years of age. In five patients who were under 17 at the time of their total nodal irradiation, full regeneration occurred in 13 out of 15 sites at risk, irrespective of the dose to those sites (from less than 30 Gy to over 40 Gy). In patients aged from 20 to 40 years at the time of irradiation, regeneration was greater than in older patients for doses lower than 40 Gy. Steere et al. (11) noted that the 3 patients showing the most rapid return to normal uptake were young males aged 15, 20, and 25. At Villejuif (Parmentier et al., unpublished data), almost complete regeneration was observed in children after total or subtotal nodal irradiation even when chemotherapy was associated with radiotherapy. However, doses in excess of 35 Gy are usually associated with inhibition of irradiated bone growth, whereas doses less than 25 Gy have only a mild effect (29). The concentration of active bone marrow in the pelvic region with age helps to explain the lower tolerance of elderly patients to extended irradiation.

The Time Course for Bone Marrow Regeneration. Several groups have investigated the chronology of regeneration and found that it varies markedly among patients. Rubin et al. (12,27), using ^{99m}Tc colloid, noted the onset of regeneration at 1-2 years; after 5 years they claimed that 50% of the patients achieved complete regeneration while an additional 35% achieved partial return to function. Steere et al. (11) showed wide variations from patient to patient. In some patients the iron uptake in the marrow returned to normal levels in 2-3 years, while in others the uptake remained suppressed after 7-8 years. Out of 19 areas scanned 2 years or more after radiotherapy, 15 showed at least 40% of the normal uptake, while only 3 showed no appreciable uptake. Sacks et al. (13) reported a very slight increase in the mean regeneration score correlating with increasing time after irradiation. Knospe et al. (10), using a ^{52}Fe scan, reported that regeneration takes place within 24 months after irradiation. However, Parmentier et al. (8) have documented by sequential study persistent unchanged hypoplasia in some patients after periods extending up to 13 years.

Tubiana and Lalanne (30) reported that 3 months after total body irradiation, up to a dose of 4-5 Gy as a preparation for kidney transplant, tolerance to further irradiation was noticeably decreased, suggesting that after this period the stem cell pool was still markedly reduced.

These data on the slow regeneration of the bone marrow reserve after irradiation are consistent with the experimental data of Knospe et al. (31,32) and Croizat et al. (33). The latter showed that 6-18 months after a total or partial body irradiation of the mouse, the bone marrow multipotential stem cell pool is still reduced and the hemopoietic activity of the irradiated territories never recover completely. Experimental data have also documented the effect of irradiation on irradiated and nonirradiated bone marrow. Croizat et al. (34,35) showed that after iterative partial body irradiation the number of CFU-S in the nonirradiated areas diminished progressively, probably due to the differentiation of stem cells, until a plateau was reached. Hendry and Lajtha (36) have shown that repeated sublethal irradiation produces a progressive decline in the size of the bone marrow CFU-S population. In conclusion, both experimental and human data suggest that regeneration takes place mainly during the first 1-2 years after irradiation and probably reaches a plateau thereafter.

Ineffective Erythropoiesis. In contrast to what is observed in mice (33), ferrokinetics did not demonstrate ineffective erythropoiesis in irradiated or nonirradiated areas. When the plasma iron turnover rate was increased shortly after radiotherapy, suggesting an ineffective erythropoiesis, it returned to normal values after a long follow-up (8).

Splenectomy. The peripheral cell count has been shown to be less depressed in splenectomized irradiated patients than in patients with their spleen intact (2). However, a splenectomy does not seem to induce any modification in the pattern of bone marrow regeneration (8,12). This point deserves further investigation. Radiation-induced splenic atrophy has been reported after radiotherapy including the delivery of 40 Gy to thc spleen (37). In one case the patient died of a spontaneous pneumococcal sepsis comparable to that observed in patients with asplenia, and the authors felt that splenic irradiation was not a benign alternative to splenectomy. At the Institut Gustave-Roussy, 18 patients were studied by splenic scintiscan. Four years after completion of radiotherapy the spleen image was reduced to 30-95% of its pretreatment surface, and it thereafter remained constant up to 10 years, in 17 of them. However, in the case of patient 18, radiation-induced splenic atrophy was discovered (Parmentier et al., unpublished data).

Influence of Patients' Sex. In the series of patients studied by Steere et al. (11), there is some suggestion of a more rapid recovery of erythropoietic function in males than in females.

3. Compensatory Mechanisms

A paradox that was reported in the late 1950s is the disparity between the early (1-3 months) recovery of the peripheral blood cell count after irradiation or even in some patients its constancy under irradiation on the one hand, and the depression of the hemopoietic activity in the irradiated areas on the other hand (38). This demonstrates the existence of compensatory mechanisms that require discussion.

As early as 1959, Tubiana et al. (38), studying ferrokinetics with ^{59}Fe, were able to show that immediately after the completion of a radiotherapy course there was a marked increase in the iron uptake and turnover in the unirradiated bone marrow areas while the iron uptake was totally suppressed in the irradiated bones. Moreover, the plasma turnover and the total incorporation of iron in the red blood cells remained unchanged, demonstrating the existence of fine tuning of the erythropoietic activity. A large body of isotopic data, obtained since that time with radioiron, supports the importance of compensatory hyperactivity in the unirradiated marrow (8,11). Parmentier et al. (8) showed that this hyperactivity of unirradiated bone marrow persists unchanged for up to 13 years after radiotherapy.

Another compensatory mechanism is the extension of hemopoietic activity to previously inactive areas of the skeleton, which was demonstrated by Rubin and co-workers (12,27) using radioactive colloid. This was reported to occur at the end of the first year following total nodal irradiation, and its frequency seems to increase until the fourth year (39). It is therefore a relatively late phenomenon (8). It is more frequent after a total nodal irradiation (13) than after a mantle irradiation (8), and it is not observed in all patients. Steere et al. (11) observed extension in only 1 out of 22 patients. Knospe et al. (10) and Rubin et al. (12) claimed that bone marrow extension may regress in direct response to the amount of in-field regeneration.

Among patients studied with radioiron, extramedullary erythropoiesis in the spleen and the liver was observed by Parmentier et al. (7,8) but not by Steere et al. (11). There is, therefore, some discrepancy with regard to both the incidence and the nature of hemopoietic extension.

4. Recovery of Granulopoiesis

The amount of data concerning the recovery of granulopoiesis after extended-field radiotherapy is smaller than that for erythropoiesis. However, in 9 patients (5 after mantle field and 4 after total nodal irradiation), the numbers of granulocyte-macrophage progenitor cells (GM-CFC) in the irradiated and nonirradiated bone marrow were assayed after a follow-up ranging from 1 to 6 years after treatment (40). The data suggest that granulopoiesis follows a pattern of regeneration similar to that of erythropoiesis. The frequency of granulopoietic progenitors is reduced in irradiated areas, but it is significantly higher following total nodal irradiation than after mantle-field irradiation alone. It is elevated in nonirradiated bone marrow. The total number of GM-CFCs in the body can be calculated (41) and was found to be normal or subnormal after treatment by mantle field alone and reduced after total nodal irradiation. It is further reduced in patients treated by a combination of chemotherapy and radiotherapy. The granulocyte blood count can be normal despite the reduction in the GM-CFC compartment. Assay of the number of progenitor cells per metamyelocyte showed an increase in the amplification factor in the compartment of differentiation and proliferation (41) in both irradiated and nonirradiated bone marrow. This mechanism of compensation, which is also observed in experimental animals, may explain how normal granulocyte production can be obtained despite a reduced progenitor pool.

Curran and Johnson (42) have examined tolerance of the granulocytic series to chemotherapy in a group of patients developing relapse of disease after primary treatment with radiotherapy. They reported that tolerance to chemotherapy improves slowly with time after irradiation and concluded that the return to the normal granulocyte reserve extends well beyond 6 months after irradiation.

D. Pathophysiologic Mechanisms

The bone marrow depression observed in the irradiated areas is easy to understand, but four observations require some discussion: (1) the stimulation of unexposed areas, (2) the abscopal effect on unirradiated bone marrow, (3) the mechanism of bone marrow regeneration in the irradiated marrow, and (4) bone marrow extension.

1. Stimulation of Unexposed Areas

In mice it has been shown that the number of multipotential stem cells (CFU-S) in the irradiated areas decreases slowly, probably due to differentiation, during the hours following subtotal irradiation (43). A few hours later the unirradiated stem cells are triggered into proliferation (34,43). These data are consistent with those obtained following the injection of a drug killing cells specifically in S phases such as [^{3}H] thymidine or hydroxyurea. These drugs have no direct effect on multipotential stem cells, which are noncycling, yet within a few hours they trigger their differentiation and proliferation (44). These sets of data strongly suggest the presence of long-range stimulating factors released shortly after irradiation. Their presence was brought into evidence by in vitro studies where it was demonstrated that irradiated bone marrow releases humoral factors that are able to trigger quiescent CFU-S into proliferation (28 and Chapter 1). Moreover, this factor was also found in the serum of irradiated mice (35). Other groups observed after irradiation an increased level of serum colony-stimulating factor (CSF), which stimulates the GM-CFC (45,46). Morley et al. (47) and Nothdurft et al. (48) found the leukocyte count in mice and in dogs, respectively, to be inversely correlated with the serum CSF activity. However, Chan and Metcalf (49) discussed the role of inhibitors other than CSF and found a radiation-induced alteration of the feedback control mechanisms (50).

The existence of a high amplification factor from progenitor cells in the bone marrow of patients long after irradiation suggests that other factors also influence the number of cell divisions in the proliferating and differentiating compartment (40,41). It should be recalled that in experimental animals the reduction of the stem cell pool can be compensated by changes in amplification due to a shortening of the intermitotic time and/or to an increase in the transit time through the maturation compartment so that more mitoses are inserted and the number of mature cells in the progeny of one stem cell is increased (51).

In conclusion, comparisons with experimental data suggest that in human beings also, irradiated bone marrow releases stimulating factors that act on the unexposed bone marrow. The early increase in the activity of unexposed bone marrow (38) shows that this release starts very early after irradiation. The persistence of compensatory hyperactivity of the unirradiated marrow over a decade after irradiation suggests that the serum level of the stimulating factor or factors remains high all during this period. When an immunoassay of human GM-CSF is available it will be of interest to follow the time course of its serum level after extended radiotherapy. However, it is not yet clear whether this release of stimulating factors is regulated only by the insult to the bone marrow or also by the level of the peripheral blood cell count. Whatever the regulatory mechanism, it is apparent that normal blood cell production can be achieved in a large proportion of patients despite a marked reduction in the size of the bone marrow cell pool, which in itself underlines the efficacy of the regulation of hemopoiesis.

2. Abscopal Effect on Unirradiated Bone Marrow

After the irradiation of 40-50% of the bone marrow, the fall in the granulocyte count is generally much greater than 50%. This observation led Tubiana and Frindel to undertake experiments in which mice were subjected to single or repeated sessions of partial body irradiation (52). Decreased cellularity as well as a reduction in the uptake of radioiron was observed in the protected bone marrow (23). Moreover, soon after the exposure the number of CFU-S fell considerably in the shielded area (34,53), and the magnitude of this fall increased with the dose to the irradiated bone marrow (43). As an indirect killing effect is unlikely, this diminution can be the consequence of an increased rate of migration and/or an increased rate of differentiation. Migration from unirradiated hemopoietic sites, with consequent seeding in the irradiated bone marrow or spleen, has been demonstrated in mice for CFU-S and other bone marrow cells (54,55). This concept concerning migration is extensively discussed in several papers (39, 56,57); however, its magnitude is small, and CFU-S migration does not increase with dose (57). Differentiation is therefore the more likely explanation for this loss of CFU-S. In the case of external irradiation, the depletion of the CFU-S compartment is followed by the recruitment of most of the previously quiescent CFU-S, and 8 hr after irradiation the CFU-S in the protected leg are triggered into proliferation. In human beings the number of circulating GM-CFC has been reported to be temporarily and markedly increased during recovery after intensive chemotherapy (58-60). The results of GM-CFC assays in the irradiated bone marrow of patients with breast or prostatic carcinoma were interpreted as compatible with increased hemopoietic migration (61). However, the data obtained in patients with lymphoma treated by radiotherapy (62) are not consistent with these observations, and the role of stem cell migration in human beings remains debatable.

3. Mechanisms of Bone Marrow Regeneration

Local regeneration depends on two factors: a sufficient number of multipotential stem cells and an appropriate microenvironment (63-65). The stromal cells probably play an important role in the microenvironment. Damage to stromal cells due to an irradiation could reduce the ability of the soil to host bone marrow regeneration. Indeed it was shown in patients (9) that after doses equal to 40 Gy there was no repopulation of the irradiated bones following an autologous bone transplant, whereas after doses up to 15 Gy a satisfactory repopulation was observed following a bone marrow allograft. For doses between 15 and 40 Gy the extent of regeneration is probably influenced by both environmental damage and the number of stem cells.

The radiosensitivity of hemopoietic stem cells and progenitor cells is discussed in Chapter 5 and in several comprehensive reviews (66-68). One of the main experimental results is that the radiosensitivity of hemopoietic cells is independent of dose rate. The radiosensitivity of human multipotential stem cells cannot be measured directly. It can generally be assumed to be in the same range as that of the other mammalian stem cells, but some observations suggest quite different properties. Clinical data obtained after splenic irradiation and large-field irradiation in chronic lymphocytic leukemia show that a severe and long-standing aplasia can be induced by very low doses of irradiation (2 $\times$ 12.5 cGy per session up to a total dose of 1-1.5 Gy) (69). In order to interpret this observation, one has to assume that (1) the pool of multipotential stem cells is extremely small in these patients and/or (2) the radiosensitivity of these stem cells is very high with a D_0 that should be as low as 0.2-0.3 Gy. In experimental animals after bone marrow irradiation, the self-renewal capacity of the surviving stem cells appears to be markedly reduced (70-72). This effect may play a role in the long-term effects of radiotherapy in patients.

The bone marrow stroma is a complex cellular environment (73) with multiple extracellular matrix components. Interactions occur between the different stromal cells and the stem cells in steady state (74). Environmental alterations after high doses of radiation are well documented (75-77). In a series of experiments, Knospe et al. (31,32) showed the importance of the sinusoidal vascular matrix to the maintenance of hemopoiesis. Moreover, hemopoietic tissue transplanted to ectopic sites can function only after a stromal matrix has developed (63,78); this is in good agreement with preliminary results suggesting the specific adhesion of human hemopoietic progenitor cells to the fibroblastic extracellular matrix (79) and with data on stromal-cell-associated hemopoiesis (74,80). The in vitro culture assay for bone marrow fibroblastic colony-forming units (CFU-F) is well standardized

(81-83). The bone marrow CFU-F produce fibronectin as well as type I and III collagens and are generally considered to be the precursors of bone marrow fibroblasts, which are one of the important components of the hemopoietic environment. In mice, in contrast to hemopoietic stem cells, their radiosensitivity is dose-rate-dependent (84). At a dose rate of 140 cGy/min (i.e., the dose rate commonly used for lymphomas), the D_0 is 170 ± 20 cGy, with $n = 1$; at a dose rate of 4.5 cGy/min (i.e., the usual dose rate in total body irradiation for bone marrow allografts), the D_0 is 260 ± 40 cGy with $n = 1$. The D_0 value of human CFU-F was found by Laver et al. 985) to be equal to 130 cGy with $n = 1.3$ These results are consistent with other published data (86-88). A relative radioresistance in CFU-F from patients with acute nonlymphocytic leukemias was reported by Greenberg et al. (89).

The above discussion strongly suggests that local regeneration is influenced by long-range stimulatory factors. After large-field irradiation the unirradiated tissues are unable to achieve sufficient cell production. This probably contributes to the release of stimulatory factors that have an impact on the local regeneration of the irradiated tissues and on the proliferation of stem cells and progenitors. However, it is not known whether stimulatory factors can also act on the microenvironment.

Besides activators, bone marrow also secretes inhibitors (90,91), and the proliferation kinetics of hemopoiesis are probably regulated by both long-range and short-range humoral factors (74,92,93). Long-term bone marrow culture has provided information about cell-to-cell interactions and the release of factors after irradiation (94,95). The role of T lymphocytes in erythropoietic recovery is also being studied (96). However, further investigations are required to assess the role of the various cellular types and the structural features of the bone marrow in hemopoietic regeneration after extended-field radiotherapy.

4. Bone Marrow Extension

Migration of stem cells and heterotypic transformation of pluripotential cells in the Haversian canals of the cortex could explain the bone marrow expansion after extended-field radiotherapy. Scarantino et al. (39) showed the importance of this phenomenon.

II. LONG-TERM BONE MARROW DAMAGE INDUCED BY CHEMOTHERAPY

A. The Role of Chemotherapy in the Treatment of Lymphoma

In patients with early stages of Hodgkin's disease without systemic symptoms and/or elevated erythrocyte sedimentation rate and one or two involved sites, extended radiotherapy (mantle plus inverted Y or paraaortic plus spleen treatment) is the main treatment advisable. Total nodal irradiation or a combination of radiotherapy and chemotherapy become mandatory for patients with four or more involved sites or splenic involvement and/or systemic symptoms (97-100).

In advanced stages the usual treatment is chemotherapy alone or combined with an iceberg radiotherapy. MOPP [mechlorethamine, Oncovin (vincristine), procarbazine, prednisone] (101) is the most frequently used combination chemotherapy. Therapeutic trials are trying to define a chemotherapy as effective as MOPP but less toxic. This will be discussed later.

In non-Hodgkin's lymphomas, patients with stage I, whatever their histological type, can be treated by radiotherapy alone. For stage II patients with a favorable histological type, radiotherapy can be used alone, but the association of radiotherapy and chemotherapy is indicated in cases with unfavorable histology. In patients with stages III and IV with a favorable histological type, the treatment strategy is debated. Relapses are frequent whatever the initial treatment. In patients with stages III and IV of unfavorable histology the prognosis is poor, and aggressive combination chemotherapy, including the use of anthracyclines, is mandatory. Children with non-Hodgkin's lymphomas are treated by very aggressive chemotherapy, often associated with an autologous bone marrow transplant.

B. Effect of Chemotherapy on the Bone Marrow

The cytological effects of chemotherapy on the bone marrow are studied in Chapters 3 and 4. As with radiotherapy, toxic effects are inflicted on the stem cells and the microenvironment. For example, busulfan causes a severe decrease in CFU-S in mice, even when the blood count remains normal. The surviving stem cells have a reduced capacity for self-renewal, and a severe bone marrow hypoplasia can occur (70,102-104). Other drugs, such as cyclophosphamide, seem to damage the microenvironment as well as the stem cells (105).

In human beings, when moderate chemotherapy is associated with extended-field radiotherapy, the regenerative pattern of the bone marrow does not seem to differ from that observed after radiotherapy alone (8,11).

After extensive chemotherapy for non-Hodgkin's lymphomas in children and in adults, the compartment of GM-CFC is reduced and contrasts with a normal or subnormal blood leukocyte count (106,107). These data suggest a mitotic amplification occurring in cell populations between the GM-CFCs and the leukocytes (108). However, a longer follow-up is needed to assess whether this situation is corrected. Functional studies have not been carried out in relapse-free patients for an extended period after aggressive multichemotherapy. Despite normal or subnormal blood counts, marked quantitative bone marrow defects probably exist as shown by the reduced tolerance to further treatment. This should be documented by further investigations.

C. Secondary Leukemias

Leukemias after cytotoxic treatment are described in Chapter 7. Only the incidence and types of acute leukemias occurring after lymphoma treatment will be discussed briefly here. Acute nonlymphocytic leukemias (ANLL) and other cancers developing after radiotherapy and/or chemotherapy for Hodgkin's disease can be preceded by a phase of dysmyelopoiesis (109,110). There is virtually no risk of developing leukemia after treatment with irradiation alone (100). The risk of ANLL has been recently quantified on the basis of the late results of EORTC clinical trials (111,112). After radiotherapy alone, the cumulative proportion of ANLL at 10 years was found to be 0.7% whereas it was 2.7% in the group of patients treated by a combined modality treatment. Compared to the general population, the relative risk of ANLL was not found to be significantly increased for patients treated by radiotherapy alone. In contrast, an increased risk, greater than 200% ($p < 0.001$) was found in patients treated by a combined modality treatment. In the NCI experience (113) concerning 473 patients treated by MOPP and/or radiotherapy, the 10-year estimated risk of ANLL is 0% for radiotherapy alone, 2% for chemotherapy alone, 6% for initial combined radiotherapy-chemotherapy, and 9% for salvage combined radiotherapy-chemotherapy. Comparable results were reported by other groups (114-119). With regard to patients treated by chemotherapy alone, higher risks (6%) have been reported (120). It is possible that some of these discrepancies could be explained by differences in toxicity of the chemotherapy used. For example, the Milan group (118) emphasizes the absence of ANLL after ABVD (adriamycine, bleomycine, vincristine, dacarbazine), but this conclusion is contested by other authors (121) and longer follow-up is needed.

Morphological and cytogenetic aspects of the secondary ANLL treatment for lymphoma are beginning to be documented (122-124), but many points remain debatable. This topic was reviewed during the Fourth International Workshop on Chromosomes in Leukemia (125) and in a recent paper by Hossfeld and Weh (126). All types of leukemias have been observed but with a predominance of M2 and M6 in the FAB classification (127). Moreover, about 10% of the secondary ANLL do not fit the FAB classification and are very similar to an acute myelodysplastic syndrome. Structural and/or numerical anomalies (128) are found in 80-100% of the cases. Hypo- and pseudodiploidy exist in 70-80% of the patients. Partial or total loss of chromosomes numbers 5 and 7 are the most commonly stressed anomalies, but chromosomes numbers 3 and 17 can also be involved (see Chapter 7). Marker chromosomes (essentially double minute), multiclonality, karyotypic instability, and karyotypic changes during the course of the disease have been reported. The specificity of these karyotypical anomalies for secondary ANLL is not clearly established, since they have been reported in patients who had received neither radiotherapy nor chemotherapy. However, two points must be stressed:

1. The Fourth International Workshop on Chromosomes in Leukemia confirmed the greater frequency of the −5/5q− and/or −7/7q− aberrations in secondary ANLL as opposed to de novo leukemias, except in children, in whom these anomalies are rare. Analysis of the patient's history with de novo ANLL often reveals an exposure to potentially mutagenic agents in patients with these aberrations.
2. The karyotypes observed in patients with acute leukemias appearing during the course of chronic myeloid leukemias or polycythemia vera differ from those found in ANLL as a consequence of radiotherapy or chemotherapy.

There is no obvious relationship between the type of treatment and the karyotypical anomalies. However, it has been suggested that the involvement of chromosomes numbers 7 and 17 was more frequent than that of chromosomes 3 and 5 in ANLL secondary to radiotherapy and/or chemotherapy (124). Similarly, a cooperative study group (129) found that the incidence of monosomy 7 was higher in leukemia occurring after treatment of malignant lymphoma than after treatment of solid tumors and that anomalies of chromosome number 17 were more frequent in patients previously exposed to occupational hazards than in those treated for a malignant disease.

Finally, recent data (130,131) show a partial deletion of the short arm of chromosome number 12 (12p−) in ANLL and show that chromosome number 7 is more frequently involved while chromosome number 5 is less frequently involved in secondary ANLL than in de novo ANLL with complex chromosome abnormalities.

III. SUMMARY

The standardization of protocols allowed interesting conclusions about the long-term bone marrow damage due to radiotherapy, summarized in Table 1.

After 40 Gy in 4 weeks, bone marrow regeneration can partially occur in the irradiated areas but is modulated by different factors. The main regulating factor is the target volume. When the irradiated volume is moderate (mantle field 20-30% of the bone marrow volume), the regeneration is almost nonexistent. After total nodal irradiation (60-70% of the bone marrow), the bone marrow regeneration becomes significant. The younger the patient, the higher the regeneration level.

Three main compensatory mechanisms have to be stressed.

1. Hyperactivity of the irradiated bone marrow is the earliest and the main compensatory mechanism. It can persist longer than a decade after irradiation of a large bone marrow volume.

Table 1 Summary of the Main Results Found After Radiotherapy for Malignant Lymphomas

	Compensatory mechanisms			
Bone marrow regeneration	Hyperactivity of the unirradiated bone marrow	Bone marrow extension	Extramedullary hemopoiesis	Mitotic amplification
Conditioned by the irradiated bone marrow volume (higher after mantle plus inverted Y field than after mantle field alone) (7,8,13). Progressive, taking months to reach a steady state (8,10-12) Higher in young patients (13) Related to dose (9,13,24) Explained by the radio-sensitivity of the hemo-poietic stem cells but also by the alteration of the stroma (9)	Early mechanism (38) Long-lasting after very extended radiotherapy (7,8,11,12)	Can occur at the end of the first year and can increase perhaps until the fourth year (12) Can regress in direct response to the amount of in-field regeneration (10,12) Can persist more than 10 years after a TNI with poor bone marrow regeneration (8)	Can be observed in patients with long follow-up (8)	Suggested by granulocyte-macrophage progenitor cell cultures (40)

2. Bone marrow extension is an inconstant and later compensatory mechanism.
3. Extramedullary hemopoiesis in the spleen and in the liver have been described.

The establishment of hematological steady state needs months and probably years.

The threshold above which bone marrow becomes unable to regenerate is generally accepted to be 25-30 Gy at a rate of 10 Gy/week, but this point remains debatable.

Toxic effects on the bone marrow due to chemotherapy are inflicted on the hemopoietic stem cells but probably also on those of the microenvironment. Moderate chemotherapy associated with extended-field radiotherapy does not seem to affect the regenerative pattern of the bone marrow. Extensive chemotherapy is able to reduce the bone marrow stem cell compartment which can be corrected by mitotic amplification.

There is virtually no risk of secondary acute nonlymphocytic leukemias (ANLL) after radiotherapy alone. This risk is not negligible after chemotherapy alone or after combined radiotherapy/chemotherapy. Cytogenetic studies on secondary ANLL have demonstrated the involvement of chromosomes numbers 5 and 7 and also chromosomes numbers 3, 12, and 17.

The main problems remaining debatable in this field are:

The precise shape of the dose-effect curve following irradiation of the bone marrow.

The importance and the duration of the bone marrow defect resulting from the various chemotherapy protocols used in clinical trials.

The importance of mitotic amplification as a compensatory mechanism.

The relative importance of the reduction in the number of hemopoietic stem cells and of stromal alterations in bone marrow regeneration.

The precise description and the significance of the karyotypic anomalies found in secondary ANLL.

Besides long-range factors, the importance of cell-cell interaction in bone marrow regeneration as well as in the establishment and maintenance of compensatory mechanisms after aggressive therapy for lymphomas.

REFERENCES

1. Gilbert, R. La roentgenthérapie de la granulomatose maligne. *J. Radiol. Electrol. 9*, 509-514 (1925).
2. Kaplan, H. S. Radiotherapy. In: *Hodgkin's disease.* Kaplan, H. S. (Ed.). Harvard University Press, Cambridge, MA, Chapter 9, pp. 366-441 (1980).
3. Woodward, H. Q., Holodny, E. A summary of the data of Mechanik on the distribution of bone marrow. *Phys. Med. Biol. 5*, 57-59 (1960).

4. Ellis, R. E. The distribution of active bone marrow in the adult. *Phys. Med. Biol. 5,* 255-258 (1961).
5. Tubiana, M., Rambert, P., Laugier, A., Lalanne, C. M. Les irradiations étendues dans la maladie de Hodgkin. *Nouv. Rev. Fr. Hématol. 6,* 164-174 (1966).
6. Cristy, M. Active bone marrow distribution as a function of age in humans. ORNL-DWG 79-18505 (1979).
7. Morardet, N., Parmentier, C., Flamant, R. Etude par le fer 59 des effets de la radiothérapie étendue des hématosarcomes sur l'érythropoièse. *Biomedicine 18,* 228-234 (1973).
8. Parmentier, C., Morardet, N., Tubiana, M. Late effects on human bone marrow after extended field radiotherapy. *Int. J. Radiat. Oncol. Biol. Phys. 9,* 1303-1311 (1983).
9. Parmentier, C., Morardet, N., Schlumberger, M., Hayat, M., Pico, J. L., Tibi, M., Tubiana, M. Erythropoietic recovery in human after extended field radiotherapy. Ferrokinetic studies of patients treated by radiotherapy followed by autologous bone marrow transplantation and of patients treated by moderate doses (20 Gy) of radiotherapy. *Radiother. Oncol. 3,* 257-265 (1985).
10. Knospe, W. H., Rayudu, M. S., Cardello, M., Friedman, A. M., Fordham, E. W. Bone marrow scanning with ^{52}iron (^{52}Fe). Regeneration and extension of marrow after ablative doses of radiotherapy. *Cancer 37,* 1432-1442 (1976).
11. Steere, H. A., Lillicrap, S. C., Clink, H. M., Peckham, M. J. The recovery of iron uptake in erythropoietic bone marrow following large field radiotherapy. *Brit. J. Radiol. 52,* 61-66 (1979).
12. Rubin, P., Landman, S., Mayer, E., Keller, B., Ciccio, S. Bone marrow regeneration and extension after extended field irradiation in Hodgkin's disease. *Cancer 32,* 699-711 (1973).
13. Sacks, E. L., Goris, M. L., Glatstein, E., Gilbert, E., Kaplan, H. S. Bone marrow regeneration following large field radiation. Influence of volume, age, dose and time. *Cancer 42,* 1057-1065 (1978).
14. Chaudhuri, T. K., Ehrardt, J. C., De Gowin, R., Christie, J. H. ^{59}Fe wholebody scanning. *J. Nucl. Med. 15,* 667-673 (1974).
15. Aubert, B., Kahn, E., Parmentier, C., Di Paola, R. Physical requirements of a ^{59}Fe bone marrow distribution digital scanning study. *Eur. J. Nucl. Med. 8,* 162-166 (1983).
16. Ferrant, A., Rodhain, J., Leners, N., Cogneau, M., Verwilghen, R. L. Quantitative assessment of erythropoiesis in bone marrow expansion areas using ^{52}Fe. *Brit. J. Haematol. 62,* 247-255 (1986).
17. Thomson, R. A. E., Corriveau, O. J., Rubin, P. ^{59}Fe labelling in bone. *J. Nucl. Med. 15,* 161-163 (1974).
18. Nelp, W. B., Gohil, M. N., Larson, S. M., Bower, R. E. Longterm effects of local irradiation of the marrow on erythron and red cell function. *Blood 36,* 617-622 (1970).
19. Hill, D. R., Price, D. C., Kane, L. J., Phillips, T. L. Effect of single dose and fractionated radiation on rabbit bone marrow. *Radiology 106,* 695-698 (1973).

20. Colonna, P., Rain, J. D., Pecking, A., Brière, J., Najean, Y. La double scintigraphie médullaire aux colloides de technetium et à la transferrine-indium dans la splénomégalie myéloide. *Nouv. Rev. Fr. Hematol. 20,* 455-464 (1978).
21. Parmentier, C., Therain, F., Charbord, P., Aubert, P., Morardet, N. Comparative study of ^{111}In and ^{59}Fe bone marrow scanning. *Eur. J. Nucl. Med. 2,* 89-92 (1977).
22. Abbatucci, J., Dutreix, A., Harichaux, P., Peyroux, J. C., Surmont, J., Tubiana, M. Etude des modifications hématologiques consécutives à certaines techniques radiothérapiques. *Ann. Radiol. 1,* 365-379 (1958).
23. Tubiana, M., Frindel, E., Croizat, H. Hematological effects of partial body irradiation: clinical and experimental data. In: *Biological aspects of radiation protection.* Sugahara, T., Hug, O. (Eds.). Igaku Shoin, Ltd, Tokoy, pp. 53-63 (1971).
24. Sykes, M. P., Chu, F. C. H., Savel, H., Bonadonna, G., Mathis, H. The effects of varying dosages of irradiation upon sternal-marrow regeneration. *Radiology 83,* 1084-1088 (1964).
25. Slanina, J., Musshoff, K., Rahner, T., Stiasny, R. Long-term side effects in irradiated patients with Hodgkin's disease. *Int. J. Radiat. Oncol. Biol. Phys. 2,* 1-19 (1977).
26. Bajsogolov, G. D., Siskin, I. P., Choptynskaja, S. K., Kolesnikova, A. I., Misanskaja, N. I. Spate bestrahlungsfolgen der zustand des stromas in bestrahlten und intakten abschnitten des menschlichen knochenmarks. *Radiobiol. Radiother. 23,* 31-35 (1982).
27. Rubin, P., Scarantino, C. The bone marrow organ: the critical structure in radiation-drug interaction. *Int. J. Radiat. Oncol. Biol. Phys. 4,* 3-23 (1978).
28. Frindel, E., Croizat, H., Vassort, F. Stimulating factors liberated by treated bone marrow. In vitro effect on CFU kinetics. *Exp. Hematol. 4,* 56-61 (1976).
29. Donaldson, S. S., Kaplan, H. S. Complications of treatment of Hodgkin's disease in children. *Cancer Treatment Rep. 66,* 977-989 (1982).
30. Tubiana, M., Lalanne, C. M. Evolution hématologique des malades soumis à une irradiation totale pour transplantation d'organes. *Ann. Radiol. 6,* 561-580 (1963).
31. Knospe, W. H., Blom, J., Crosby, W. H. Regeneration of locally irradiated bone marrow. I. Dose dependent long-term changes in rat bone marrow with particular emphasis upon vascular and stromal defects. *Blood 28,* 398-415 (1966).
32. Knospe, W. H., Blom, J., Crosby, W. H. Regeneration of locally irradiated bone marrow. II. Induction or regeneration in permanently aplastic medullary cavities. *Blood 31,* 400-405 (1968).
33. Croizat, H., Frindel, E., Tubiana, M. Long term radiation effects on the bone marrow stem cells of C3H mice. *Int. J. Radiat. Biol. 36,* 91-99 (1979).
34. Croizat, H., Frindel, E., Tubiana, M. Proliferative activity of the stem cells in the bone marrow of mice after single and multiple irradiations (total- or partial-body exposure). *Int. J. Radiat. Biol. 18,* 347-358 (1970).

35. Croizat, H., Frindel, E. Study of a CFU-s stimulating factor liberated by bone marrow cells after total and partial body irradiation. *Exp. Hematol. 8,* 185-191 (1980).
36. Hendry, J. H., Lajtha, L. G. The response of hemopoietic colony-forming units to repeated doses of X-rays. *Radiat. Res. 52,* 309-315 (1972).
37. Dailey, M. O., Coleman, C. N., Kaplan, H. S. Radiation induced splenic atrophy in patients with Hodgkin's disease and non-Hodgkin's lymphomas. *New Engl. J. Med. 4,* 215-217 (1980).
38. Tubiana, M., Bernard, C. I., Lalanne, C. Modification de l'érythropoièse après radiothérapie pelvienne. *Acta Radiol. 52,* 321-335 (1959).
39. Scarantino, C. W., Rubin, P., Constine, L. S., III. The paradoxes in patterns and mechanism of bone marrow regeneration after irradiation. I. Different volumes and doses. *Radiother. Oncol. 2,* 215-225 (1984).
40. Morardet, N., Parmentier, C., Hayat, M., Charbord, P. Effects of radiotherapy on the bone marrow granulocytic progenitor cells (CFUc) of patients with malignant lymphomas. II. Long-term effects. *Int. J. Radiat. Oncol. Biol. Phys. 4,* 853-857 (1978).
41. Parmentier, C., Droz, J. P., Tubiana, M. Ways of expressing results of human bone marrow progenitor cell culture. *Brit. J. Haematol. 40,* 105-109 (1978).
42. Curran, R. E., Johnson, R. E. Tolerance to chemotherapy after prior irradiation for Hodgkin's disease. *Ann. Intern. Med. 72,* 505-509 (1970).
43. Croizat, H., Frindel, E., Tubiana, M. Abscopal effect of irradiation on hematopoietic stem cells of shielded bone marrow. Role of migration. *Int. J. Radiat. Biol. 30,* 347-358 (1976).
44. Vassort, F., Winterholer, M., Frindel, E., Tubiana, M. Kinetic parameters of bone marrow stem cells using in vivo suicide by tritiated thymidine, or by hydroxyurea. *Blood 41,* 789-796 (1973).
45. Sodicoff, M., Binhammer, R. Leukocytosis-inducing factor in the blood of X-irradiated rats. *Radiat. Res. 33,* 82-93 (1968).
46. Hall, B. M. The effect of whole-body irradiation on serum colony stimulating factor and in vitro colony-forming cells in the bone marrow. *Brit. J. Haematol. 17,* 553-561 (1969).
47. Morley, A., Richard, K., Howard, D., Stohlman, F., Jr. Studies on the regulation of granulopoiesis. IV. Possible humoral regulation. *Blood 37,* 14-22 (1971).
48. Nothdurft, W., Steinbach, K. H., Fliedner, T. M. Dose and time related quantitative and qualitative alteration in the granulocyte/macrophage progenitor cell (GM-CFC) compartment of dogs after total-body irradiation. *Radiat. Res. 98,* 332-344 (1984).
49. Chan, S., Metcalf, D. Local and systemic control of granulocytic and macrophage cell regeneration after irradiation. *Cell Tissue Kinet. 6,* 185-197 (1973).
50. Chervenick, P. A., Boggs, D. R. In vitro growth of granulocytic and mononuclear cells from blood of normal individuals. *Blood 39,* 131-135 (1971).
51. Lamerton, L. F., Blackett, N. H. A comparison of proliferative characteristics of bone marrow and tumors and responses to cytotoxic agents. In: *Control of proliferation in animal cells.* Clarkson, B., Baserga, R. (Eds.). Cold Spring

Harbor Conferences on Cell Proliferation. Cold Spring Harbor Laboratory, Cold Spring Harbor, NY, pp. 973-984 (1974).

52. Tubiana, M., Frindel, E. Effets sur les tissues hématopoiétiques et les cellules sanguines d'irradiation subtotale par séances quotidiennes répétées pendant un mois. *C.R. Acad. Sci. 254,* 183-185 (1962).

53. Gidali, J., Lajtha, L. G. Regulation of haemopoietic stem cell turnover in partially irradiated mice. *Cell Tissue Kinet. 5,* 147-157 (1972).

54. Tubiana, M., Frindel, E., Kozinetz, G. L., Dalle-Chavaudra, N. Migration des cellules hématopoiétiques médullaires chez les souris irradiées et normales. *Nouv. Rev. Fr. Etud. Clin. Biol. 9,* 742-745 (1964).

55. Hanks, G. In vivo migration of colony forming units from shielded bone marrow in the irradiated mouse. *Nature (London) 203,* 1393-1395 (1964).

56. Lajtha, L. G., Pozzi, L. V., Schofield, R., Fox, M. Kinetic properties of haemopoietic stem cells. *Cell Tissue Kinet. 2,* 39-49 (1969).

57. Croizat, H., Frindel, E., Tubiana, M. The effect of partial body irradiation on haemopoietic stem cell migration. *Cell Tissue Kinet. 13,* 319-325 (1980).

58. Lohrmann, H. P., Schreml, W., Fliedner, T. M., Heimpel, H. Reaction of human granulopoiesis to high-dose cyclophosphamide therapy. *Blut 38,* 9-16 (1979).

59. Richman, C. M., Weiner, R. S., Yankel, R. S. Increase of circulating stem cells following chemotherapy in man. *Blood 47,* 1031-1039 (1976).

60. To, L. B., Haylock, D. N., Kimber, R. J., Juttner, C. A. High levels of circulating haemopoietic stem cells in very early remission from acute non-lymphoblastic leukemia and their collection and cryopreservation. *Brit. J. Haematol. 58,* 399-410 (1984).

61. Hörnsten, P., Wahren, B., Esposti, P. L. Granulocytopoietic precursor cells and regulatory factors in irradiated human bone marrow. *Int. J. Radiat. Oncol. Biol. Phys. 11,* 783-789 (1985).

62. Droz, J. P., Parmentier, C., Morardet, N., Maraninchi, D., Tubiana, M. Effects of radiotherapy on the bone marrow granulocytic progenitor cells (CFUc) of patients with malignant lymphomas. I. Short term effects. *Int. J. Radiat. Oncol. Biol. Phys. 4,* 845-851 (1978).

63. Patt, H. M., Maloney, M. A. Evolution of marrow regeneration as revealed by transplantation studies. *Exp. Cell. Res. 71,* 307-312 (1972).

64. Trentin, J. J., Rauchwerger, J. M., Gallagher, M. T. Regulation of hemopoietic stem cell differentiation and proliferation by hemopoietic inductive microenvironment. In: *Control of proliferation in animal cells.* Clarkson, B., Baserga, R. (Eds.). Cold Spring Harbor Conferences on Cell Proliferation. Cold Spring Harbor Laboratory, Cold Spring Harbor, NY, pp. 927-932 (1974).

65. Wolf, N. S. The haemopoietic enviornment. *Clin. Haematol. 8,* 469-500 (1979).

66. Hendry, J. H., Lord, B. I. The analysis of the early and late response to cytotoxic insults in the hematopoietic cell hierarchy. In: *Cytotoxic insult to tissue (Effects on cell lineages).* Henry, J. H. (Ed.). Churchill Livingstone, Edinburgh, pp. 1-66 (1983).

67. Hendry, J. H. The cellular basis of long-term marrow injury after irradiation. *Radiother. Oncol. 3,* 331-338 (1985).
68. Hendry, J. H. Review: survival curves for normal-tissue clonogens: a comparison of assessments using in vitro, transplantation, or in situ techniques. *Int. J. Radiat. Biol. 47,* 3-16 (1985).
69. Parmentier, C., Chauvel, P., Hayat, M., Bok, B., Tubiana, M. La radiothérapie dans la leucémie lymphoide chronique: l'irradiation splénique. *Nouv. Rev. Fr. Hematol. 14,* 737-754 (1974).
70. Hellman, S., Otnick, L. E. Stem cell depletion: an explanation of the late effects of cytotoxins. *Int. J. Radiat. Biol. 2,* 181-184 (1977).
71. Sainteny, F., Guigon, M., Mary, J. Y. Decrease in the ability of CFU-s in shielded marrow to be recruited into cell cycle after multiple irradiations: experimental results and computer simulation. *Cell Tissue Kinet. 17,* 387-400 (1984).
72. Schofield, R. Assessment of cytotoxic injury to bone marrow. *Brit. J. Cancer 53* (*Suppl. VII*), 115-125 (1986).
73. Singer, J. W., Keating, A., Wright, T. N. The human haematopoietic environment. In: *Recent advances in haematology.* Hoffbrand, A. (Ed.). Churchill Livingstone, Edinburgh, pp. 1-24 (1985).
74. Dexter, T. M. Stromal cell associated haemopoiesis. *J. Cell. Physiol. Suppl. 1,* 87-94 (1982).
75. Elbadawi, N., Rubin, P., Thomson, R. A. E. Histopathological appearance of irradiated bone marrow following single and fractionated dose exposures (Abstract). *Radiat. Res. 59,* 52 (1974).
76. Werts, E. D., Johnson, M. J., De Gowin, R. L. Abscopal suppression of bone marrow erythropoiesis. *Radiat. Res. 76,* 206-218 (1978).
77. Wathen, L. M., Knapp, S. A., De Gowin, R. L. Suppression of marrow stromal cell and microenvironmental damage following sequential radiation and cyclophosphamide. *Int. J. Radiat. Oncol. Biol. Phys. 7,* 935-941 (1981).
78. Tavassoli, M., Crosby, W. H. Transplantation of bone marrow to extramedullary sites. *Science 161,* 54-56 (1968).
79. Parmentier, C., Coulombel, L., Caillou, B., Gaillard, N., Talbot, M., Pauzie, N., Bayet, S., Morardet, N., Bayle, C., Leroy, C., Gospodarowicz, D. Increased adhesion of hematopoietic precursor cells on extracellular-matrix (ECM) coated dishes. *Exp. Hematol. 13,* 462 (1985).
80. Tsai, S., Sieff, C. A., Nathan, D. G. Stromal cell-associated erythropoiesis. *Blood 67,* 1418-1426 (1986).
81. Friedenstein, A. J., Petrakova, K. V., Kuralesova, A. I., Frolova, G. B. Heterotopic transplants of bone marrow. Analysis of precursor cells for oestogenic and hematopoietic tissues. *Transplantation 6,* 220-239 (1968).
82. Xu, C. X., Hendry, J. H., Testa, N. G., Allen, T. D. Stromal colonies from mouse bone marrow: characterisation of cell types, optimisation of plating efficiency and its effect on radiosensitivity. *J. Cell. Sci. 61,* 453-466 (1983).
83. Castro-Malaspina, H., Gay, R. E., Jhanvar, S. C., Resnick, G., Kapoor, N., Meyers, P. A., Chiarieri, D., McKenzie, S., Broxmeyer, H. E., Moore, M. A. S.

Characteristics of bone marrow fibroblast colony-forming cells (CFU-F) and their progeny. *Blood 56,* 289-301 (1980).
84. Hendry, J. H., Wang, S. B., Testa, N. G. Greater sparing of stromal progenitor cells than of haemopoietic stem cells in irradiated mouse marrow using low dose-rates. *Biomed. Pharmacother. 38,* 356-358 (1984).
85. Laver, J., Ebell, W., Castro-Malaspina, H. Radiobiological properties of the human hematopoietic microenvironment: contrasting sensitivities of proliferative capacity and hematopoietic function to in vitro irradiation. *Blood 6,* 1090-1097 (1986).
86. Chamberlin, W., Barone, J., Kado, A., Fried, W. Lack of recovery of murine hematopoietic stromal cells after irradiation induced damage. *Blood 44,* 385-392 (1974).
87. Cox, R., Masson, W. K. Radiosensitivity in cultured human fibroblasts. *Int. J. Radiat. Biol. 38,* 575-576 (1980).
88. Tavassoli, M. Radiosensitivity of stromal cells responsible for in vitro maintenance of hemopoietic stem cell in continuous long term marrow culture. *Exp. Hematol. 10,* 435-443 (1982).
89. Greenberg, B. R., Wilson, D. W., Woo, L., Klein, K., Rosenblatt, L. S. Increased in vitro radioresistance of bone marrow fibroblastic progenitors (CFU-F) from patients with acute non-lymphocytic leukemia. *Leuk. Res. 8,* 267-273 (1984).
90. Lord, B. I., Mori, K. J., Wright, E. G., Lajtha, L. G. An inhibitor of stem cell proliferation in normal bone marrow. *Brit. J. Haematol. 34,* 441-445 (1976).
91. Frindel, E., Guigon, M. Inhibition of CFU entry into cycle by a bone marrow extract. *Exp. Hematol. 5,* 74-76 (1977).
92. Till, J. E., Price, J. B., Serm, J. S., McCulloch, E. A. Cell interactions in the control of hemopoiesis. In: *Growth kinetics and biochemical regulation of normal and malignant cells.* Drewinko, B., Humphrey, R. M. (Eds.). Williams and Wilkins, Baltimore, pp. 223-235 (1977).
93. Dexter, T. M., Spooncer, E., Hendry, J. H., Lajtha, L. G. Stem cells in vitro. In: *Hemopoietic cell differentiation* (ICN-UCLA Symp. Mol. Cell. Biol.). Golde, D. W., Metcalf, D., Cline, M. J., Fox, F. (Eds.). Academic Press, New York, pp. 163-173 (1978).
94. Greenberger, J. S., Klassen, V., Kase, K., Shadduck, R. K., Sakaleeny, B. S. Effects of low dose rate irradiation on plateau phase bone marrow stromal cells in vitro: demonstration of a new form of non-lethal, physiological damage to support of hematopoietic stem cells. *Radiat. Oncol. Biol. Phys. 10,* 1027-1037 (1984).
95. Naparstek, E., Donnelly, T., Shadduck, R. K., Waheed, A., Wagner, K., Kase, K. R., Greenberger, J. S. Persistent production of colony-stimulating factor (CSF-1) by cloned bone marrow stromal cell line D2XR11 after X-irradiation. *J. Cell. Physiol. 126,* 407-413 (1986).
96. Dygai, A. M., Goldberg, E. D., Agafonov, V. I. Regeneration of hematopoiesis during local irradiation. *Bull. Exp. Biol. Med. 96,* 1614-1616 (1983).

97. Carbone, P. P., Kaplan, H. S., Musshoff, K., Smithers, W., Tubiana, M. Reports of the Committee on Hodgkin's disease classificiation. *Cancer Res. 31,* 1860-1861 (1971).
98. Tubiana, M., Carde, P., Burgers, J. M. V., Cosset, J. M., Van Glabbeke, M., Somers, R. Non Hodgkin's lymphoma. *Cancer Surv. 4,* 377-398 (1985).
99. Tubiana, M., Henry-Amar, M., Hayat, M., Burgers, M., Qasim, M., Somers, R., Sizoo, W. The EORTC treatment of early stages of Hodgkin's disease: the role of radiotherapy. *Int. J. Radiat. Oncol. Biol. Phys. 10,* 197-210 (1984).
100. Hoppe, R. T., Horning, S. J., Rosenberg, S. A. The concept evolution and preliminary results of the current Stanford clinical trials for Hodgkin's disease. *Cancer Surv. 4,* 459-475 (1985).
101. De Vita, V. T., Jr., Serpick, A., Carbone, P. P. Combination chemotherapy in the treatment of advanced Hodgkin's disease. *Ann. Intern. Med. 73,* 881-895 (1970).
102. Testa, N. G., Hendry, J. H., Molineux, G. Long term bone marrow damage in experimental systems and in patients after radiation or chemotherapy. *Anticancer Res. 5,* 101-110 (1985).
103. Morley, A., Blake, J. An animal model of chronic aplastic marrow failure. I. Late marrow failure after busulphan. *Blood 44,* 49-56 (1974).
104. Morley, A., Trainor, K., Black, J. A primary cell lesion in experimental chronic hypoplastic marrow failure. *Blood 45,* 681-688 (1975).
105. Molineux, G., Xu, C., Hendry, J., Testa, N. G. A cellular analysis of long-term haematopoietic damage in mice after repeated treatment with cyclophosphamide. *Cancer Chemother. Pharmacol. 18,* 11-16 (1986).
106. Parmentier, C., Maraninchi, D., Morardet, N., Droz, J. P., Charbord, P. Effects of treatment of malignant lymphomas on the granulocytic progenitor cells (CFUc). *Recent Res. Cancer Res. 65,* 181-187 (1978).
107. Hartmann, O., Parmentier, C., Lemerle, J., Gout, M., Schweisguth, O. Sequential study of the bone marrow granulocytic progenitor cells (CFC) in children treated by chemotherapy for non-Hodgkin malignant lymphomas. *Nouv. Rev. Fr. Hematol. 21,* 239-250 (1979).
108. Parmentier, C., Tchernia, G., Subtil, E., Diakhate, L., Morardet, N. In vitro medullary granulocytic progenitor (CFUc) cultures from 6 cases of granulocytopenias. *Scand. J. Haematol. 21,* 19-23 (1978).
109. Arseneau, J. C., Canellos, G. P., Johnson, R. Risk of new cancers in patients with Hodgkin's disease. *Cancer 40,* 1912-1916 (1977).
110. De Vita, T. D. The consequences of the chemotherapy of Hodgkin's disease: the 10th David A. Karnofsky memorial lecture. *Cancer 47,* 1-13 (1981).
111. Henry-Amar, M. Second cancers after radiotherapy and chemotherapy for early stages of Hodgkin's disease. *J. Natl. Cancer Inst. 71,* 911-916 (1983).
112. Henry-Amar, M. Second cancers after treatment in two successive cohorts of patients with early stages of Hodgkin's disease in malignant lymphomas and Hodgkin's disease: experimental and therapeutic advances. In: *Proceedings of the Second International Conference on Malignant Lymphomas,*

Lugano, Switzerland, June 13-16, 1984, Cavalli, F., Bonadonna, G., Rozencweig, M. (Eds.). Martinus Nijhoff, Boston, pp. 417-428 (1985).

113. Tester, W. S., Kinsella, T. G., Waller, B., Makuch, R. W., Kelley, P. A., Gladstein, E., De Vita, V. T. Second malignant neoplasms complicating Hodgkin's disease: the National Cancer Institute experience. *J. Clin. Oncol. 2,* 762-769 (1984).
114. Boivin, J. F., Hutchinson, G. B. Leukemias and other cancers after radiotherapy and chemotherapy for Hodgkin's disease. *J. Natl. Cancer Inst. 67,* 751-760 (1981).
115. Coleman, C. N., Kaplan, H. S., Cox, R., Varghese, A., Butterfield, P., Rosenberg, S. A. Leukemias, non-Hodgkin's lymphomas and solid tumours in patients treated for Hodgkin's disease. *Cancer Surv. 1,* 733-744 (1982).
116. Glicksman, A. S., Pajak, T. F., Gottlieb, A. Second malignant neoplasms in patients successfully treated for Hodgkin's disease: a cancer and leukemia group B study. *Cancer Treat. Rep. 66,* 1035-1044 (1982).
117. Pedersen-Bjegaard, J., Larsen, S. O. Incidence of acute nonlymphocytic leukemia, preleukemia and acute myeloproliferative syndrome up to 10 years after treatment of Hodgkin's disease. *New Engl. J. Med. 307,* 965-971 (1982).
118. Valagussa, P., Santoro, A., Bellini, F., Francji, F., Banfi, A., Bonadonna, G. Absence of treatment induced second neoplasms after ABVD in Hodgkin's disease. *Blood 59,* 488-494 (1982).
119. Piga, A., Ambrosetti, A., Todeschini, G., Cetto, G., Perona, G., Cellerino, R. Doxorubicin, bleomycin, vinblastine and docarbazine (ABVD) salvage of mecloretamine, vincristine, prednisone and procarbazine (MOPP) resistant advanced Hodgkin's disease. *Cancer Treat. Rep. 68,* 947-951 (1984).
120. Coltman, C. A., Dixon, A. O. Second malignancies complicating Hodgkin's disease: a southwest oncology group 10 year follow up. *Cancer Treat. Rep. 66,* 1023-1033 (1982).
121. Papa, G., Mavro, F. R., Anselmo, A. P., et al. Acute leukemia in patients treated for Hodgkin's disease. *Brit. J. Haematol. 58,* 43-52 (1984).
122. Rowley, J. D., Colomb, H. M., Vardiman, J. Nonrandom chromosomal abnormalities in acute non-lymphocytic leukemia in patients treated for Hodgkin's disease and non Hodgkin lymphomas. *Blood 50,* 759-770 (1977).
123. Berger, R., Bernheim, A., Daniel, M. T., Valensi, F., Flandrin, G. Leucémias induites. Aspect cytogénétique et cytologique. Comparaison avec des leucémies primitives. *Nouv. Rev. Fr. Hématol. 23,* 275-284 (1981).
124. Sandberg, A. A., Abe, S., Kowalczyk, J. R., Zedgenidze, A., Takeuchi, J., Kakati, S. Chromosomes and causation of human cancer and leukemia: The cytogenetics of leukemias complicating other diseases. *Cancer Genet. Cytogenet. 7,* 95-136 (1982).
125. The Fourth International Workshop on Chromosomes in Leukemia, 1982, *Cancer Genet. Cytogenet. 11,* 249-360 (1984).
126. Hossfeld, D. K., Weh, H. J. Chromosome findings in secondary acute leukemias. In: *Tumor aneuploidy.* Büchner, T., Bloomfield, C. D., Hiddeman, W., Hossfeld, D. K., Schumann, J. (Eds.). Springer-Verlag, Berlin, pp. 29-33 (1985).

127. Bennett, J. M., Catovsky, D., Daniel, M. T., Flandrin, G., Galton, D. A. G., Gralnick, H. R., Sultan, C. Proposals for the classification of the acute leukemias. *Brit. J. Haematol. 33,* 451-458 (1976).
128. ISCN: An international system for human cytogenetic nomenclature. *Cytogenet. Cell. Genet. 21,* 309-314 (1978).
129. Groupe Français de cytogénétique hématologique. Chromosome analysis of 63 cases of secondary non lymphoid blood disorders: a cooperative study. *Cancer Genet. Cytogenet. 12,* 95-104 (1984).
130. Berger, R., Bernheim, A., Le Coniat, M., Vecchione, D., Pacot, A., Daniel, M. T., Flandrin, G. Abnormalities of the short arm of chromosome 12 in acute non lymphocytic leukemia and dysmyelopoietic syndrome. *Cancer Genet. Cytogenet. 19,* 281-289 (1986).
131. Levin, M., Le Coniat, M., Bernheim, A., Berger, R. Complex chromosomal abnormalities in acute nonlymphocytic leukemia. *Cancer Genet. Cytogenet. 22,* 113-119 (1986).

14
Long-Term Hemopoietic Damage After Cytotoxic Drug Therapy for Solid Tumors

HANS-PETER E. LOHRMANN
Kreiskrankenhaus, Lemgo, Federal Republic of Germany

WOLFGANG SCHREML
Kreiskrankenhaus, Günzburg, Federal Republic of Germany

I. INTRODUCTION

The use of cytotoxic drugs in the treatment of hematological malignancies and solid tumors has been increasing over the past three decades, leading to a greater appreciation of the occurrence of long-term effects after cytotoxic treatment. These effects are particularly important in the clinical setting of adjuvant chemotherapy. Cytotoxic agents are administered more and more in routine treatment following surgery in an attempt to eradicate clinically undetectable micrometastatic disease (1). We expect at least some of the patients so treated to become long-term survivors; obviously, these patients are particularly at risk of developing long-term damage following exposure to cytotoxic drugs.

The potential long-term effects of repeated exposure to cytotoxic agents are now well defined. Persistent chromosomal aberrations (2), irreversible damage to various organs (3), and increased risk of secondary acute leukemias (4-6) are well known (see Chapters 7, 10, and 13). In contrast to these well-characterized sequelae of cytotoxic drug treatment, the possibility of long-term damage to self-renewal tissues has only recently gained attention. Here we review experimental and clinical evidence for the existence of long-term damage to the hemopoietic system.

II. THE STEM CELL COMPARTMENT

A short discussion of the present concept of an age structure in the hemopoietic stem cell compartment seems appropriate. Hemopoietic stem cells are not a homogeneous cell population. This is true not only with respect to physical features such as cell size and density, but also with respect to their self-replication potential. Hemopoietic stem cells display a wide continuous spectrum of self-replication capacity (7). The stem cells that are out of cycle possess the greatest potential for self-replication. As these stem cells gradually lose proliferative potential, their proliferative activity increases. Evidence indicates that under steady-state conditions the demand for stem cell input into the hemopoietic cell lineages is mostly fulfilled by such "older" stem cells with lowered proliferative potential. By this mechanism, "young" hemopoietic stem cells with high proliferative potential are protected, as they are only occasionally called upon to maintain the equilibrium between the hemopoietic compartments that is necessary for the life long maintenance of the hemopoietic system.

III. EFFECTS OF CYTOTOXIC DRUGS ON STEM CELLS

In theory, cytotoxic drugs could induce permanent damage to the hemopoietic stem cell compartments in two ways that do not necessarily exclude each other:

1. They could permanently reduce the size of the stem cell compartment (i.e., the number of hemopoietic stem cells).
2. They could alter the age structure of the hemopoietic stem cell compartment by a shift toward "older" stem cells (i.e., by a relative depletion of "young" stem cells with high proliferative potential).

There is evidence for the existence of both of these mechanisms.

Animal experiments provide ample evidence that acute exposure to cytotoxic drugs causes changes in the size of the pluripotent stem cell compartment; some cytotoxic drugs deplete this compartment considerably, whereas others affect it only slightly (8). A number of variables are known to affect the pattern of depletion and replenishment of the stem cell compartment: Dose, schedule of administration, and proliferative state of the stem cells at the time of drug administration are all relevant; however, the most important variables are the type of cytotoxic drug and its mode of action. Following exposure to most cytotoxic agents, the size of the stem cell compartment is reduced, but it recovers rapidly to pretreatment size. This is achieved by a transiently increased proliferative activity of those stem cells that survived exposure to the drug. Some cytotoxic drugs, however—for example, busulfan and the nitrosoureas—deplete the stem cell compartment for a prolonged period of time (8,9). It is easily conceivable that premature readministration of these drugs before numerical normalization will lead to cumulative toxicity, i.e., to progressive loss of hemopoietic stem cells.

Return of the hemopoietic stem cell compartment to pretreatment size following exposure to a cytotoxic agent does not necessarily indicate a complete restoration, since changes in the age structure of the stem cell population may persist even after normalization of the number of cells. There is experimental evidence for the existence of such qualitative defects within the pluripotent stem cell compartment after cytotoxic drug exposure in vivo. Measuring the capacity of murine pluripotent stem cells (CFU-S) for self-replication within individual spleen colonies, Schofield (10) observed a decrease in this parameter after busulfan treatment. Botnick and co-workers used the capacity to repopulate the marrow of lethally irradiated mice in serial bone marrow transfer experiments as a measure of the pluripotent stem cells' potential for proliferation and self-replication and observed a decreased repopulating capability in bone marrow after treatment of the original bone marrow donors with busulfan or phenylalanine mustard (11,12). These authors also demonstrated "aging" (i.e., loss of proliferative potential) of pluripotent stem cells after exposure to these two drugs by determining the capacity of CFU-S to replicate within the femur of irradiated recipients (13). Repopulation of the CFU-S compartment in the bone marrow was delayed after transfer of syngeneic marrow from cyclophosphamide-pretreated donors into irradiated recipients (14), indicating a decreased proliferative potential of stem cells following exposure to cyclophosphamide.

Taken together, these data support the conclusion that stem cells may lose some of their proliferative potential and thus "age" following treatment with a number of cytotoxic agents. The depletion of the hemopoietic stem cell compartment may act as a trigger for young surviving stem cells to divide repeatedly in an effort to replenish the compartment to its original size. This may use up some of the total capacity of these young stem cells for cellular division (7,15). Schofield has proposed a different mechanism; he suggested that under normal conditions (i.e., in the unperturbed bone marrow) only young stem cells (with high proliferative potential) occupy (nutritional?) "niches" (10). Following destruction of such stem cells by cytotoxic drugs, other, older stem cells with lower proliferative potential can move into the now empty niches. Thus, the average proliferative capacity of the stem cells (i.e., the capacity of pluripotent stem cells located in the niches to produce committed stem cells) will be reduced following cytotoxic drug treatment. Both hypotheses imply that proliferative potential continually decreases with repeated cytotoxic injury to pluripotent stem cells and that such loss of potential is irreversible: stem cells can lose but not regain the capacity for self-replication.

Physiologically, the proliferative potential of pluripotent stem cells decreases during fetal life but remains constant throughout extrauterine life (16). Under normal conditions, there is no recognizable aging of the hemopoietic stem cell population after birth. If, however, repeated administration of cytotoxic drugs causes perturbation of the hemopoietic stem cell pool, cumulative loss of proliferative potential, with failure of the hemopoietic stem cell compartment as the extreme result, could ensue. Such stem cell failure, of course, would mean hemopoietic failure. Again, this consideration is supported by experimental findings.

IV. EXPERIMENTAL LONG-TERM DAMAGE

Under appropriate experimental conditions, late bone marrow failure follows cytotoxic drug treatment (17-20). After short-term treatment with busulfan, mice apparently recovered hematologically but developed bone marrow hypoplasia some time later. Overt bone marrow aplasia was preceded by a phase of "latent aplasia," characterized by normal mature hemopoietic cell compartments but a progressively shrinking stem cell compartment. There was little if any defect of the hemopoietic microenvironment in this situation. These findings were later extended: Residual bone marrow damage occurred after biscloroethylnitrosourea (BCNU), chlorambucil, phenylalanine mustard, and mitomycin C (21,22), but not after cytosine arabinoside (23) or bleomycin (24). Whenever late hemopoietic damage after cytotoxic drug exposure was observed, it could be demonstrated most clearly in the pluripotent stem cell compartment either as a size reduction (14,18,21,25) or as a qualitative defect (12,14). It is of some interest that busulfan and BCNU cause the greatest degree of stem cell aging (7) and the most severe late marrow failure, whereas antimetabolites fail to exert either effect. Such differences may be explained by the different actions of these drugs: Antimetabolites, killing cells preferentially or exclusively during certain phases of the cell cycle, act on proliferating cells; they will therefore preferentially kill the older, more actively cycling, stem cells whose proliferation capacity is less. Because antimetabolites spare the resting young stem cells, which possess the highest proliferation potential, they have little adverse effect on the age structure of the stem cell compartment. In contrast, alkylating agents, especially the cycle-independent drugs busulfan and BCNU, act on resting cells and may thus seriously injure young hemopoietic stem cells.

V. PERSISTENT DAMAGE IN PATIENTS

There is limited evidence for the existence of persistent cytotoxic drug-induced damage to the hemopoietic system in human beings. Normally, the hemopoietic system recovers rather promptly and predictably following cytotoxic drug therapy for hematological malignancies and solid tumors. However, it is well known to oncologists (although poorly documented) that the hemopoietic system of heavily pretreated patients is often unusually sensitive to further administration of cytotoxic agents. This sensitivity may manifest itself as unusually low nadir values of granulocytes and/or platelets and/or delayed or incomplete recovery to pretreatment values. In clinical practice, this often requires dose reduction and/or longer time intervals between successive treatment courses. Cumulative toxicity to the hemopoietic system is encountered with particular frequency during intermittent chemotherapy incorporating nitrosoureas (26-29) or mitomycin C. The cumulative toxicity of the latter manifests itself primarily in the megakaryocyte/platelet system.

We have shown that the sensitivity of the progenitors of granulocytes and macrophages (GM-CFC) to cytotoxic agents remains unchanged after repeated exposure in vivo in patients who receive adriamycin repeatedly (30). An increased hemotoxicity following repeated administration of cytotoxic drugs in vivo is therefore most likely the expression of irreversible damage to the hemopoietic stem cell compartment caused by the preceding cytotoxic treatment.

A number of observations that indicate a long-lasting defect of the hemopoietic system in human beings after cytotoxic chemotherapy (see Table 1) are discussed in the following paragraphs.

1. Decreased Bone Marrow Granulocyte Reserve. Between 8 and 21 months following treatment for primary breast cancer with phenylalanine mustard, the bone marrow granulocyte reserve was reported to remain decreased in 3 of 7 patients tested with the prednisolone stimulation test (31). It is remarkable that in all these patients the bone marrow was considered to be hypocellular (20-55% of normal cellularity), whereas the cellular composition of the bone marrow was normal.

2. Slow Regeneration of Bone Marrow GM-CFC. In 15 patients with small-cell lung cancer, regeneration of bone marrow GM-CFCs was studied following the first and fourth administrations of a chemotherapy regimen consisting of adriamycin, cyclophosphamide, and vincristine, given every 3 weeks (32). The incidence of bone marrow GM-CFCs was lower before the fourth than before the first treatment course (difference statistically not significant). Moreover, the pattern of regeneration was considerably altered by the chemotherapy: Following the first treatment, the incidence of GM-CFCs decreased, but it recovered to greater than pretreatment values by the 14th day and remained supranormal by the 22nd day. In contrast, pretreatment values were not reached by days 14 or 22 following the fourth cytotoxic drug treatment. This impaired regeneration of GM-CFCs was paralleled by decreasing peripheral blood granulocyte counts between treatment courses 1-4.

3. Long-Lasting (Permanent?) Cytotoxic Drug-Induced Defect of the Granulocytic System. Following six courses of adjuvant chemotherapy for primary breast cancer with the combination of adriamycin (50 mg/m^2) and cyclophosphamide (500 mg/m^2), we observed long-lasting and possibly permanent damage at all levels of the human granulopoietic system (34,35). The peripheral blood granulocyte concentration was significantly reduced for 6-8 months after cessation of chemotherapy. The regeneration of GM-CFCs in the bone marrow was slower during the sixth than during the first treatment cycle. Fifty-five days after cessation of chemotherapy, the incidence of GM-CFCs appeared to be reduced compared with pretreatment values (differences not significant).

A persisting cytotoxic drug-induced defect of the granulopoietic system could be demonstrated most clearly and reproducibly by measuring the peripheral blood

Table 1 Observations Indicating Long-Lasting Damage to the Hemopoietic System Due to Cytotoxic Drug Therapy

Diagnosis	Drugs (dose, schedule)	Parameter measured	Type of damage	Permanence of damage	Ref.
	Mitomycin C, repeated	Blood count	Thrombocytopenia	Long-lasting, reversible	—
Gastric cancer	Nitrosoureas, intermittent	Blood count	Neutropenia, thrombocytopenia	Long-lasting	—
Brain tumor	Me-CCNU 120 mg/m^2 q 3 wk	Blood count	Severe myelosuppression	Long-lasting	36
Gastric cancer metastatic	BCNU or Me-CCNU (repeated)	Peripheral blood GM-CFC	Almost complete disappearance	Long-lasting	9
Gastric cancer adjuvant treatment	BCNU or Me-CCNU (repeated)	Bone marrow GM-CFC	Reduction, severe	Long-lasting (persisting?) after regeneration of peripheral blood granulocytes	9

Primary breast cancer, adjuvant treatment	L-Phenylalanine mustard (repeated)	Bone marrow granulocyte reserve	3 of 7 patients: PMN reserve reduced, marrow hypocellular	8-21 months after cessation of chemotherapy	31
Small-cell lung cancer	Adriamycin + cyclophosphamide + vincristine, q 3 wk	Bone marrow GM-CFC	Delayed regeneration after repeated chemotherapy	Studied during 1st and 4th course; no later follow-up	32
Primary breast cancer, adjuvant treatment	Adriamycin ($50 mg/m^2$) + cyclophosphamide ($500 mg/m^2$), ×6 q 4 wk	Peripheral blood granulocytes	Decrease	For 6-8 months after chemotherapy	34,35
		Bone marrow GM-CFC	Delayed regeneration during 6th cycle		
			Reduced relative numbers (N.S.)	55 days after chemotherapy	
		Peripheral blood GM-CFC	Reduced	For at least 5 years after chemotherapy	
	CMF	Peripheral blood GM-CFC	Reduced	More than 1 year	35

Table 2 Circulating Neutrophilic Granulocytes (PMN), Committed Granulopoietic (GM-CFC), and Erythropoietic (BFU-E) Progenitor Cells Before and After Adjuvant Chemotherapy with Adriamycin (50 mg/m^2 X 6) + Cyclophosphamide (500 mg/m^2 X 6) (Median Values)

	PMN/μl	GM-CFC/liter	BFU-E/liter
Controls before chemotherapy	4500	22,400	130,000
Days after chemotherapy			
50	2650[a]	4,000[c]	–
150-250	2830[b]	8,000[c]	–
250-350	3150	7,200[c]	–
350-450	3350	4,400[c]	53,000
450-550	3500	8,700[c]	112,000
550-650	3250	5,900[c]	166,000
650-750	5100	8,000[c]	115,000
750-850	3650	6,500[c]	120,000
850-950	4550	6,400[c]	99,000
950-1150	4950	10,900[c]	125,000
1150-1350	4950	9,700[c]	121,000
1350-1550	4700	11,400[a]	139,000
1550-1850	5100	13,100	148,000

[a] $p < 0.01$
[b] $p < 0.05$
[c] $p < 0.001$

GM-CFC pool size (GM-CFC/liter blood) (Table 2). It is noteworthy that the GM-CFCs in peripheral blood were reduced as late as 5 years after completion of chemotherapy; since determinations at later times were not performed, we have to speculate as to whether this defect will ultimately be repaired or whether it is irreversible.

It is worth noting that the pool of GM-CFCs in the peripheral blood—which probably reflects to some degree the size of the bone marrow pool—was reduced postchemotherapy even in the absence of a reduction in peripheral blood granulocyte numbers. Apparently the defect at the level of the committed granulopoietic cells is compensated for by regulatory processes (increased number of cellular divisions?) in the more mature granulocytic compartments. It is noteworthy that a similar defect could not be demonstrated in the erythropoietic

Table 3 Circulating Neutrophilic Granulocytes (PMN), Committed Granulopoietic (GM-CFC), and Erythropoietic (BFU-E) Progenitor Cells Before and After Adjuvant Chemotherapy with CMFX6 (Median Values)

	PMN/μl	GM-CFC/liter	BFU-E/liter
Controls before chemotherapy	4200	21,200	127,000
Days after chemotherapy			
50	2850[a]	4,000[c]	–
100	2670[b]	13,600[c]	114,000
100-200	2700[b]	8,100[b]	89,000
200-300	3700	5,000[b]	115,000
300-400	2700	9,900[b]	70,000
400-500	3420	–	70,000
500-600	3130	–	–

[a] $p < 0.05$
[b] $p < 0.01$
[c] $p < 0.001$

system: BFU-E in the peripheral blood were found to be normal as early as 1 year after cessation of chemotherapy (earlier measurements were not performed).

It is of interest, and also of some concern, that these changes in human beings qualitatively resemble those described during the phase of latent aplasia in busulfan-treated mice that precedes overt marrow aplasia (17).

We have demonstrated a similar defect of the granulopoietic system following adjuvant chemotherapy with CMF (cyclophosphamide, methotrexate, and 5-fluorouracil) (Table 3; Ref. 35) during an observation period of more than 1 year following cessation of chemotherapy. Again, circulating GM-CFCs but not circulating BFU-E did reflect persistent drug-induced damage to the hemopoietic system in these patients.

4. Long-Lasting Marrow Failure Following Nitrosoureas. In 7 of 17 patients treated for malignant brain tumors with postoperative cranial irradiation and subsequent methyl-CCNU (120 mg/m^2 every 3 weeks), protracted severe myelosuppression developed, requiring red cell transfusion support in 6 of 7 patients (36 and Table 1). The total dose of methyl-CCNU in these patients was greater than 1200 mg/m^2. A more detailed analysis of the hemopoietic system was not performed in these patients.

This clinical report of a long-lasting hemopoietic compromise may find its explanation in the long-lasting depletion of the granulopoietic progenitor cell compartments in bone marrow and peripheral blood that we have described after both BCNU and methyl-CCNU (9). Following administration of both nitrosoureas, GM-CFCs disappeared completely from the peripheral blood for a prolonged period of time. Similarly, bone marrow GM-CFCs dropped to low levels and remained at these low levels without any of the signs of regeneration that are usually seen after day 10 following administration of other cytotoxic agents (8). Finally, the proliferative and maturing granulocytic compartments reflected similar long-lasting depressions. It is important to note, however, that the incidence of GM-CFCs in the bone marrow and in the peripheral blood continued to be low at the time of recovery of the peripheral blood granulocyte concentration from nitrosourea-induced toxicity that occurred after day 35. Thus, normalization of peripheral blood granulocyte counts does not necessarily indicate normalization from cytotoxic-drug-induced damage in more immature granulopoietic compartments; this may explain the development of cumulative hemopoietic damage with repeated cytotoxic drug therapy.

VI. EVALUATION OF THE PERSISTENT DAMAGE

The clinical importance of a long-lasting defect of the human hemopoietic system following at least some forms of cytotoxic treatment remains to be determined. As mentioned earlier, this question is of particular importance and concern in the context of adjuvant chemotherapy. Some of these patients may be cured of their malignancy; from the data discussed above, development of late bone marrow failure appears as a serious possibility. To our knowledge, no reports of marrow failure following adjuvant chemotherapy have appeared so far; however, it may well be that such cases will be observed as more time goes by.

It may also be that residual marrow damage following cytotoxic treatment does not proceed to overt marrow failure per se, but that these patients are at risk of developing marrow failure when they are exposed to environmental factors that normally induce little stem cell toxicity. A normal marrow may be able to cope with such factors without recognizable impact on blood cell production; when the same factors act on marrow with a preexisting cytotoxic drug-induced defect, marrow failure may ensue. Experimental data (37) suggest unrecognized damage of the hemopoietic system as a possible cause of marrow failure; thus, these considerations are not merely hypothetical.

Finally, persistent marrow damage may become clinically manifest in situations of hemopoietic stress. This was experimentally demonstrated during erythropoietic (23) but not during granulopoietic stress (25).

Patients may relapse following adjuvant chemotherapy. One might expect salvage chemotherapy in this situation to be more difficult to administer if damage to the hemopoietic system persists from previous (adjuvant) chemotherapy. Fortunately, the available evidence does not support this consideration.

Information on the late effects of chemotherapy on the hemopoietic system is scarce both in animal systems and in clinical situations. This may change, however, as more patients become long-term survivors of cytotoxic treatment. For the clinician, it is important to realize not only that cytotoxic drugs may induce short-term and reversible damage to the hemopoietic system, but also that long-term and possibly permanent hemopoietic defects may result from such treatment.

REFERENCES

1. Jones, S. E., Salmon, S. E. *Adjuvant therapy of cancer,* Vol. II. Springer, Berlin (1979).
2. Miller, R. C., Hill, R. B., Nichols, W. W., Meadows, A. T. Acute and long-term cytogenetic effects of childhood cancer chemotherapy and radiotherapy. *Cancer Res. 38,* 3241-3246 (1978).
3. Schein, P. S., Winokur, W. H. Immunosuppressive and cytotoxic therapy: long-term complications. *Ann. Intern. Med. 82,* 84-95 (1975).
4. Reimer, R. R., Hoover, R., Fraumeni, J. F., Young, R. C. Acute leukemia after alkylating-agent therapy of ovarian cancer. *New Engl. J. Med. 297,* 177-180 (1977).
5. Sieber, S. M., Adamson, R. H. Toxicity of antineoplastic agents in man: chromosomal aberrations, antifertility effects, congenital malformations, and carcinogenic potential. *Adv. Cancer Res. 22,* 57-155 (1975).
6. Louie, S., Schwartz, R. S. Immunodeficiency and the pathogenesis of lymphoma and leukemia. *Semin. Hematol. 15,* 117 (1978).
7. Botnik, L. E., Hannon, E. C., Hellman, S. Nature of the hemopoietic stem cell compartment and its proliferative potential. *Blood Cells 5,* 195-206 (1979).
8. Lohrmann, H.-P., Schreml, W. Cytotoxic drugs and the granulopoietic system. *Rec. Res. Cancer Res. 81,* (1982).
9. Lohrmann, H.-P., Lepp, K., Schreml, W. 5-Fluorouracil, 1,3-bis(chloroethyl)-1-nitrosourea, and 1-(2-chloroethyl)-3-(4-methylcyclohexyl)-1-nitrosourea: effect on the human granulopoietic system. *J. Natl. Cancer Inst. 68,* 541-547 (1982).
10. Schofield, R. The relationship between the spleen colony-forming cell and the haemopoietic stem cell. A hypothesis. *Blood Cells 4,* 7-25 (1978).
11. Botnick, L. E., Hannon, E. C., Hellman, S. Limited proliferation of stem cells surviving alkylating agents. *Nature 162,* 68-70 (1976).
12. Botnick, L. E., Hannon, E. C., Hellman, S. Multisystem stem cell failure after apparent recovery from alkylating agents. *Cancer Res. 38,* 1942-1947 (1978).
13. Hellman, S., Botnick, L. E., Hannon, E. C., Vigneulle, R. M. Proliferative capacity of murine hematopoietic stem cells. *Proc. Natl. Acad. Sci. USA 75,* 490-494 (1978).

14. Fried, W., Barone, J. Residual marrow damage following therapy with cyclophosphamide. *Exp. Hematol. 8,* 610-614 (1980).
15. Hellman, S., Botnick, L. E. Stem cell depletion: an explanation of the late effects of cytotoxins. *Int. J. Radiat. Oncol. Biol. Phys. 2,* 181-184 (1977).
16. Micklem, H. S., Ogden, D. A. Ageing of haematopoietic stem cell populations in the mouse. In: *Stem cells of renewing cell populations,* Cairnie, Lala, Osmond, (Eds.). Academic, New York, pp. 331-341 (1976).
17. Morley, A., Blake, J. An animal model of chronic aplastic marrow failure. I. Late marrow failure after busulfan. *Blood 44,* 49-56 (1974).
18. Morley, A., Blake, J. Haemopoietic precursor cells in experimental hypoplastic marrow failure. *Aust. J. Exp. Biol. Med. Sci. 52,* 909-914 (1974).
19. Morley, A., Trainor, K., Blake, J. A primary stem cell lesion in experimental chronic hypoplastic marrow failure. *Blood 45,* 681-688 (1975).
20. Morley, A. A., Trainor, K. J., Seshadri, R. S. Chronic hypoplastic marrow failure and residual injury. *Blood Cells 4,* 253-266 (1978).
21. Trainor, K. J., Morley, A. A. Screening of cytotoxic drugs for residual bone marrow damage. *J. Natl. Cancer Inst. 57,* 1237-1239 (1976).
22. Trainor, K. J., Seshadri, R. S., Morley, A. A. Residual marrow injury following cytotoxic drugs. *Leuk. Res. 3,* 205-210 (1979).
23. Braunschweiger, P. G., Schenken, L. L., Schiffer, L. M. Adriamycin-induced delayed erythropoietic injury expressed following anemia stress. *Cancer Res. 40,* 2257-2262 (1980).
24. Nowrousian, M. R., Schaefer, U. W., Öhl, S., Boecker, W. R., Schmidt, C. G. Effekte der zytostatischen Langzeittherapie mit Bleomycin auf die Hämopoese. *Blut 41,* 320 (1980).
25. Fitchen, J. H., Cline, M. J. The effect of granulopoietic stress in mice with "latent" bone marrow failure. *Exp. Hematol. 8,* 788-794 (1980).
26. Fewer, D., Wilson, C. B., Boldrey, E. B., Enot, J. K. Phase II study of 1-(2-chloroethyl)-3-cyclohexyl-1-nitrosourea (CCNU; NSC-79037) in the treatment of brain tumors. *Cancer Chemother. Rep. 56,* 421-427 (1972).
27. Rosenblum, M. L., Reynolds, A. F., Smith, K. A., Rumack, B. H., Walker, M. D. Chloroethyl-cyclohexyl-nitrosourea (CCNU) in the treatment of malignant brain tumors. *J. Neurosurg. 39,* 306-314 (1973).
28. Ward, H. W. C. Central nervous system tumors of childhood treated with CCNU, vincristine, and radiation. *Med. Pediat. Oncol. 4,* 315-320 (1978).
29. Young, R. G., Walker, M. D., Canellos, G. P., Schein, P. S., Chabner, B. A., DeVita, V. T. Initial clinical trials with methyl-CCNU, 1-(2-chloroethyl)-3-(4-methylcyclohexyl)-1-nitrosourea (MeCCNU). *Cancer 31,* 1164-1169 (1973).
30. Lohrmann, H.-P., Schreml, W. Sensitivity of human granulopoiesis in vitro to adriamycin before and after exposure in vivo. *Cancer Res. 39,* 527-530 (1979).
31. Corder, M. P., Jochimsen, P. R., Dick, F. R. Abnormal peripheral neutrophil and white cell stimulation in patients treated for regional carcinoma of the breast with adjuvant chemotherapy. *Clin. Res. 37,* 383 (1979).

32. Nowrousian, M. R., Niederle, N., Schaefer, U. W., Krischke, W., Schmidt, C. G. Einfluss der zytostatischen Chemotherapie auf das Regenerationsverhalten der granulopoetisch determinierten Stammzellen (CFU-C) in Blut und Knochenmark bei Patienten mit kleinzelligem Bronchialkarzinom. *Onkologie 4,* 285 (1981).
33. Lohrmann, H.-P., Schreml, W., Lang, M., Betzler, M., Fliedner, T. M., Heimpel, H. Changes of granulopoiesis during and after adjuvant chemotherapy of breast cancer. *Brit. J. Haematol. 40,* 369-381 (1978).
34. Schreml, W., Lohrmann, H.-P. Hematotoxicity of adjuvant therapy. In: *Adjuvant therapy of cancer,* Vol. II. Jones, X.X., Salmon, X. (Eds.). Grune and Stratton, New York, pp. 63-70 (1979).
35. Schreml, W., Lohrmann, H.-P., Anger, B. Stem cell defects after cytoreductive therapy in man. *Exp. Hematol. 13* (*Suppl. 16*), 31-42 (1985).
36. Osband, M., Cohen, H., Cassady, J. R., Faffe, N. Severe and protracted bone marrow dysfunction following long-term therapy with methyl-CCNU. *Proc. Am. Ass. Cancer Res. 18,* 303 (1979).
37. Morley, A., Trainor, K., Remes, J. Residual marrow damage: possible explanation for idiosyncrasy to chloramphenicol. *Brit. J. Haematol. 32,* 525-531 (1976).

15

Hemopoietic Engraftment and Differentiation After Bone Marrow Transplantation

STEPHEN G. EMERSON
University of Michigan Medical Center, Ann Arbor, Michigan

ROBERT PETER GALE
University of California–Los Angeles School of Medicine, Los Angeles, California

I. INTRODUCTION

Bone marrow transplantation is increasingly used to treat individuals with leukemia, solid tumors, and hematological, genetic, and immune disorders (1). The principle underlying this approach is to administer very high doses of cytotoxic drugs and radiation followed by "rescue" with histocompatible bone marrow cells. The latter provide a source of hemopoietic stem cells that permanently replace recipient hemopoiesis in most instances.

One requirement for the success of bone marrow transplantation is that the donor bone marrow contain adequate numbers of pluripotent hemopoietic stem cells to permit complete and sustained recovery of hemopoiesis in the recipient. Donor-derived red blood cells, granulocytes, platelets, and lymphocytes usually reach normal levels between 3 and 6 months following successful transplantation. As we will discuss, however, levels of mature cells in the blood may not accurately reflect the state of the stem cell pool in the bone marrow.

The establishment and expansion of grafts of bone-marrow-derived hemopoietic stem cells, although commonly observed, is poorly understood. The fact that bone marrow transplants can succeed indicates that donor-derived self-renewing pluripotent stem cells engraft and expand. However, the mechanisms by which this occurs are not known. From a clinical standpoint this is a critical problem because not all bone marrow transplants are successful in reconstituting hemopoiesis in the recipient. In fact, nonengraftment or engraftment followed by graft failure are major problems in some clinical settings such as HLA-haplotype mismatched transplants and transplants of T-lymphocyte-depleted bone marrow (2).

In addition to clinical issues, bone marrow transplantation represents a unique opportunity to study human hemopoietic stem cell differentiation. Presently, the only in vitro assays of undifferentiated bone marrow function measure the behavior of relatively late committed cells called progenitors. We lack in vitro assays that analyze the processes of committment to differentiation, self-renewal, and lineage selection. Observations on hemopoiesis following bone marrow transplant, however, can be informative in this context.

In this chapter we review data related to hemopoietic progenitor cells and recovery of hemopoiesis following bone marrow transplantation in humans. We focus on three features: homing of stem cells to the bone marrow, hemopoietic growth factor production by accessory cells, and suppression of hemopoiesis by regulatory cells.

II. IN VITRO ANALYSIS OF HUMAN HEMOPOIETIC STEM CELL DIFFERENTIATION

Hemopoietic differentiation is a complex process in which undifferentiated pluripotent stem cells evolve into committed progenitor cells that are more differentiated and have less self-renewal capacity. The first descendants of pluripotent stem cells, termed progenitor cells, are committed to one or more hemopoietic lineages; human progenitor cells are marked by the presence of surface HLA-DR (3) and My10 antigens (4). Although the molecular events triggering stem cells to divide and differentiate to progenitor cells are not known, the subsequent stages in which the committed progenitor cells differentiate to recognizable precursor cells and finally to mature myeloid and lymphoid cells are beginning to be understood.

Four hormones that influence myeloid differentiation have been described in the mouse (data summarized in Table 1): granulocyte-colony-stimulating factor (G-CSF), which induces the terminal differentiation of committed granulocytic progenitors (5); monocyte-macrophage colony-stimulating factor (M-CSF), which induces monocyte progenitors to differentiate (6); granulocyte-macrophage colony-stimulating factor (GM-CSF), which induces granulocyte, monocyte, and bipotent granulocyte-macrophage progenitors as well as eosinophilic and, to a limited extent, erythroid progenitors (7); and Multi-CSF or interleukin-3 (IL-3), which induces all classes of myeloid progenitor cells as well as mast cells, megakaryocytic progenitors, and possibly pre-B cells (8). IL-3, GM-CSF, and probably M-CSF are normal, inducible T cell products; the physiological source of G-CSF is unknown. The genes for two of these molecules have been cloned, and their protein products have been expressed and purified and their activities confirmed (9,10).

Human analogs to these four growth factors have been identified, and their encoding genes have been molecularly cloned. These data are summarized in

Table 1 Activities of Hemopoietic Growth Factors

Species	Hormone[a]	Progenitors induced
Mouse	G-CSF	Granulocyte
	M-CSF	Monocyte-macrophage
	GM-CSF	Granulocyte Monocyte-macrophage Granulocyte-monocyte Eosinophil Erythrocyte
	IL-3	Granulocyte Monocyte-macrophage Granulocyte-monocyte Multipotential granulocyte-erythrocyte-monocyte-megakaryocyte Erythrocyte Pre-B lymphocyte
Man	G-CSF	Granulocyte
	M-CSF	Monocyte-macrophage
	GM-CSF	Granulocyte Monocyte-macrophage Granulocyte-monocyte Eosinophil Erythrocyte Multipotential granulocyte-erythrocyte-monocyte
	IL-3	Granulocyte Monocyte Granulocyte-monocyte Erythrocyte Multipotential granulocyte-erythrocyte-monocyte

[a]G-CSF, granulocyte colony-stimulating factor; M-CSF, monocyte colony-stimulating factor; GM-CSF, granulocyte-monocyte colony-stimulating factor; IL-3, interleukin-3.

Table 1. Human GM-CSF was initially described as a restricted granulocyte and monocyte inducer with some granulocyte-activating features (11). Recent data indicate that GM-CSF also stimulates erythroid and multipotent erythroid-myeloid progenitors in vitro (12) and is functionally active in primates in vivo (13,14). GM-CSF also stimulates the growth of myeloid leukemia progenitor cells in vitro, although the comparative responsiveness of normal and leukemic progenitor cells is not yet known. Human M-CSF, or CSF-1, has likewise been purified and molecularly cloned (15). A third molecule produced by a bladder carcinoma cell line with multiple trophic activities and termed pluropoietin (16) has recently been described. The protein product expressed from this gene has properties similar to those of murine G-CSF. The human analog to murine IL-3 gene has also recently been molecularly cloned. The protein product has pluripoietic myeloid colony-stimulating activity (17). The two human hormones with the broadest spectrum of hemopoietic activities are GM-CSF and IL-3. These data are summarized in Table 1.

These hemopoietic growth factors are produced by mature cells in the bone marrow, termed accessory cells. Accessory cells include fibroblasts, which produce GM-CSF and perhaps M-CSF and G-CSF (18,19); endothelial cells, which produce GM-CSF (20); T lymphocytes, which produce GM-CSF, M-CSF, and IL-3 (11,17); and perhaps natural killer cells (21,22) as well as other cells. Accessory cells secrete these hormones at very low basal levels; the amounts secreted are increased by mitogenic stimulation (11) and by products of activated monocytes (20). These data are summarized in Table 2. Since production of these growth factors is absolutely required for hemopoietic differentiation, toxic effects or developmental defects that inhibit the accessory cells could profoundly depress hemopoiesis even in the absence of direct toxicity to hemopoietic progenitor cells.

Although hemopoietic growth factors are essential for stem cell differentiation, they are not sufficient. A key additional requirement is the localization of the undifferentiated cells to fixed geometric niches that maintain cell-cell contact of progenitor daughter cells. This is observed in vitro as the requirement for a semisolid matrix such as agar or methylcellulose, without which progenitor division and differentiation cease after three or four divisions. In vivo this requirement

Table 2 Accessory Cells Producing Hemopoietic Growth Factors

Accessory cells	Hemopoietic growth factor	Inducer
T lymphocytes	G-CSF	
	M-CSF	
	GM-CSF	
	IL-3	Interleukin-2, phytohemaglutinin
Fibroblasts, endothelial cells	G-CSF	
	M-CSF	Interleukin-1, tumor necrosis factor
	GM-CSF	
Monocytes	?	?
NK cells	?	?

is apparent from the geographic limitation of hemopoiesis to the bone marrow or spleen, or rarely the liver.

One of the important molecular determinants of the geographic localization of hemopoiesis appears to be the presence of membrane receptors for extracellular matrix proteins on hemopoietic precursors. Reticulocytes possess membrane receptors for fibronectin; the receptors are lost coincident with bone marrow egress of mature erythrocytes (23,24). This receptor is present in all defined precursor stages of erythropoiesis and on a subset of erythroid progenitor cells in the bone marrow (25,26).

Similarly, myeloid precursor cells appear to bind to a different, distinct extracellular matrix protein termed hemonectin (27). Whether myeloid progenitor cells themselves bind to hemonectin or whether this specificity appears during differentiation is unknown.

There is increasing evidence that lineage-specific differentiation occurs within local biochemical niches defined by the presence of specific extracellular matrix proteins. This finding may furthermore explain one unusual aspect of hemopoietic physiology, namely, the presence of progenitors and stem cells in peripheral blood: BFU-E, GM-CFC, Mix-CFC, and even pluripotent stem cells are found in peripheral blood mononuclear cells at nearly the same frequency as in bone marrow (28), although recognizable precursor cells are absent. One possibility is that as circulating stem cells differentiate, they acquire matrix protein receptors and so adhere following passage through the bone marrow interstitium. Whether these adhesive interactions are random or are facilitated by chemoattractive signals released by the bone marrow is not known.

Hemopoietic differentiation begins in appropriate bone marrow niches under the influence of positive trophic hemopoietic hormones. Under these circumstances proliferation of progenitor cells appears to be regulated by autoregulatory suppressor cells. Suppressor cells have been detected in some patients with monoclonal proliferations of T cells (29) and have been generated in vitro by IL-2 stimulation of T cells (30). Hemopoietic suppressor T cells can be directly generated by autologous non-T cells (31); as such they appear to be normal inducible elements of the T cell repertoire. Under certain circumstances, increased numbers or activity of these cells can lead to cytopenias (29).

III. EXPERIMENTAL ANALYSIS OF ENGRAFTMENT—STEM CELLS, MICROENVIRONMENT, AND GENETIC RESISTANCE

Diverse elements including hemopoietic growth factors, lineage-specific extracellular matrix proteins, and hemopoietic suppressor cells are likely to play roles in hemopoietic engraftment and differentiation following bone marrow transplantation.

Ford and co-workers (32) and Vos et al. (33) first demonstrated that the regenerating hemopoietic system posttransplant is derived from donor cells. Subsequent experiments in mice, rats, and dogs have established that hemopoietic engraftment depends on the number and source of infused donor cells as well as on their regulation by the host environment.

Murine pluripotent stem cells (CFU-S) occur in high frequency in the bone marrow, 500 CFU-S per 10^5 nucleated cells. Spleen and fetal liver have a lower frequency of CFU-S. They are not detectable in lymph node and thymus (34). Splenic hemopoietic colonies can be detected 8-10 days after the injection of 10^4-10^5 bone marrow cells into lethally irradiated syngeneic mice. (See Chapter 1.) A dose of 10^5 cells or greater is required for full engraftment as determined by survival; presumably lower doses could reconstitute hemopoiesis, but death supervenes because of profound bone marrow suppression. CFU-S derived from infused donor spleen cells are more typically erythroid than are CFU-S following bone marrow transplants, which are more often granulocytic (35). Spleen cells are threefold less effective at protecting irradiated hosts than bone marrow cells (36). Thus stem cells from different sites behave qualitatively and quantitatively differently in the setting of transplantation.

The hemopoietic microenvironment of the host also influences both quantitative and qualitative stem cell differentiation. The Steel mutant mouse has a hereditary form of anemia related to a stromal defect; this defect can be cured by transplantation of spleen-derived stromal cells from normal littermates (37, 38). Moreover, in normal mice, stromal cells derived from different organs exert diverse regulatory effects. For example, in the mouse, erythroid differentiation predominates in spleen stroma and myeloid differentiation in bone marrow stroma (39). Single CFU-S, which develop on the border of bone marrow spicules artificially implanted into the spleen, show erythroid growth on the splenic, myeloid growth on the bone marrow sides of the spicule border (40).

Genetic histocompatibility between donor and host also plays an important role in engraftment. Mice immunosuppressed with 8 Gy total body radiation require 60 times more H-2-incompatible donor bone marrow cells for engraftment than recipients of syngeneic transplants. Twice as many H-2-matched, minor histocompatible antigen-mismatched donor bone marrow cells are needed (41,42).

Engraftment is impaired even when parental bone marrow cells are transplanted into F_1 recipients, a situation in which there are no mismatched donor histocompatibility antigens as a target of graft rejection. Radiated recipients of certain murine strains reject parental bone marrow grafts despite their acceptance of other grafted tissues from the same donor. This phenomenon, termed hybrid resistance, has been investigated in considerable detail. Hybrid resistance appears to be mediated by natural killer (NK) cells. Hybrid resistance in mice is thymus-independent, requires no prior immunization (43), is relatively radioresistant (43,44), and can be overcome by treatment with silica or carageenan (47) or by increasing the dose of donor bone marrow cells. Strains that are genetically resistant to endogenous virally induced leukemias, such as C57Bl/6, have high levels of both in vitro NK activity and in vivo F_1 hybrid resistance to bone marrow grafts (45,46). Moreover, treatments that suppress NK function without inhibiting other known immune mechanisms abrogate their ability to reject parental bone marrow grafts (47-49). Partially purified NK cells dramatically suppress CFU-S growth when incubated with bone marrow prior to transplantation (50). The concept of hybrid resistance extends beyond the parent to the F_1 hybrid transplant setting and has in some instances been termed genetic resistance. The genetic loci responsible for this phenomenon have been partially mapped and are termed Hh, or hemopoietic histocompatibility, loci. NK cells have been implicated in transplant rejection in humans in some but not all studies (51), and while NK cells with NK phenotype are prevalent posttransplant, classic cytotoxic T lymphocytes may actually be more prominent in human graft rejection than NK cells (52).

IV. HEMOPOIESIS FOLLOWING BONE MARROW TRANSPLANTATION IN HUMANS

Evaluation of engraftment in humans is complex because of the diverse settings in which transplants are performed. Pretransplant conditioning regimens vary among leukemia, aplastic anemia, immunodeficiency, and genetic disorders. The hemopoietic microenvironment of the recipient may be influenced by disease or by the conditioning regimen. Notwithstanding these complexities, clinical data have suggested certain principles that form the basis for future investigation.

Circulating nucleated red blood cells and immature myeloid cells are detectable in buffy coat preparations 7-10 days posttransplant. These cells are probably the progeny of circulating committed progenitor cells infused in the bone marrow inoculum (53). Granulocyte production increases after 2-3 weeks and, in the absence of infections or severe graft-versus-host disease, normalizes within 1-2 months. The rate of myelopoietic recovery is related to the dose of GM-CFC in the donor bone marrow in some but not all studies (54-56). Reticulocytes reach maximal levels by 4-8 weeks posttransplant. Platelets normalize in some patients within 1-3 months. In many patients, however, adequate megakaryopoiesis is never achieved; in others it decreases after initially achieving normal platelet levels. Platelet production may be suppressed by chronic graft-versus-host disease, and persistent thrombocytopenia posttransplant indicates a poor prognosis (57). For reasons that are uncertain, megakaryopoiesis is less adequately restored posttransplant than other cell lineages. This does not appear to be related to histocompatibility differences, since similar observations have been made in autotransplants in syngeneic grafts. Also, it does not appear to be related to damage induced by cryopreservation, since transplants of noncryopreserved cells show a similar pattern.

Although granulocytes usually reach normal levels within 1-2 months, the pool of committed myeloid progenitors responsible for maintaining this pool may be reduced in number as well as function. Gale and co-workers initially reported severely reduced bone marrow GM-CFC density 2 months and 8 years, respectively, following transplantation for aplastic anemia and acute leukemia (58,63). This deficiency in GM-CFCs following transplantation has been recently confirmed (56). Decreased frequencies of GM-CFCs are not invariably detected in the first 3 months posttransplant (59) and may be more apparent later (60). The decline in number of GM-CFCs may be due to a proliferative defect (61) or to a greater reliance on Mix-CFC proliferation at later intervals posttransplant (62).

Quantitative and qualitative deficiencies in progenitor cells posttransplant may be related to three sources: decreased numbers of hemopoietic stem cells, activation of suppressor cells, and abnormal function of accessory cells that produce hemopoietic growth factors. Li and co-workers found that GM-CFCs derived from both peripheral blood and bone marrow in transplant recipients were markedly reduced in number compared to normal bone marrow donor (blood $5 \pm 1/10^6$ versus $37 \pm 4/10^6$; bone marrow, $23 \pm 5/2 \times 10^5$ versus $170 \pm 21/2 \times 10^5$ cells) (63). Depletion of T cells from recipient bone marrow by E rosette formation resulted in normalization of GM-CFC values. These investigators suggested that the decreased cloning efficiency of GM-CFC posttransplant might be related to a suppressive effect of autologous T cells. Suppression of GM-CFC-derived colony formation in vitro has also been reported by Raghavachar and co-workers, predominantly in patients with acute GVHD (64).

Production of hemopoietic growth factors by T cells may be deficient following bone marrow transplantation. Emerson and co-workers used a successive fractionation technique to distinguish production of burst-promoting activity (BPA), which stimulates early erythroid progenitor cells, and colony-stimulating activity (CSA probably containing more than one type of CSF) by adherent cells, NK cells, and T cells (65). They found that although adherent cells often function normally after transplantation, NK cells and T cells produced little if any BPA or CSA. Northern blot analyses of NK and T cells from these patients confirmed that T cell GM-CSF mRNA levels were greatly decreased or absent. These observations suggest that normalization of hemopoiesis posttransplant may depend on growth factors produced by accessory cells, or possibly by stromal cells.

Nakao and co-workers reported that circulating T cells obtained within 3 weeks following bone marrow transplant augment BFU-E-derived colony formation; cells obtained later were inactive (66). This observation is consistent with the notion that T cells that support initial hemopoiesis are infused in the transplant inoculum and that T cells that subsequently develop in the recipient are less effective. Recently Mitsuyasu et al. reported decreased in vitro T lymphocyte colonies (CFU-TL) in transplant recipients (67). This defect appeared to

Table 3 Evidence for Abnormal Hemopoiesis Following Bone Marrow Transplantation

Authors (Ref.)	Abnormalities
Li et al. (63)	Decreased GM-CFC ? Myeloid suppressor T cells
Arnold et al. (56)	Decreased GM-CFC, BFU-E
Raghavachar et al. (64)	Decreased GM-CFC Myeloid suppressor T cells (patients with GVHD only)
Barrett and Adams (61)	Decreased GM-CFC proliferation
Mitsuyasu et al. (67)	Decreased CFU-TL
Nakao et al. (66)	Loss of BPA-producing T cells
Emerson et al. (65)	Decreased BPA/CSA-producing T cells and NK cells

be intrinsic to CFU-TL, since addition of normal T cells from the donor did not correct the defect or lead to suppression of donor CFU-TL. The abnormalities that may affect hemopoiesis following transplantation are summarized in Table 3.

V. T CELL DEPLETION AND GRAFT FAILURE

Recently, transplants of T-cell-depleted grafts have been performed as a method of preventing graft-versus-host disease (GVHD) (for review, see 68). Although this approach is successful in reducing GVHD, it is associated with an increased risk of graft failure: 10-20% in T-cell-depleted transplants versus <1% in conventional transplants. The mechanism underlying the graft failure in this setting follows two patterns; in one there is no evidence of initial engraftment; in the second, initial engraftment is followed by subsequent graft failure. The cause of this increase in graft failure is unknown. Several possibilities exist: (1) immune-mediated graft rejection; (2) damage to hemopoietic stem cells by the process of T cell depletion; (3) abnormalities in cells that regulate hemopoiesis posttransplant; and (4) suppression by residual leukemic cells. Immune-mediated graft rejection has been hypothesized to mediate graft failure for theoretical reasons that appear to be confirmed by recent studies. While the dose of chemotherapy and radiation used in pretransplant conditioning regimens are usually lethal, they are not high enough to destroy all recipient myeloid and lymphoid cells. Although residual recipient cells are rarely detected in mice following conventional allogeneic transplants, both residual myeloid and lymphoid cells are readily detected months after T-cell-depleted bone marrow transplants performed at identical cell doses (69). Butturini and colleagues have confirmed that human recipient T lymphocytes can survive pretransplant conditioning and are readily detected prior to the infusion of the donor marrow inoculum (70). These data imply that it is the removal of donor T cells that permits the survival and proliferation of residual recipient hemopoietic cells.

If the residual recipient T cells are not killed by donor T cells, it seems plausible that they could recognize and eventually destroy donor stem cells. As yet there have been no clearly documented cases of residual T-cell-mediated graft failure. However, two recent trials confirm that intravenous posttransplant therapy with specific monoclonal anti-T-cell antibodies can lead to decreased incidence of graft failure in T-cell-depleted bone marrow transplants (71,72).

Damage to stem cells by the process of T cell depletion could certainly cause graft failure. Indeed, the earliest trials of monoclonal antibody bone marrow treatment for ALL autotransplants were complicated by persistent thrombocytopenia, and recent attempts to treat stage IV neuroblastoma by autotransplant following antineuroblastoma antibody plus complement have also encountered problems with graft failure. However, in these situations the donor/recipient bone marrow had already been heavily treated, so stem cell damage may have preceded the transplant procedure. For T-cell-depleted allogeneic marrow grafts, however, the donor bone marrow has received no prior chemotherapy. In addition, increased graft failure has been observed with a variety of physical and immunologic techniques of T cell depletion. It is therefore unlikely that each of these techniques also damages stem cells.

Alterations in the function of donor hemopoietic regulatory cells that differentiate in the recipient have been well described, but their impact on graft failure is unknown. Autologous suppressive T lymphocytes have been described in two studies (63,64), and decreased T cell hemopoietin production in one other (65), but all of these patients were fully engrafted. Moreover, in one of the studies demonstrating T cell suppression, significant effects were seen only in patients with GVHD. T cell depletion clearly reduces GVHD, however, so the relevance of this in vitro finding to the pathogenesis of graft failure in T-cell-depleted marrow transplantation may be limited. Even if these mechanisms were important, proving their relevance to clinical graft failure would be extremely difficult. To demonstrate their role in grafts that never began would require performing experiments with vanishingly few cells. In cases of late graft rejection, experiments would need to be performed as the graft was being lost, a very narrow window in time that could easily be missed.

Suppression of normal donor hemopoiesis by residual leukemic cells is a final potential mechanism of graft failure in T-cell-depleted marrow transplants. Donor T cells probably can detect and destroy residual leukemic cells, just as they remove normal clonogenic myeloid and lymphoid cells; this is referred to as graft-versus-leukemia (GVL). Removal of donor T cells from marrow transplant inocula could lead to increased leukemic relapse. A recent literature review indicates that the leukemic relapse rate increases from 5-20% in recipients of untreated grafts to 20-40% in recipients of T-cell-depleted grafts (68). This trend has also been confirmed in a randomized trial (73).

Residual leukemic cells could theoretically lead to suppression of donor hemopoiesis and graft failure, even before or without overt relapse. Leukemic cells secrete unusually high levels of iron-binding proteins (lactoferrins, acidic isoferritins) that inhibit normal hemopoiesis (reviewed in 74). Residual leukemic cells, present in too small a number to be conclusively detected by bone marrow aspiration, could therefore suppress normal hemopoiesis. Since the incidence and numbers of such cells would be expected to be increased in T-cell-depleted transplants, the risk of leukemic cell-mediated marrow suppression would also be higher. Perhaps the concurrent deficiency of normal hemopoietic accessory cell activity would accentuate the sensitivity of donor marrow stem cells to the effects of these inhibiting molecules.

Overall the present data suggest that graft failure is most likely mediated by immune rejection. However, another, related, possibility is that radiation of recipient bone marrow stromal cells might temporarily decrease their ability to secrete hemopoietic growth factors. If donor T cells are removed, the few infused adherent bone marrow fibroblasts and endothelial cells might be inadequate to support hemopoiesis. This is particularly true if residual cytotoxic T cells of recipient origin reject transplanted donor stem cells. Whether or not donor-derived hemopoietic stem cells engraft would thus be determined by the balance among active accessory cells of donor or recipient origin supporting engraftment, residual recipient cytotoxic T cells that react against the grafts, residual leukemic cells secreting inhibitory molecules, and donor suppressor T cells, which can also inhibit hemopoiesis.

VI. FUTURE DIRECTIONS

Assays of helper and suppressor cell functions, target cell specificity, and growth factor production exist in sufficient variety and sensitivity for a careful analysis of the regulation of hemopoiesis following bone marrow transplantation. Given the substantial problem of nonengraftment in T-cell-depleted transplants, investigators might focus attention on problems specific to or accentuated in these patients. These might include serum levels of GM-CSF and IL-3, fibroblast and T cell GM-CSF and IL-3 production, donor cytotoxic or suppressor T cells, and expression of extracellular matrix protein receptors on progenitor cells.

In addition, experiments to distinguish T cell subsets that cause GVHD from those that are responsible for GVL are essential. While as yet no such separation has been convincingly demonstrated, recent experiments by Krensky et al. suggest that tumor-specific T cells may constitute a unique, separable subset (75). Isolation of these cells in humans would be a major advance.

In summary, the reestablishment of hemopoiesis following bone marrow transplantation occurs via imperfectly understood physiologic processes. Recent advances in our understanding of the cellular and molecular regulation of hemopoiesis permit detailed analyses of these events. These analyses may result in an understanding of the abnormalities that eventuate in graft failure, particularly in recipients of T-cell-depleted bone marrow grafts. Data from these studies may improve results of bone marrow transplantation and provide important insights into the regulation of normal hemopoiesis.

REFERENCES

1. Gale, R. P., Champlin, R. E. (Eds.). *Bone marrow transplantation: recent advances and future directions.* Liss, New York (1987).
2. O'Reilly, R. J., Brochstein, J., Kirkpatrick, D., et al. Transplantation of histocompatible, soybean lectin (SBA) separated, E-rosette depleted marrow for severe combined immunodeficiency (SCID) and leukemia: MHC-related graft resistance in leukemic transplant recipients. *Blood 62* (*Suppl.*), 227a (1983).
3. Linch, D. C., Nadler, L. M., Luther, E. A., Lipton, J. Discordant expression of human Ia-like antigens on hematopoietic progenitor. *J. Immunol. 132,* 2324-2329 (1984).
4. Civin, C. I., Strauss, L. C., Brovall, C., Fackler, J. M., Schwartz, J., Shapen, J. A. A hematopoietic progenitor cell surface antigen defined by a monoclonal antibody raised against KG-Ia cells. *J. Immunol. 133,* 157-165 (1984).
5. Nicola, N. A., Metcalf, D., Matsumoto, M., Johnson, G. R. Purification of a factor inducing differentiation in murine myelomonocytic leukemia cells. *J. Biol. Chem. 258,* 9017-9021 (1983).
6. Stanley, E. R., Heard, P. M. Factors regulating macrophage production and growth. *J. Biol. Chem. 252,* 4305-4312 (1977).
7. Burgess, A. W., Camarkis, J., Metcalf, D. Purification and properties of colony-stimulating factor from mouse lung-conditioned medium. *J. Biol. Chem. 252,* 1998-2003 (1977).
8. Ihle, J. N., Keller, J., Henderson, L., Klein, F., Palaszynshi, E. Procedures for the purification of interleukin 3 to homogeneity. *J. Immunol. 129,* 2431-2436 (1982).
9. Gough, N. M., Gough, J., Metcalf, D., Kelso, A., Graie, D., Nicola, N. A., Burgess, A. W., Dunn, A. R. Molecular cloning of cDNA encoding a murine haematopoietic growth regulator, granulocyte-macrophage colony stimulating factor. *Nature 309,* 763-767 (1984).
10. Fung, M. C., Hapel, A. J., Ymer, S., Cohen, D. R., Johnson, R. M., Campbell, H. D., Young, I. G. Molecular cloning of cDNA for murine interleukin-3. *Nature 307,* 233-237 (1984).

11. Wong, G. G., Witek, J. S., Temple, P. A., Wilkens, K. M., Leary, A. C., Luxenberg, D. P., Jones, S. S., Brown, E. L., Kay, R. M., Orr, E. D., Shoemaker, C., Golde, D. W., Kaufman, R. J., Hewick, R. M., Wang, E. A., Clark, S. C. Human GM-CSF: molecular cloning of the complementary DNA and purification of the natural and recombinant proteins. *Science 228,* 810-815 (1985).
12. Emerson, S. G., Sieff, C. A., Wang, E. A., Wong, G. G., Clark, S. C., Nathan, D. G. Purification of fetal hematopoietic progenitors and demonstration of recombinant multipotential colony-stimulating activity. *J. Clin. Invest. 76,* 1286-1290 (1985).
13. Donahue, R., Wang, E. A., Emerson, S. G., Sehgal, P., Wong, G. G., Clark, S. C., Nathan, D. G. *Blood 66* (*Suppl.*), 479a (1985).
14. Donahue, R. E., Wang, E. A., Stone, D. K., Kamen, R., Wong, G. G., Sehgal, P. K., Nathan, D. G., Clark, S. C. Stimulation of haematopoiesis in primates by continuous infusion of recombinant human GM-CSF. *Nature 321,* 872-875 (1986).
15. Kawasaki, E. S., Ladner, M. B., Wang, A. M., Arsell, J. V., Warren, M. K., Corpe, M. Y., Schweickert, V. L., Lee, M. T., Wilson, K. J., Boosman, A., Stanley, E. R., Ralph, P., Mark, D. F. Molecular cloning of a complementary DNA encoding human macrophage-specific colony-stimulating factor (CSF-1). *Science 230,* 291-296 (1985).
16. Walte, K., Platzer, E., Lu, L., Gabrilove, J. L., Levi, E., Mertelsmann, R., Moore, M. A. S. Purification and biochemical characterization of human pluripotent hematapoietic colony-stimulating factor. *Proc. Natl. Acad. Sci. USA 82,* 1526-1530 (1985).
17. Yang, Y. C., Ciarletta, A. B., Temple, P. A., Chung, M. P., Kovacic, S., Witek-Gianotti, J. S., Leary, A. C., Kriz, R., Donahue, R. E., Wong, G. G., Clark, S. C. Human IL-3 (multi-CSF): identification by expression cloning of a novel hematopoietic growth factor related to murine IL-3. *Cell 47,* 3-10 (1986).
18. Tsai, S., Emerson, S. G., Sieff, C. A., Nathan, D. G. Isolation of a human stromal cell strain secreting hemopoietic growth factors. *J. Cell. Physiol. 127,* 137-145 (1986).
19. Zucali, J. R., Dinarello, C. A., Oblon, D. J., Gross, M. A., Anderson, L., Weiner, R. S. Interleukin 1 stimulates fibroblasts to produce granulocyte-macrophage colony-stimulating activity and prostaglandin E_2. *J. Clin. Invest. 77,* 1857-1863 (1986).
20. Zuckerman, K. S., Bagby, G. C., McCall, E., Sparks, B., Wells, J., Patel, V. R., Goodrum, D. A monokine stimulates production of human erythroid burst-promoting activity by endothelial cells in vitro. *J. Clin. Invest. 75,* 722-729 (1985).
21. Linch, D. C., Lipton, J. M., Nathan, D. G. Identification of three accessory cell populations in human bone marrow with erythroid burst-promoting properties. *J. Clin. Invest. 75,* 1278-1284 (1985).
22. Pistoia, V., Ghio, R., Nocera, A., Leprini, A., Perata, A., Ferrarine, M. Large granular lymphocytes have a promoting activity on human peripheral blood erythroid burst-forming units. *Blood 65,* 464-472 (1985).

23. Patel, V. P., Ciechanover, A., Platt, O., Lodish, H. F. Mammalian reticulocytes lose adhesion to fibronectin during maturation to erythrocytes. *Proc. Natl. Acad. Sci. USA 82,* 440-444 (1985).
24. Patel, V. P., Lodish, H. F. Loss of adhesion of murine erythroleukemia cells to fibronectin during erythroid differentiation. *Science 224,* 996-998 (1984).
25. Tsai, S., Sieff, C. A., Patel, V. P., Lodish, H. F. Differential binding of primitive erythroid and myeloid progenitors to fibroblasts and fibronectin. *Blood 68 (Suppl.),* 495 (1986).
26. Vuillet, M. H., Leroy, C., Parmentier, C., Tchernia, G., Coulombel, L. Lineage- and stage-specific adhesion of human hematopoietic precursor cells (HPC) to extracellular matrices (ECM). *Blood 68 (Suppl.),* 500 (1986).
27. Campbell, A. D., Wicha, M. S., Long, M. Extracellular matrix promotes the growth and differentiation of murine hematopoietic cells in vitro. *J. Clin. Invest. 75,* 2085-2090 (1985).
28. McCarthy, D. M., Goldman, J. M. Transfusion of circulating stem cells. *CRC Crit. Rev. Clin. Cal. Sci. 20,* 1-25 (1984).
29. Lipton, J. M., Nadler, L. M., Cannellos, G. P., Kudisch, M., Reiss, C. S., Nathan, D. G. Regulation of de novo purine synthesis in human bone marrow mononuclear cells by hypoxanthine. *J. Clin. Invest. 72,* 965-970 (1983).
30. Burdach, S., Falardo, L., Shatsky, M., Wagenhast, B., Levitt, L. Interleukin-2 inhibition of erythropoiesis is mediated by sequential lymphokine-target cell interactions and is restricted to CD3 triggered T cells. *Blood 68 (Suppl.),* 523 (1986).
31. Harada, M., Nakao, S., Kondo, K., Odaka, K., Ueda, M., Shiobara, S., Matsue, K., Mori, T., Matsuda, T. Effect of activated lymphocytes on the regulation of hematopoiesis: enhancement and suppression of in vitro BFU-E growth by T cells stimulated by autologous non-T cells. *Blood 67,* 1143-1147 (1986).
32. Ford, C. E., Hamerton, J. L., Barnes, D. W. H., Loutit, J. F. Cytological identification of radiation-chimaeras. *Nature 177,* 452-454 (1956).
33. Vos, O., Davids, J. A. G., Weyzen, W. W. H., van Bekkum, D. W. Evidence for the cellular hypothesis in radiation protection by bone marrow cell. *Acta Physiol. Pharmacol. Neer. 4,* 482-488 (1956).
34. Gallagher, M. T. Experimental basis. In: *Clinical bone marrow transplantation.* Blume, K. G., Petz, L. D. (Eds.). Churchill Livingstone, New York, pp. 33-64 (1983).
35. Wolf, N. S., Jenkins, V. K., Trentin, J. J. Increase in proportion of erythropoietic spleen colonies in mice injected with spleen cells as compared with bone marrow cells. *Exp. Hematol. 22,* 37-45 (1972).
36. Kretchmar, A. L., Conover, W. R. A difference between spleen-derived and bone marrow-derived colony-forming units in ability to protect lethally irradiated mice. *Blood 36,* 772-776 (1970).
37. Bernstein, S. E., Russel, E. S., Keighley, G. Two hereditary mouse anemias (SL/SL^d and W/W^v) deficient in response to erythropoietin. *Ann. N.Y. Acad. Sci. 149,* 475-485 (1968).

38. Gallagher, M. T., McGarny, M. P., Trentin, J. J. Defect of splenic stroma (hematopoietic inductive microenvironments) in genetic anemia of SL/SL^d mice. *Fed. Proc. 30,* 684 (abstr.) (1971).
39. Trentin, J. J. Determination of bone marrow stem cell differentiation by stromal hemopoietic inductive microenvironments (HIM). *Amer. J. Pathol. 65,* 621-628 (1971).
40. Trentin, J. J. Hemopoietic colony studies: V. Effect of hemopoietic organ stroma on differentiation of pluripotent stem cells. *J. Exp. Med. 127,* 205-214 (1968).
41. Vriesendorp, H. M., van Bekkum, D. W. In: *The canine as a biomedical research model.* Shifrine, M., Wilson, F. D. (Eds.). U.S. Department of Energy, Washington, DC, pp. 153-172 (1980).
42. Wolff, N. S., Trentin, J. J. Linearity of counts of endogenous and exogenous colonies in mouse bone marrow. *Exp. Hematol. 3,* 54-56 (1975).
43. Cudowicz, G., Bennett, M. Peculiar immunobiology of bone marrow allografts: I. Graft rejection by irradiated responder mice. *J. Exp. Med. 134,* 83-102 (1971).
44. Rauchwerger, J. M., Gallagher, M. T., Trentin, J. J. Role of the hematopoietic inductive microenvironment (HIM) in xenogeneic bone marrow transplantation. *Proc. Soc. Exp. Biol. Med. 143,* 145-154 (1973).
45. Lotzova, E., Gallagher, M. T., Trentin, J. J. Involvement of macrophage in genetic resistance to bone marrow grafts. Studies with two specific antimacrophage agents carrageenan and silica. *Biomedicine 22,* 387-392 (1975).
46. Gallagher, M. T., Lotzova, E., Trentin, J. J. Genetic resistance to marrow transplantation as a leukemia defense mechanism. *Biomedicine 25,* 1-4 (1976).
47. Kaplan, H. S. On the natural history of the murine leukemias. Presidential address. *Cancer Res. 27,* 1325-1332 (1967).
48. Kiessling, R., Hochman, P. S., Haller, O., Shearer, G. M., Wigzell, H., Cudowicz, G. Evidence for a similar or common mechanism for natural killer cell activity and resistance to hemopoietic grafts. *Eur. J. Immunol. 7,* 655-663 (1977).
49. Datta, S. K., Gallagher, M. T., Trentin, J. J. Apparent identity of mechanisms of genetic resistance to marrow transplantation and natural killer cell activity. *Biomedicine 31,* 62 (1979).
50. Holmberg, L. A., Miller, B. A., Ault, K. A. The effect of natural killer cells on the development of syngeneic hematopoietic progenitors. *J. Immunol. 133,* 2933-2937 (1984).
51. Goss, G. D., Wittever, M. A., Bezwoda, W. R., Herman, J., Rabson, A., Seymour, L., Derran, D. P., Mendelow, B. Effect of natural killer cells on syngeneic bone marrow: in vitro and in vivo studies demonstrating graft failure due to NK cells in an identical twin treated by bone marrow transplantation. *Blood 66,* 1043-1046 (1985).
52. O'Reilly, R. J., Collins, N. H., Kernan, N., Brochstein, J., Dinsmore, R., Kirkpatrick, D., Siena, S., Keever, C., Jordan, B., Shank, B., Wolf, L., DuPont, B.,

Reisner, Y. Transplantation of marrow-depleted T cells by soybean lectin agglutination and E-rosette depletion: major histocompatibility complex-related graft resistance in leukemic transplant recipients. *Transplant. Proc. 17,* 455-459 (1985).
53. Koeffler, P. H., Gale, R. P., Golde, D. W. Myeloid colony-forming cell kinetics in man. *Exp. Hematol. 8,* 271-277 (1980).
54. Faille, A., Maraninchi, D., Gluckman, E., Devergie, A., Balitrand, N., Ketels, F., Dresch, C. Granulocyte progenitor compartments after allogeneic bone marrow grafts. *Scand. J. Haematol. 26,* 202-214 (1981).
55. Spitzer, G., Verma, D. S., Fisher, R., Zander, A., Vellekoop, L., Litam, J., McCredie, K. B., Dicke, K. A. The myeloid progenitor cell—its value in predicting hematopoietic recovery after autologous bone marrow transplantation. *Blood 55,* 317-323 (1980).
56. Arnold, R., Schmeiser, T., Heit, W., Frickhofen, N., Pabst, G., Heimpel, H., Kubanek, B. Hemopoietic reconstitution after bone marrow transplantation. *Exp. Hematol. 14,* 271-277 (1986).
57. First, L. R., Smith, B. R., Lipton, J. M., Nathan, D. G., Parkman, R. P., Rappeport, J. M. The prognostic significance of thrombocytopenia following bone marrow transplantation. *Blood 62* (*Suppl.*), 221a (1983).
58. Gale, R. P., Li, S., Fitchen, J. H. Hematopoietic reconstitution following bone marrow transplantation: absent or decreased myeloid progenitor cells. *Exp. Hematol. 10* (*Suppl. 11*), 31 (1982).
59. Atkinson, K., Norrie, S., Chan, P., Biggs, J. Bone marrow cellularity and blood and marrow myeloid and erythroid stem cell colony growth during the first three months after allogeneic marrow transplantation for severe aplastic anemia or acute leukemia. *Exp. Hematol. 10* (*Suppl. 11*), 34 (1982).
60. Arnold, R., Heit, W., Heimpel, H., Frickhofen, N., Schneiser, T., Kubanek, B. The reconstitution of haemopoietic precursors after bone marrow transplantation. *Exp. Hematol. 10* (*Suppl. 10*), 79-82 (1982).
61. Barrett, A. J., Adams, J. A proliferative defect of human bone marrow after transplantation. *Brit. J. Haematol. 49,* 159-164 (1981).
62. Fauser, A. A., Messner, H. A. Proliferative state of human pluripotent hemopoietic progenitors (CFU-GEMM) in normal individuals and under regenerative conditions after bone marrow transplantation. *Blood 54,* 1197-1200 (1979).
63. Li, S., Champlin, R., Fitchen, J. H., Gale, R. P. Abnormalities of myeloid progenitor cells after "successful" bone marrow transplantation. *J. Clin. Invest. 75,* 234-241 (1985).
64. Raghavachar, A., Frickhofen, N., Arnold, R., Schmeiser, T., Porzsolt, F., Heimpel, H. Hematopoietic colony formation after allogeneic bone marrow transplantation: enhancement by cyclosporin A and anti-γ-(immune) interferon antiserum in vitro. *Exp. Hematol. 14,* 621-625 (1986).
65. Emerson, S. G., Sieff, C. A., Gross, R. G., Rozans, M. T., Miller, R. A., Rappeport, J. R., Nathan, D. G. *Exp. Hematol. 15,* 1013-1021 (1987).
66. Nakao, S., Harada, M., Ueda, M., Knodo, K., Odaka, K., Ohtake, S., Matsue, K., Shiobara, S., Mari, T., Matsuda, T. Enhancement of in vitro erythro-

poiesis 13 by peripheral blood mononuclear cells from allogenic marrow recipients. *Scand. J. Haematol. 36,* 180-185 (1986).
67. Mitsuyasu, R. T., Li, S. N., Champlin, R. E., Gale, R. P. Abnormal T-lymphocyte colonies (CFU-TL) following bone marrow transplantation and immunotherapy: use of monoclonal antibodies. *Exp. Haematol. 14,* 1049-1055 (1986).
68. Fahey, J. L., Sarna, G., Gale, R. P., Seeger, R. Immune interventions in disease. *Ann. Int. Med. 106,* 257-274 (1987).
69. Ferrara, J., Lipton, J., Helman, S., Burakoff, S. J., Mauch, P. The role of cell dose in T cell depleted bone marrow transplantation in the mouse. *Transplantation* in press.
70. Butturini, A., Seeger, R. C., Gale, R. P. Recipient immune-competent T lymphocytes can survive intensive conditioning for bone marrow transplantation. *Blood 68,* 954-956 (1986).
71. Fisher, A., Griscelli, C., LeDeist, F., Blanche, S., Verber, F., Lopez, M., Delaage, M., Olive, D., Mawas, C., Janossy, G. Prevention of graft failure by an anti-LFA-1 monoclonal antibody in HLA-mismatched bone-marrow transplantation. *Lancet 2,* 1058-1061 (1986).
72. Cobbold, S. P., Martin, G., Qin, S., Waldmann, H. Monoclonal antibodies to promote marrow engraftment and tissue graft tolerance. *Nature 323,* 164-165 (1986).
73. Mitsuyasu, R. T., Champlin, R. E., Gale, R. P., Ho, W., Lenarsky, C., Winston, D., Selch, W., Elashoff, R., Giorgi, J. V., Wells, J., Terasaki, P., Billing, R., Feig, S. Treatment of donor bone marrow with monoclonal anti-T-cell antibody and complement for the prevention of graft-versus-host disease. *Ann. Intern. Med. 105,* 20-26 (1986).
74. Broxmeyer, H. E. Biomolecule-cell interactions and the regulation of myelopoiesis. *Int. J. Cell Cloning 4,* 378-405 (1986).
75. Clayberger, C., Koller, C., Carroll, W., Link, M., Smith, S., Levy, R., Krensky, A. Submitted. 1987.

16

The Origin of Bone Marrow Stroma After Transplantation

Implications for Graft Failure

DONNA PRZEPIORKA* and BEVERLY TOROK-STORB
Fred Hutchinson Cancer Research Center and University of Washington, Seattle, Washington

PAUL J. SIMMONS
Fred Hutchinson Cancer Research Center, Seattle, Washington

I. INTRODUCTION

The observation that hemopoiesis in vivo is limited to specific organs despite the fact that pluripotent stem cells can be found in the circulation has led to the theory that effective hemopoiesis in vivo requires both pluripotent stem cells and a localized, supportive milieu termed the microenvironment. Experimental evidence suggests that the ME has at least two functions in vivo: to direct homing of circulating hemopoietic stem cells (1) and to regulate proliferation and differentiation of the stem cells (2). Efforts to define functional components of the hemopoietic microenvironment have been greatly facilitated by the development of an in vitro culture system by Dexter and co-workers (3). In this long-term bone marrow culture (LTBMC) system, the presence of marrow-derived adherent cells and unobstructed contact with the stem cells were shown to be required for maintenance of hemopoiesis (4). Further studies indicated that the adherent cell layer has an affinity for stem cells (5) and produces factors that stimulate (6,7) or inhibit (8,9) the proliferation and differentiation of committed progenitors. These properties parallel the functions of the microenvironment in vivo and thus suggest that the adherent cell layer in LTBMCs is an appropriate in vitro model of the microenvironment. The validity of this assumption is supported by the success of therapeutic maneuvers directed by results of in vitro manipulations of LTBMCs from patients with failed hemopoiesis (10).

**Present affiliation*: University of Pittsburgh and Montefiore Hospital, Pittsburgh, Pennsylvania.

On the basis of morphologic, cytochemical, biochemical, and immunologic data, it has been shown that the adherent cell layer of LTBMCs from humans (11) and mice (12,13) consists of macrophages and a nonhematological population termed stromal cells comprised of fibroblastoid cells, adipocytes, and endothelial cells. Current evidence suggests that the adipocytes (5) or the endothelial cells (14) are involved in adhesion of the stem cells, while both the macrophages (15) and the stromal cells (16) have been implicated as sources of hemopoietic regulatory factors. The control of factor production by cells of the various types in the adherent cell layer and the interactions between them are currently subjects of intense investigation. The tremendous heterogeneity of the adherent cell layer is clearly a problem, but the study of single cell types using in situ hybridization, cloned cell lines, flow microfluorimetry, and other physical separation techniques should make it possible to dissect this system in the near future.

II. ORIGIN OF STROMAL CELLS AFTER TRANSPLANTATION

A. Murine System

While there is ample evidence that transfused pluripotent stem cells can home to and repopulate hemopoietic organs, studies of the transplantability of stromal cells with similar homing and repopulating properties have produced inconsistent conclusions (11,17-25). Several investigators have studied LTBMCs established from marrow transplant recipients to determine whether stromal cells are donor in origin. However, the inevitable presence of donor-derived macrophages in the adherent cell layer of LTBMCs presents a considerable problem. Thus, only methods whereby both the cell type and host or donor origin could be ascertained simultaneously would be considered valid. To this end, Marshall et al. (22) fractionated adherent cells of LTBMCs from radiochimeric mice by magnetic separation of carbonyliron-ingesting macrophages and then analyzed each fraction for the host or donor allotype of the enzyme glucose phosphate isomerase. Although they found that 70% of the enzyme was donor type in the nonphagocytic fraction and concluded that stromal cells were transplantable, they also admitted that they were unable to completely deplete this fraction of macrophages. In addition, the macrophage had a higher level of enzyme per cell, so their calculated percentage of donor type could be grossly overestimated. Furthermore, these investigators were unable to recover donor stromal cells from spleen or marrow when cultured stromal cells were transplanted into a lethally irradiated mouse.

Piersma et al. (21) utilized cytogenetic analysis of fibroblast colony-forming units (CFU-F) from radiochimeric mice transplanted from a donor with a cytogenetic marker and found that 44-63% of the CFU-F were donor in origin 1-94 days after injection of a large inoculum of cells. However, Maloney et al. (23) pointed out that the total CFU-F recovered by Piersma et al. was only 10% of normal, so that even if donor stromal cells were present, they did not appear to effect significant repopulation. This was supported in part by a subsequent study by Piersma et al. (24) wherein they suggested that a disproportionate number of donor CFU-F were recovered in vitro because host CFU-F had lost the capacity to proliferate in vitro as a result of radiation.

More recently, Lennon and Micklem (25) used the alloenzyme technique to analyze specific subpopulations of the adherent layer of LTBMCs from mice 12 months after transplantation. The adherent cells were sorted into four subpopulations on the basis of autofluorescence and phagocytosis. One population was clearly granulocytic. A second was donor in origin, expressed the T200 antigen, was enriched for CFU-S and GM-CFC, and morphologically consisted of blast cells. The third population was easily characterized as donor macrophages. The last population appeared to be fibroblastoid, contained alkaline phosphatase, was host in origin, and remained host in origin during 5 months of a continuous culture. Thus, the preponderance of published data suggest that in the murine system transfused stromal cells do not repopulate the transplant recipient.

B. Human System

It was widely believed that stromal cells were not transplantable in humans either (18) until Keating et al. (20) published their observation that host stromal cells in LTBMCs from transplant recipients decreased in proportion with time after transplantation. In this study, the host-donor pairs were sex-mismatched, and the genotype of the stromal cells was determined by quinacrine staining for Y bodies. The utility of this technique is limited by the lack of specificity and sensitivity. The specific identification of the Y body in an interphase cell by quinacrine staining relies on the presence of a Y chromosome with an adequate length of heterochromatin in the long arm and the absence of extensive heterochromatic material in the satellites of the autosomes (26). Clearly, this ideal is not always met. In fact, Keating et al. (20) reported a sensitivity of only 66%, and their specificity of 99% was based on only three negative controls. Furthermore, it was not clear that macrophages and stromal cells could still be distinguished morphologically once they had undergone preparation for quinacrine staining. The conclusion of these investigators that stromal cells are transplantable in humans is thus called into question by the limited reliability of the methodology employed.

In a recent study, we have overcome the problems of genotype identification by using in situ hybridization with a DNA probe specific for a repetitive sequence in the Y chromosome (27). After extensive testing, we have found that this procedure has essentially 100% sensitivity and specificity and does not interfere with morphological identification of the cells. Using this approach, we have studied the adherent cells from LTBMCs established 28-1073 days after transplantation from 14 patients who received HLA-matched transplants and 8 patients who received HLA-mismatched transplants. Two populations of cells were clearly identified morphologically in Wright-stained preparations of adherent cells from these cultures (Fig. 1). One consisted of macrophages that each had a small, round,

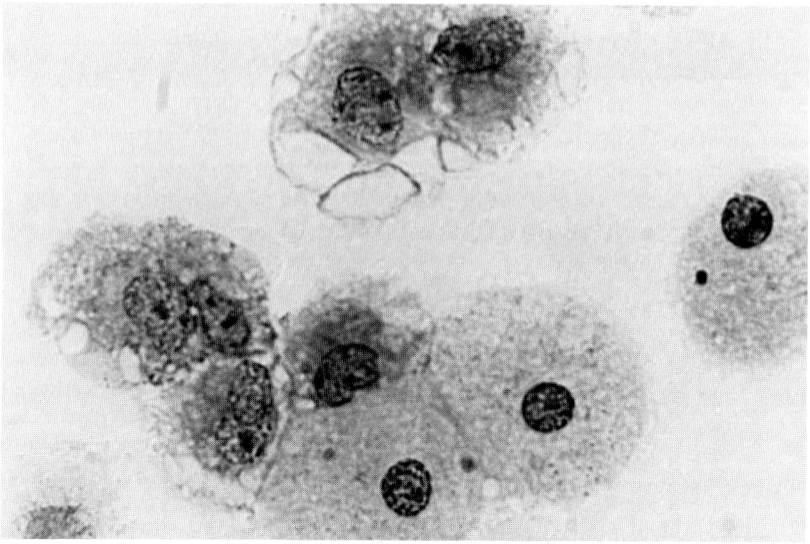

Figure 1 Wright-stained cytospin preparation of adherent cells from LTBMC.

homogeneous nucleus, abundant light blue cytoplasm, and a low nuclear/cytoplasmic (N/C) ratio. The other consisted of stromal cells, each with an oval or irregularly shaped nucleus having a coarse chromatin pattern and two or more nucleoli, granular dark blue cytoplasm (with obvious vesicles in the adipocytes), and a higher N/C ratio. A distinction between the two populations was confirmed by staining for nonspecific esterases (Fig. 2). The proportion of macrophages in the trypsinized preparations from different cultures varied from 0 to 100% and depended to a large extent on the length of exposure to trypsin. Detachment of stromal cells required longer trypsinization. Since the characteristic morphology of the cells was preserved through the hybridization procedure, the identification of cell type by morphology and genotype by in situ hybridization could easily be determined simultaneously (Fig. 3). In all 22 cases studied, the stromal cells were exclusively of host genotype. Our findings have recently been confirmed by Laver et al., who established the source of the stromal cells by HLA typing the adherent cells from LTBMC of patients who had received HLA-mismatched transplants (R. O'Reilly, personal communication). Thus, it appears that stromal cells infused intravenously do not effectively home to and repopulate the marrow in humans using the standard conditioning regimens for allogeneic marrow transplantation.

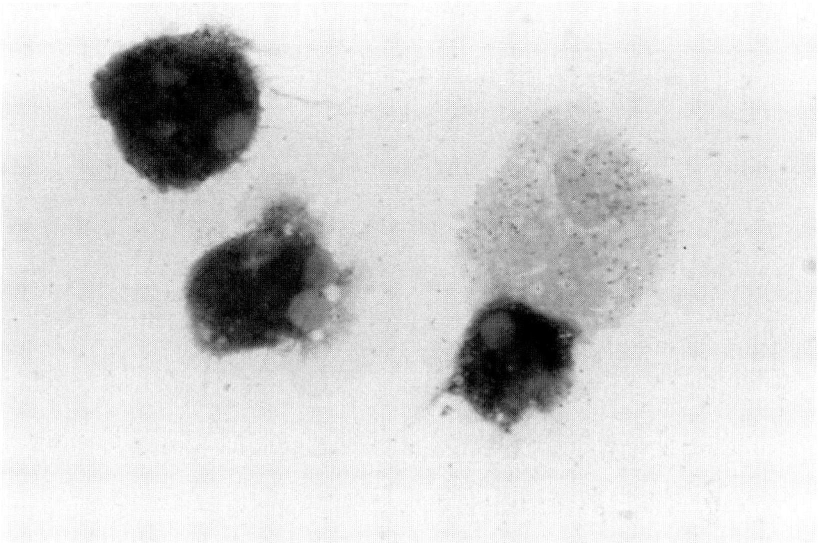

Figure 2 Adherent cells from LTBMC stained for nonspecific esterase.

III. IMPLICATIONS FOR GRAFT FAILURE

Failure to engraft or loss of a graft occurs in <5-38% of patients after bone marrow transplantation (28-32). While the majority of these cases are due to relapse or host-derived immune-mediated mechanisms, as evidenced by the detection of host cells in the blood or marrow, we have encountered several patients with pancytopenia after bone marrow transplantation whose peripheral blood mononuclear cells did not display antidonor activity and in whom persisting host cells were not detected (33). Since it is unlikely that damage to the hemopoietic stem cells occurred during marrow harvest or infusion, dysfunction of the microenvironment arises as an alternative explanation for graft failure in these patients. As we have shown above, stromal cells infused with the marrow do not repopulate the microenvironment and probably do not contribute significantly to hemopoiesis after bone marrow transplantation. The residual host stromal cells bear the responsibility for support of hemopoiesis. Thus, primary or acquired damage of the host microenvironment could play a significant role in graft failure, and there are several ways by which this might happen.

A. Primary Dysfunction of the Microenvironment

While dysfunction of the microenvironment has long been hypothesized as one of several etiologies of aplastic anemia in humans, support for this idea relied

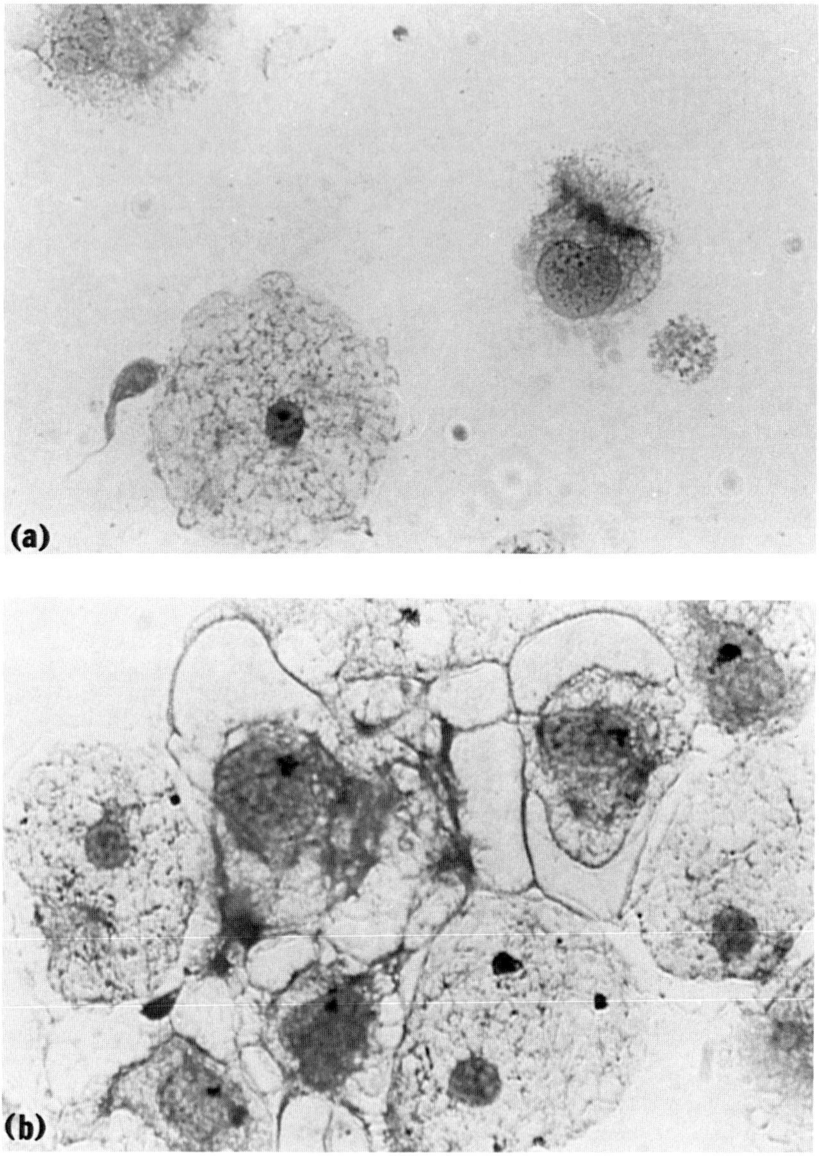

Figure 3 Adherent cells from long-term cultures of marrow from a female recipient of male marrow (*a*) and a male recipient of female marrow (*b*) hybridized in situ for the Y chromosome. Note the black intranuclear dot in the macrophage in (*a*) and in the stromal cells in (*b*).

solely on indirect evidence; that is, there were patients with aplastic anemia whose marrow grew normally in soft agar assays for progenitors of granulocytes and macrophages (GM-CFC) despite obvious marrow hypoplasia (10,34). Direct evidence was first reported by Ershler et al. (35), who found that bone fragments from a patient with congenital anemia did not support erythropoiesis in liquid culture despite the fact that progenitors of erythroid cells (CFU-E and BFU-E) from the marrow aspirates were normal. With the introduction of the methodology for LTBMCs, the function of the adherent cells could be assessed directly. Using this technique, Hotta et al. (36) reported three patients with aplastic anemia whose adherent cells did not support the growth of marrow progenitors. This obviously raises the question of whether sustained marrow engraftment could be achieved in patients with aplastic anemia due to primary microenvironment dysfunction.

Gordon and Gordon-Smith (37) found that normal marrow fibroblasts secrete a factor that enhances the activity of granulocyte-macrophage colony-stimulating factor (GM-CSF), but marrow fibroblasts from 3 of 6 patients with aplastic anemia produced subnormal levels of the enhancing activity. One of these patients successfully underwent allogeneic bone marrow transplantation, and the CSF-enhancing activity of the marrow fibroblasts posttransplant was normal. This was interpreted to suggest that the initial dysfunction was overproduction of an inhibitor rather than impaired production of a stimulating factor. Although these patient data could also be interpreted to suggest that some initial signal normally produced by macrophages and required for inducing stromal cell factor production was missing and subsequently provided by donor macrophages posttransplant (16), production of an inhibitor of hemopoiesis by adherent cells from long-term cultures of normal marrow has been reported (10,38). Overproduction of an inhibitor of hemopoiesis has recently been postulated as an underlying defect in the Sl/Sl^d murine model of congenital anemia (9,39). Production of the putative inhibitor in vitro by normal murine and Sl/Sl^d stromal cells was reduced by radiation (8,39). The delineation of cellular mechanisms responsible for comparable inhibitors in LTBMC established from patients with aplastic anemia, and the characterization of their sensitivity to radiation and drugs, would clearly aid in designing appropriate pretransplant conditioning regimens for patients with aplastic anemia who exhibit this type of dysfunction.

A more serious problem is presented by patients with aplastic anemia whose stromal cells fail to produce the appropriate stimulatory factors. Castro-Malaspina et al. (40) reported just such a case and have devised a novel approach to therapy. Their patient with aplastic anemia failed to engraft after two allogeneic transplants, and neither antidonor cytotoxicity nor suppressors of hemopoiesis were detected. Since functional stromal cells could not be transplanted efficiently via the intravenous route, cultured adherent marrow cells and T-cell-depleted hemopoietic cells from the same donor were injected directly into the patient's marrow cavity. The patient died from a viral infection 10 days after transplantation, but engraftment was documented histologically, and stromal cells grown from the marrow were identified as donor in origin by HLA typing.

B. Effect of Acute Leukemia

While the occurrence of cytopenias in the patient with acute leukemia whose marrow is packed with blast cells is generally attributed to the lack of space for normal hemopoiesis, this cannot explain the pancytopenia seen in patients with "oligoleukemia" and hypocellular marrow. Whether or not active leukemia adversely affects the microenvironment was addressed to some extent by Nagao et al. (41), who evaluated the cloning efficiency of CFU-F in patients with acute leukemia. These investigators observed that there was a significant decrease in CFU-F in all 6 of 6 patients studied. An increase in the CFU-F was observed when the leukemic cells were removed from the culture (41) and when the patient achieved a remission (42). Furthermore, CFU-F of normal marrow was decreased on coculture with leukemic marrow or medium conditioned by leukemic marrow. While these data suggest that leukemic cells can inhibit the proliferation of marrow fibroblasts in vitro, the effect of leukemic cells on stromal cell production of hemopoietic regulatory factors under conditions permissive for hemopoiesis has not been studied. Clinically it has been noted that in comparison to patients transplanted in remission, patients with active leukemia have a higher rate of delayed engraftment or graft failure after bone marrow transplantation, and this effect is independent of HLA matching (C. Anasetti, manuscript in preparation). This is unlikely to be due to a direct effect of the leukemic cells on the graft, since there should be relatively few viable tumor cells extant at the time of marrow infusion. Delayed engraftment may instead be a manifestation of the lag time required for repair or expansion of the stromal cell compartment after release from the inhibitory effects of leukemia.

Some degree of marrow fibrosis is frequently seen with acute leukemia or chronic myeloproliferative disorders. Although one might expect that such fibrosis could physically obstruct the functional microenvironment and thus impede cell-cell interactions necessary for effective hemopoiesis, reports of successful engraftment after bone marrow transplantation in patients with myelofibrosis have suggested otherwise (43,44). More recently, Rajantie et al. (45) found that there was a significant delay in engraftment and higher risk of graft failure in patients with severe fibrosis. They also observed that while regression of fibrosis was detected histologically in the majority of patients, it reappeared in some patients at the time of graft rejection and leukemic relapse. Thus, they were not able to distinguish between impairment of graft function due to the presence of fibrosis and that due to an effect of the underlying malignancy. The resolution of the controversy will be determined by the outcome of marrow transplantation in patients with myelofibrosis due to a benign process such as thorium dioxide exposure (46).

C. Effect of Treatment

It has long been observed that patients who received sublethal doses of radiation may experience prolonged periods of cytopenias, and this was attributed to radiation-induced stem cell damage. Marrow scans of such patients, however, revealed an absence of hemopoiesis specifically in the irradiated field, and recovery of hemopoiesis as well as resolution of the cytopenias was delayed for as much as a year, much longer than one might expect for circulating stem cells to repopulate the area (47-49). The extent of recovery varied with the radiation dose, and minimal or no hemopoiesis was seen in localized areas for many years after exposure to more than 20-30 Gy (48,49). While it was widely believed that the microenvironment was resistant to radiation, these observations suggested otherwise. Using murine models, Chamberlin et al. (50) and Friedenstein et al. (51) demonstrated that the microenvironment recovered in parallel with or slightly more slowly than the stem cell compartment and concluded that the prolonged lack of hemopoiesis was due in part to radiation-induced damage to the microenvironment.

In contrast to the irreversible effect of radiation on hemopoietic tissue, the survival curves for marrow fibroblasts reproducibly exhibit a shoulder (52), so some degree of repair of radiation-induced damage is expected. In animal models and in vitro systems, the extent and duration of the effect of radiation on the cloning efficiency or proliferative capacity of marrow fibroblasts varied with the total dose (53-55), dose rate (55-57), type of beam (photon versus neutron) (58), and use of a fractionated schedule (58). Greenberger et al. (55) have also reported that radiation of adherent cells in vitro impaired CSF production and support of hemopoiesis in LTBMCs without a cytotoxic effect, but this was seen only at a very high dose rate (2 Gy/min). The dosimetry of contemporary total body irradiation regimens is governed largely by extramedullary toxicity (especially lung and gastrointestinal tract), so graft failure due to radiation alone is clinically not a significant problem for most patients. However, in the absence of controlled radiation exposure, for example, in a nuclear accident, there is a possibility of irreversible damage to the microenvironment.

As discussed above, patients with lymphoma who received curative doses of radiation can suffer permanent impairment of hemopoiesis in the irradiated fields (49). If the field encompasses a significant volume of the marrow cavity, there is reason to expect that the additional toxicity incurred by conventional total body irradiation might delay engraftment. However, delayed engraftment has not been found in transplant recipients whose prior therapy for lymphoma included radiation with or without chemotherapy (59). The use of radiolabeled bone-seeking agents or radiolabeled antibodies to effect myeloablation without extramedullary toxicity is now being investigated. Clearly, this approach has the potential for selective extensive damage to the microenvironment. Meticulous dosimetry will be required to avoid graft failure with this type of therapy.

In contrast to radiation, conventional doses of cyclophosphamide (CY) are generally associated with only a brief period of myelosuppression. In vitro studies using 4-HP, an active form of CY, revealed that human marrow stromal progenitors were relatively resistant to this alkylating agent. Adherent cells proliferated well in LTBMCs after treatment of the marrow with up to 300 μmol/liter of 4-HP (60), which is well above levels of active metabolites achieved clinically (61), and, once established, there was no effect observed on support of hemopoiesis (60). In a murine model (62), single or multiple doses of CY at 400-500 mg/kg did impair the microenvironment for as long as 6 weeks as determined by femur implant studies, but the effect was apparently subclinical, since numbers of CFU-S were normal by 6 weeks after treatment. The effect of CY on CFU-F appeared to be synergistic with that of radiation, but again a very high dose was tested (63). Without marrow transplantation, single or multiple doses of cyclophosphamide at 120-170 mg/kg administered to humans have had little overt effect on recovery of hemopoiesis (64), and when used at 120 mg/kg in conjunction with total body irradiation for myeloablation, there has been no significant adverse effect on engraftment after allogeneic bone marrow transplantation (28). In vitro, stromal cells also appear to be relatively resistant to VP-16 as assessed by CFU-F and ability to support hemopoiesis in LTBMC (65), and there have been no reports of impaired engraftment following its use in conditioning regimens for bone marrow transplantation (66).

Like radiation, drugs such as busulfan, nitrogen mustard, and the nitrosoureas are associated with delayed recovery of hemopoiesis, and these drugs are known to have adverse effects on stromal cells (67,68). Busulfan is the best studied of these drugs. Mice treated with 70 mg/kg busulfan over 4 weeks still had subnormal numbers of CFU-F at 40 weeks (69), and marrow adherent cells were still deficient in their ability to support hemopoiesis in LTBMC when taken from mice more than 1 year after treatment with 20 mg/kg over 8 weeks (70). In clinical studies, Nagao et al. (41) demonstrated a significant decrease in marrow CFU-F in chronic myeloid leukemia (CML) patients after treatment with busulfan, and this chronic effect of busulfan raises a concern about engraftment for patients with CML treated with this drug. Thomas et al. (71) did report that, in comparison to those not treated, CML patients who had been treated with busulfan had a higher mortality after marrow transplantation, but engraftment in these patients was not discussed. Pretransplant conditioning regimens combining busulfan (8-16 mg/kg) with CY have no clinically significant effect on engraftment when used either initially (72) or for preparation for a second transplant (J. Sanders, submitted for publication). In contrast, 2 of 11 patients failed to engraft after autologous transplantation when conditioned with total body irradiation and dimethylbusulfan, a potent congener of busulfan (73).

D. Effect of Viral Infection

Pancytopenia may occur with several types of viral infections, but it is an uncommon sequela in healthy individuals (74). The pathogenesis of pancytopenia in these cases has not been fully elucidated, but infection of hemopoietic progenitors, development of suppressor cells or cytotoxic antibodies, and production of interferon have been implicated. Transplant recipients have a risk of developing hepatitis B (HBV) infections through multiple blood product exposure during conventional therapy and after transplantation, and this virus is known to infect hemopoietic cells (75,76). HBV infection of stromal cells has not been documented, but even if it did occur it does not appear to have a permanent adverse effect on the microenvironment, since patients with HBV-induced aplasia have undergone successful transplantation (77).

Cytomegalovirus (CMV) infections in transplant recipients have been observed in association with leukopenia and thrombocytopenia (78,79), but the frequency with which they cause graft failure is unknown. In studies of lymphocyte subpopulations in transplant patients, an inverted CD4/CD8 ratio is common in the first year after transplantation, but persistently high levels of CD8 + Leu-7 + lymphocytes were found in patients with CMV infections (80-82). We have recently reported that this phenotype predominates in patients with graft failure whether or not there is antidonor cytotoxic activity associated with the episode of graft failure (33). In seven patients with graft failure and no evidence of relapse, the mean CD4/CD8 ratio was 0.29, and 55% of the lymphocytes were Leu-7+. Five of the seven were culture-positive for CMV. One patient who had persistent viremia and esophageal infection developed graft failure late. When studied at 1 year after bone marrow transplantation, there was no evidence of relapse by cytogenetics or in situ hybridization, and lymphocyte surface marker analysis revealed a CD4/CD8 ratio of 0.14 with 58% positive for Leu-7. A second infusion of marrow at this time was ineffective. Stromal cells from this patient grew well in LTBMC, but they had abnormally large nucleoli (Fig. 4). We have not observed this morphology in adherent cells from 15 patients with normal graft function, but we have seen it in 2 of 6 patients with graft failure. While reminiscent of viral inclusions, it is possible that they are only reactive nucleoli, which are known to occur in highly active cells responding to injury.

CMV has been isolated from human lymphohemopoietic cells (83) but not from marrow stromal cells. It does not appear to be a problem of permissiveness, since Bowden et al. (84; personal communication) have successfully infected cultured marrow fibroblasts with CMV, albeit not under conditions that would support hemopoiesis. In a simian system, Kramvis et al. (85) found that stromal cells

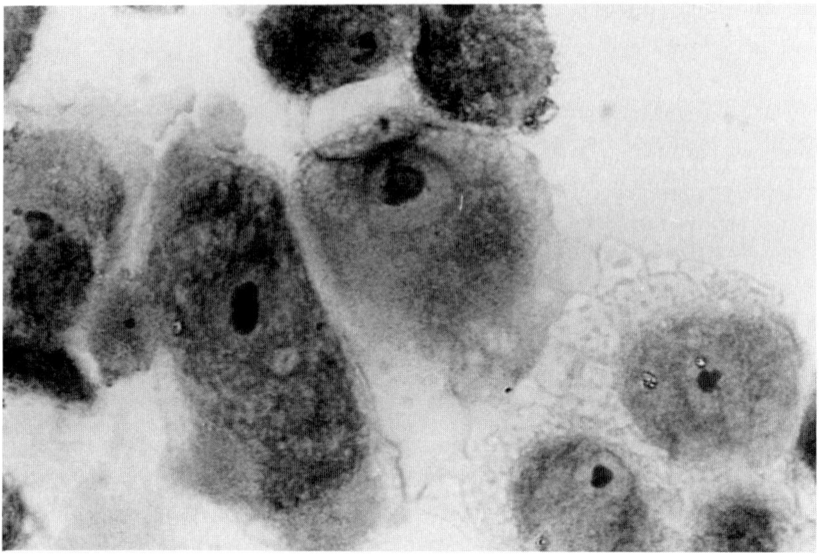

Figure 4 Adherent cells from LTBMC established from a patient with graft failure and invasive CMV infection.

did support production of low titers of simian CMV, and, interestingly, infection was associated with an increase in GM-CSF production in LTBMC. Further study will be needed to determine the role of CMV infections in graft failure after bone marrow transplantation and whether or not stromal cell dysfunction contributes to the pathogenesis.

E. Effect of Graft-Versus-Host Disease (GVHD)

Marrow hypoplasia is cited as one consequence of GVHD in murine systems, and impairment of the host microenvironment has been implicated (86). In the murine model, external signs of GVHD vary in terms of time of onset, organ system involvement and severity, and in one study these variables were associated with a specific effector cell (T cell versus non-T cell) and target antigen (major versus minor histocompatibility antigen) (87). In GVHD-related graft failure, the effector cell(s) mediating the reaction and the target antigen(s) are unknown. While it is easy to imagine that graft failure could occur on the basis of alloreactive damage to the microenvironment in HLA-mismatched transplant recipients, graft rejection due to host antidonor activity is cited more frequently. On the other hand, Sullivan et al. (88) reported problems with engraftment in 4 of 16 patients with hyperacute GVHD who had received HLA-matched transplants without prophylactic immunosuppression. In order to evaluate the question of immunologic

Table 1 In Vitro Antistromal Cell Cytotoxicity

Effector cells	Stimulation	% Specific lysis[a]
Fresh normal PBMC[b]	None	0
Cultured normal PBMC	IL-2 and PHA	27
Cultured normal PBMC	B cell line matched with target for 1 class I antigen	58
Cultured normal PBMC	B cell line matched with target for 3 class I antigens	71

[a]Four-hour ^{51}Cr-release assay at an effector/target ratio of 10:1 using as targets adherent cells from a long-term culture of marrow from a patient 28 days after bone marrow transplantation.
[b]Normal peripheral blood mononuclear cells.

damage to the microenvironment, a modified ^{51}Cr-release assay (33) was used to test for cell-mediated stromal cell cytotoxicity. As shown in Table 1, adherent cells from LTBMC could be lysed by either alloantigen-activated or lymphokine-activated mononuclear cells. Lysis by uncultured mononuclear cells, as might be mediated by natural killer cells, was not seen in this experiment, but the effector/target ratio (10:1) may not have been sufficient to detect this activity. Thus, stromal cells are susceptible to cell-mediated lysis, and more than one type of cytotoxic cell may be capable of effecting the lytic function. Further work in progress will determine if anti-host stromal cell activity can be detected in patients with graft failure and hyperacute GVHD.

IV. CONCLUSION

We have reviewed the experimental evidence for damage to the microenvironment that might compromise host microenvironmental function and result in graft failure after marrow transplantation. The mechanisms discussed could explain both primary and delayed graft failure. It is clear from in vitro studies of patients with normal engraftment that there is in fact measurable compromise of the host microenvironment early after bone marrow transplantation (89), but the effect was apparently reversible and subclinical, since normal engraftment ensued. The extent of microenvironmental damage in patients with graft failure is not well studied. For patients who have incurred moderate insults to the microenvironment, its tremendous functional reserve and repair capability should restore adequate capacity to support hemopoiesis with time. This would explain the success of second marrow infusions without reconditioning in patients with poor graft function (90). Unfortunately, since we are unable to transplant a functional microenvironment using standard techniques, treatment options for patients with irreversible damage to the microenvironment are limited. Recombinant growth factors capable of stimulating committed progenitor cells are available, but the signals that control pluripotent stem cell replication and commitment have not been identified. It is unlikely, therefore, that exogenously administered growth factors alone can replace a malfunctioning host microenvironment. Furthermore, the long-term efficacy of intramedullary transplantation of cultured stromal cells has not been determined. Thus, maintenance of a viable host microenvironment remains imperative.

ACKNOWLEDGMENTS

We are grateful to Lori Ausburn for preparation of the manuscript, to Gretchen Johnson and Lisa Sandell for technical assistance, to Dr. Claudio Anasetti and Dr. Jean Sanders for helpful discussion, and to Dr. Rainer Storb for careful review of the manuscript. The Y chromosomal probe was a gift from Dr. C. Y-F. Lau. This work was supported in part by grants CA 09515, CA 18029, CA 18221, HL 36444, and DK 34431 awarded by the National Institutes of Health.

REFERENCES

1. Till, J. E., McCulloch, G. A. A direct measurement of the radiation sensitivity of normal mouse bone marrow cells. *Radiat. Res. 14,* 213-222 (1961).
2. McCulloch, E. A., Siminovitch, L., Till, J. E., Russel, E. S., Bernstein, S. E. The cellular basis of the genetically determined hemopoietic defect in anemic mice of genotype Sl/Sl^d. *Blood 26,* 399-410 (1965).
3. Dexter, T. M., Lajtha, L. G. Proliferation of haemopoietic stem cells in vitro. *Brit. J. Haematol. 28,* 525-530 (1974).
4. Bentley, S. A. Close range cell:cell interaction required for stem cell maintenance in continuous bone marrow culture. *Exp. Hematol. 9,* 308-312 (1981).
5. Gordon, M. Y., Hibbin, J. A., Dowding, C., Gordon-Smith, E. C., Goldman, J. M. Separation of human blast progenitors from granulocytic, erythroid, megakaryocytic, and mixed colony-forming cells by "panning" on cultured marrow-derived stromal layers. *Exp. Hematol. 13,* 937-940 (1985).
6. Heard, J.-M., Fichelson, S., Varet, B. Role of colony-stimulating activity in murine long-term bone marrow cultures: evidence for its production and consumption by the adherent cells. *Blood 59,* 761-767 (1982).
7. Shadduck, R. K., Waheed, A., Greenberger, J. S., Dexter, T. M. Production of colony stimulating factor in long-term bone marrow cultures. *J. Cell. Physiol. 114,* 88-92 (1983).
8. Guraltieri, R. J., Shadduck, R. K., Baker, D. G., Quesenberry, P. J. Hematopoietic regulatory factors produced in long-term murine bone marrow cultures and the effect of in vitro irradiation. *Blood 64,* 516-525 (1984).
9. Wright, E. G., Lorimore, S. A., Lord, B. I. Regulators of stem cell proliferation in the haemopoietic tissues of W/W^v and Sl/Sl^d mice. *Leuk. Res. 9,* 491-496 (1985).

10. Abdou, N. I., Verdirame, J. D., Amare, M., Abdou, N. L. Heterogeneity of pathogenetic mechanisms in aplastic anemia. Efficacy of therapy based on in-vitro results. *Ann. Intern. Med. 95,* 43-50 (1981).
11. Simmons, P., Przepiorka, D., Thomas, E. D., Torok-Storb, B. Host origin of marrow stromal cells following allogeneic bone marrow transplantation. *Nature 328,* 429-432 (1987).
12. Allen, T. D. Haemopoietic microenvironments in vitro: ultrastructural aspects. In: *Microenvironments in haemopoietic and lymphoid differentiation* (CIBA Foundation Symposium 84). Porter, R., Whelan, J. (Eds.). Pittman Medical, London (1981).
13. Tavassoli, M., Takahashi, K. Morphological studies on long-term culture of marrow cells: characterization of the adherent stromal cells and their interactions in maintaining the proliferation of hemopoietic stem cells. *Amer. J. Anat. 164,* 91-111 (1982).
14. Chertkov, J. L. Early hemopoietic and stromal precursor cells. *Int. Rev. Cytol. 102,* 271-313 (1986).
15. Oblon, D. J., Castro-Malaspina, H., Broxmeyer, H. E. The production of colony stimulating activity of monocyte enriched fractions from murine continuous bone marrow culture adherent layers. *Brit. J. Haematol. 54,* 291-299 (1983).
16. Broudy, V. C., Zuckerman, K. S., Jetmalani, S., Fitchen, J. H., Bagby, G. C. Monocytes stimulate fibroblastoid bone marrow stromal cells to produce multilineage hematopoietic growth factors. *Blood 68,* 530-534 (1986).
17. Friedenstein, A. J., Ivanov-Smolenski, A. A., Chajlakjan, R. K., Gorskaya, U. F., Kuralesova, A. I., Lutzinik, V. N., Gerasimov, U. W. Origin of bone marrow stromal mechanocytes in radiocheimeras and heterotypic transplants. *Exp. Hematol. 16,* 440-444 (1978).
18. Golde, D. W., Hocking, W. G., Quan, S. G., Sparkes, R. S., Gale, R. P. Origin of human bone marrow fibroblasts. *Brit. J. Haematol. 44,* 183-187 (1980).
19. Bentley, S. A. Bone marrow connective tissue and the haemopoietic microenvironment. *Brit. J. Haematol. 50,* 1-6 (1982).
20. Keating, A., Singer, J. W., Killen, P. D., Striker, G. E., Salo, A. C., Sanders, J., Thomas, E. D., Thorning, O., Fialkow, P. J. Donor origin of the in vitro haematopoietic microenvironment after marrow transplantation in man. *Nature 298,* 280-283 (1982).
21. Piersma, A. H., Ploemacher, R. E., Brockbank, K. G. M. Transplantation of bone marrow fibroblastoid stromal cells in mice via the intravenous route. *Brit. J. Haematol. 54,* 285-290 (1983).
22. Marshall, M. J., Nisbet, N. W., Evans, S. Donor origin of the in vitro hematopoietic microenvironment after marrow transplantation in mice. *Experientia 40,* 385-386 (1984).
23. Maloney, M. A., Lamela, R. A., Patt, H. M. The question of bone marrow stromal fibroblast traffic. *Ann. N.Y. Acad. Sci. 459,* 190-197 (1985).
24. Piersma, A. H., Brockbank, K. G. M., Ploemacher, R. E., Ottenheim, C. P. E. Recovery of hemopoietic stromal progenitor cells after lethal total-body irradiation and bone marrow transplantation in mice. *Transplantation 40,* 198-201 (1985).

25. Lennon, J. E., Micklem, H. S. Stromal cells in long-term murine bone marrow culture: FACS studies and origin of stromal cells in radiation chimeras. *Exp. Hematol. 14,* 287-292 (1986).
26. Uchida, I. A., Lin, C. C. Quinacrine fluorescence patterns. In: *Human chromosome methodology,* 2nd ed. Yunis, J. J. (Ed.). Academic Press, New York, pp. 47-58 (1974).
27. Lau, Y.-F., Huang, J. C., Dozy, A. M., Kam, Y. W. A rapid screening test for antenatal sex determination. *Lancet 1,* 14-16 (1984).
28. Thomas, E. D., Storb, R., Clift, R. A., Fefer, A., Johnson, F. L. Neiman, P. E., Lerner, K. G., Glucksberg, H., Buckner, C. D. Bone-marrow transplantation. *New Engl. J. Med. 292,* 832-843 (1975).
29. Storb, R., Prentice, R. L., Thomas, E. D., Appelbaum, F. R., Deeg, H. J., Doney, K., Fefer, A., Goodell, B. W., Mickelson, E., Stewart, P., Sullivan, K. M., Witherspoon, R. P. Factors associated with graft rejection after HLA-identical marrow transplantation for aplastic anemia. *Brit. J. Haematol. 55,* 573-585 (1983).
30. Beatty, P. G., Clift, R. A., Mickelson, E. M., Nisperos, B. B., Flournoy, N., Martin, P. J., Sanders, J. E., Stewart, P., Buckner, C. D., Storb, R., Thomas, E. D., Hansen, J. A. Marrow transplantation from related donors other than HLA-identical siblings. *New Engl. J. Med. 313,* 765-771 (1985).
31. Hows, J. M., Yin, J. L., Marsh, J., Swirsky, D., Jones, L., Apperley, J. F., James, D. C. O., Smithers, S., Batchelor, J. R., Goldman, J. M., Gordon-Smith, E. D. Histocompatible unrelated volunteer donors compared with HLA nonidentical family donors in marrow transplantation for aplastic anemia and leukemia. *Blood 68,* 1322-1328 (1986).
32. Martin, P. J., Hansen, J. A., Torok-Storb, B., Durnam, D., O'Quigley, J., Sanders, J., Sullivan, K. M., Witherspoon, R. P., Deeg, H. J., Appelbaum, F. R., Stewart, P., Weiden, P., Doney, K., Buckner, C. D., Clift, R., Storb, R., Thomas, E. D. Graft failure in patients receiving T cell-depleted HLA-identical allogeneic marrow transplants (submitted for publication).
33. Sandell, L., Johnson, G., Przepiorka, D., Torok-Storb, B. Phenotype and function of T cells associated with marrow graft failure and rejection. In: *T cell depletion in allogeneic bone marrow transplantation.* Martelli, M. F., Reisner, Y. (Eds.). Raven Press, New York, in press.
34. Kagan, W. A., Ascensao, J. L., Fialk, M. A., Coleman, M., Valera, E. B., Good, R. A. Studies on the pathogenesis of aplastic anemia. *Amer. J. Med. 66,* 444-449 (1979).
35. Ershler, W. B., Ross, J., Finlay, J. L., Shahidi, N. T. Bone-marrow microenvironment defect in congenital hypoplastic anemia. *New Engl. J. Med. 302,* 1321-1327 (1980).
36. Hotta, T., Kato, T., Maeda, H., Yamao, H., Yamada, H., Saito, H. Functional changes in marrow stromal cells in aplastic anemia. *Acta Haematol. 74,* 65-69 (1985).
37. Gordon, M. Y., Gordon-Smith, E. C. Bone marrow fibroblast function in relation to granulopoiesis in aplastic anaemia. *Brit. J. Haematol. 53,* 483-489 (1983).

38. Zipori, D., Reichman, N., Arcavi, L., Shtalrid, M., Berrebi, A., Resnitzky, P. In vitro functions of stromal cells from human and mouse bone marrow. *Exp. Hematol. 13,* 603-609 (1985).
39. Zuckerman, K. S., Prince, C. W., Ribadeneira, M. Sl/Sl^d mouse bone marrow stroma in vitro contains an active radiation-sensitive inhibitor of normal hemopoiesis. *Blood 68,* 1201-1206 (1986).
40. Castro-Malaspina, H., Laver, J., Kushner, B. H., O'Reilly, R. J. Aplastic anemia secondary to a defective marrow microenvironment: evidence for correction by intramedullary transplantation of cultured allogeneic marrow stromal cells (MSC). *J. Cell. Biochem. 10 (Suppl.),* 239 (1986).
41. Nagao, T., Yamauchi, K., Komatsuda, M. Serial in vitro bone marrow fibroblast culture in human leukemia. *Blood 61,* 589-592 (1983).
42. Nagao, T., Yamauchi, K., Komatsuda, M., Noguchi, K., Shimizu, M., Yonekura, S., Nozaki, H. Inhibition of human bone marrow fibroblast colony formation leukemic cells. *Blood 62,* 1261-1265 (1983).
43. Rozman, C., Granena, A., Hernandez-Prieto, M., Vela, E., Brugues, R. Bone marrow transplantation for acute myelofibrosis. *Lancet 1,* 618 (1982).
44. McGlave, P. B., Brunning, R. D., Hurd, D. D., Kim, T. H. Reversal of severe bone marrow fibrosis and osteosclerosis following allogeneic bone marrow transplantation for chronic granulocytic leukemia. *Brit. J. Haematol. 52,* 189-194 (1982).
45. Rajantie, J., Sale, G. E., Deeg, H. J., Amos, D., Appelbaum, F. R., Storb, R., Clift, R. A., Buckner, C. D. Adverse effect of severe marrow fibrosis on hematologic recovery after chemoradiotherapy and allogeneic bone marrow transplantation. *Blood 67,* 1693-1697 (1986).
46. Johnson, S. A. N., Bateman, C. J. T., Beard, M. E. J., Whitehouse, J. M. A., Waters, A. H. Long-term haematological consequences of thorotrast. *Quart. J. Med. 46,* 259-269 (1977).
47. Knospe, W. H., Rayudu, V. M. S., Cardello, M., Friedman, A. M., Fordham, E. W. Bone marrow scanning with ^{52}iron (^{52}Fe). Regeneration and extension of marrow after ablative doses of radiotherapy. *Cancer 37,* 1432-1442 (1976).
48. Sykes, M. P., Chu, F. C. H., Savel, H., Bonadonna, G., Mathis, H. The effects of varying dosages of irradiation upon sternal-marrow regeneration. *Radiology 83,* 1084-1087 (1964).
49. Permentier, C., Moaradet, N., Tubiana, M. Late effects on human bone marrow after extended field radiotherapy. *Int. J. Radiat. Oncol. Biol. Phys. 9,* 1303-1311 (1983).
50. Chamberlin, W., Barone, J., Kedo, A., Fried, W. Lack of recovery of murine hematopoietic stromal cells after irradiation-induced damage. *Blood 44,* 385-392 (1974).
51. Friedenstein, A. J., Gorskaja, U. F., Kulagina, N. N. Fibroblast precursors in normal and irradiated mouse hematopoietic organs. *Exp. Hematol. 4,* 267-274 (1976).
52. Laver, J., Abell, W., Castro-Malaspina, H. Radiobiological properties of the human hematopoietic microenvironment: contrasting sensitivities of prolifer-

ative capacity and hematopoietic function to in vitro irradiation. *Blood 67,* 1090-1097 (1986).
53. Tavassoli, M. Radiosensitivity of stromal cells responsible for in vitro maintenance of hemopoietic stem cells in continuous, long-term marrow culture. *Exp. Hematol. 10,* 435-443 (1982).
54. Piersma, A. H., Ploemacher, R. E., Brockbank, K. G. M. Radiation damage to femoral hemopoietic stroma measured by implant regeneration and quantitation of fibroblastic progenitors. *Exp. Hematol. 9,* 884-890 (1983).
55. Greenberger, J. S., Klassen, V., Kase, K., Shadduck, R. K., Sakakeeny, M. A. Effects of low dose rate irradiation on plateau phase bone marrow stromal cells in vitro: demonstration of a new form of non-lethal, physiologic damage to support of hematopoietic stem cells. *Int. J. Radiat. Oncol. Biol. Phys. 10,* 1027-1037 (1984).
56. Hendry, J. H., Wang, S. B., Testa, N. G. Greater sparing of stromal progenitor cells than of haemopoietic stem cells in gamma-irradiated mouse marrow using low dose-rates. *Biomed. Pharmacol. 38,* 356-358 (1984).
57. FitzGerald, T. J., McKenna, M., Rothstein, L., Daugherty, C., Kase, K., Greenberger, J. S. Radiosensitivity of human bone marrow granulocyte-macrophage progenitor cells and stromal colony-forming cells: effect of dose rate. *Radiat. Res. 107,* 205-215 (1986).
58. Xu, C. X., Hendry, J. H., Testa, N. G. The response of stromal progenitor cells in mouse marrow to graded repeated doses of X rays or neutrons. *Radiat. Res. 96,* 82-89 (1983).
59. Sargur, M., Buckner, C. D., Appelbaum, F. R., Stewart, P., Deeg, H. J., Weiden, P. L., Sullivan, K. M., Fefer, A., Thomas, E. D. Marrow transplantation for acute nonlymphocytic leukemia following therapy for Hodgkin's disease. *J. Clin. Oncol. 5,* 731-734 (1987).
60. Siena, S., Castro-Malaspina, H., Gulati, S. C., Lu, L., Colvin, M. O., Clarkson, B. D., O'Reilly, R. J., Moore, M. A. S. Effects of in vitro purging with 4-hydroperoxycyclophosphamide on the hematopoietic and microenvironmental elements of human bone marrow. *Blood 65,* 655-662 (1985).
61. Grochow, L. B., Colvin, M. Clinical pharmacokinetics of cyclophosphamide. *Clin. Pharmacokinet. 4,* 380-394 (1979).
62. Fried, W., Kedo, A., Barone, J. Effects of cyclophosphamide and of busulfan on spleen colony-forming units and on hematopoietic stroma. *Cancer Res. 37,* 1205-1209 (1977).
63. Wathen, L. M., Knapp, S. A., DeGowin, R. L. Suppression of marrow stromal cells and microenvironmental damage following sequential radiation and cyclophosphamide. *Int. J. Radiat. Oncol. Biol. Phys. 7,* 935-941 (1981).
64. Buckner, C. D., Briggs, R., Clift, R. A., Fefer, A., Funk, D. D., Glucksberg, H., Neiman, P. E., Storb, R., Thomas, E. D. Intermittent high-dose cyclophosphamide (NSC-26271) treatment of stage III ovarian carcinoma. *Cancer Chemother. Rep. 58,* 697-703 (1974).
65. Kushner, B. H., Kwon, J.-H., Gulati, S. C., Castro-Malaspina, H. Preclinical assessment of purging with VP-16-213: key role for long-term marrow cultures. *Blood 69,* 65-71 (1987).

66. Sculier, J. P., Klastersky, J., Stryckmans, P., EORTC Lung Cancer Working Party. Late intensification in small-cell lung cancer: a phase I study of high doses of cyclophosphamide and etoposide with autologous bone marrow transplantation. *J. Clin. Oncol. 3,* 184-191 (1985).
67. Anderson, R. W., Matthews, K. I., Crouse, D. A., Sharp, J. G. In vitro evaluation of hematopoiesis in mice treated with busulfan or nitrogen mustard. *Biomedicine 36,* 149-152 (1982).
68. Greenberger, J. S., Eckner, R. J., Otten, J. A., Tennant, R. W. In vitro quantitation of lethal and physiologic effects of total body irradiation on stromal and hematopoietic stem cells in continuous bone marrow cultures from Rf mice. *Int. J. Radiat. Oncol. Biol. Phys. 8,* 1155-1165 (1982).
69. McManus, P. M., Weiss, L. Busulfan-induced chronic bone marrow failure: changes in cortical bone, marrow stromal cells, and adherent cell colonies. *Blood 64,* 1036-1041 (1984).
70. Hays, E. F., Hale, L., Villarreal, B., Fitchen, J. H. "Stromal" and hemopoietic stem cell abnormalities in long-term cultures of marrow from busulfan-treated mice. *Exp. Hematol. 10,* 383-392 (1982).
71. Thomas, E. D., Clift, R. A., Fefer, A., Appelbaum, F. R., Beatty, P., Bensinger, W. I., Buckner, C. D., Cheever, M. A., Deeg, H. J., Doney, K., Flournoy, N., Greenberg, P., Hansen, J. A., Martin, P., McGuffin, R., Ramberg, R., Sanders, J. E., Singer, J., Stewart, P., Storb, R., Sullivan, K., Weiden, P. L., Witherspoon, R. Marrow transplantation for the treatment of chronic myelogenous leukemia. *Ann. Intern. Med. 104,* 155-163 (1986).
72. Santos, G. W., Tutschka, P. J., Brookmeyer, R., Saral, R., Beschorner, W. E., Bias, W. B., Braine, H. G., Burns, W. H., Elfenbein, G. J., Kaizer, H., Mellits, D., Sensenbrenner, L. L., Stuart, R. K., Yeager, A. M. Marrow transplantation for acute nonlymphocytic leukemia after treatment with busulfan and cyclophosphamide. *New Engl. J. Med. 309,* 1347-1353 (1983).
73. Kanfer, E. J., Petersen, F. B., Buckner, C. D., Stewart, P., Storb, R., Hill, R. S., Appelbaum, F. R., Clift, R. A., Doney, K. C., Shulman, H. M., Thomas, E. D. Phase I study of high-dose dimethylbusulfan followed by autologous bone marrow transplantation in patients with advanced malignancy. *Cancer Treat. Rep. 71,* 101-102 (1987).
74. Young, N., Mortimer, P. Viruses and bone marrow failure. *Blood 63,* 729-737 (1984).
75. Romet-Lemonne, J. L., Elfassi, E., Haseltine, W., Essex, M. Infection of bone marrow cells by hepatitis B virus. *Lancet 2,* 732 (1983).
76. Zeldis, J. B., Mugishima, H., Steinberg, H. N., Nir, E., Gale, R. P. In vitro hepatitis B virus infection of human bone marrow cells. *J. Clin. Invest. 78,* 411-417 (1986).
77. The Royal Marsden Hospital Bone-Marrow Transplantation Team. Failure of syngeneic bone-marrow graft without preconditioning in post-hepatitis marrow aplasia. *Lancet 2,* 742-745 (1977).
78. Quinnan, G. V., Kirmani, N., Rook, A. H., Manischewitz, J. F., Jackson, L., Moreschi, G., Santos, G. W., Saral, R., Burns, W. H. Cytotoxic T cells in cytomegalovirus infection. *New Engl. J. Med. 307,* 7-13 (1982).

79. Rook, A. H., Quinnan, G. V., Frederick, W. J. R., Manischewitz, J. F., Kirmani, N., Dantzler, T., Lee, B. B., Currier, C. B. Importance of cytotoxic lymphocytes during cytomegalovirus infection in renal transplant recipients. *Amer. J. Med. 76,* 385-392 (1984).
80. Schroff, R. W., Gale, R. P., Fahey, J. L. Regeneration of T cell subpopulations after bone marrow transplantation: cytomegalovirus infection and lymphoid subset imbalance. *J. Immunol. 129,* 1926-1930 (1982).
81. Favrot, M., Janossy, G., Tidman, N., Blacklock, H., Lopez, E., Bofill, M., Lampert, I., Morgenstein, G., Powles, R., Prentice, H. G., Hoffbrand, A. V. T cell regeneration after allogeneic bone marrow transplantation. *Clin. Exp. Immunol. 54,* 59-72 (1983).
82. Wursch, A. M., Gratama, J. W., Middledorp, J. M., Nissen, C., Gratwohl, A., Speck, B., Jansen, J., D'Amaro, J., The, T. H., DeGast, G. C. The effect of cytomegalovirus infection on T lymphocytes after allogeneic bone marrow transplantation. *Clin. Exp. Immunol. 62,* 278-287 (1985).
83. Rice, G. P. A., Schrier, R. D., Oldstone, M. B. A. Cytomegalovirus infects human lymphocytes and monocytes: virus expression is restricted to immediate-early gene products. *Proc. Natl. Acad. Sci. USA 81,* 6134-6138 (1984).
84. Bowden, R. A., McGavren, L., Hayward, A. R., Levin, M. J. Use of bone marrow fibroblasts to prepare targets for an HLA restricted-cytotoxicity assay system. *J. Clin. Microbiol. 20,* 696-700 (1984).
85. Kramvis, A., Garnett, H. M., Sadan, Y. Replication of simian cytomegalovirus (SCMV) in Vervet monkey bone marrow stromal cells. *10th international herpesvirus workshop,* Ann Arbor, MI, pp. 233-234 (1985).
86. Hirabayashi, N. Studies on graft versus host (GvH) reactions. I. Impairment of hemopoietic stroma in mice suffering from GvH disease. *Exp. Hematol. 9,* 101-110 (1981).
87. O'Kunewick, J. P., Meredith, R. F., Raikow, R. B., Buffo, M. J., Jones, D. L. Possibility of three distinct and separable components to fatal graft-vs-host reaction. *Exp. Hematol. 10,* 277-291 (1982).
88. Sullivan, K. M., Deeg, H. J., Sanders, J., Klosterman, A., Amos, D., Shumlman, H., Sale, G., Martin, P., Witherspoon, R., Appelbaum, F., Doney, K., Stewart, P., Meyers, J., McDonald, G. B., Weiden, P., Fefer, A., Buckner, C. D., Storb, R., Thomas, E. D. Hyperacute graft-v-host disease in patients not given immunosuppression after allogeneic marrow transplantation. *Blood 67,* 1172-1175 (1986).
89. Da, W.-M., Ma, D. D. F., Biggs, J. C. Studies of hemopoietic stromal fibroblastic colonies in patients undergoing bone marrow transplantation. *Exp. Hematol. 14,* 266-270 (1986).
90. Bolger, G. B., Sullivan, K. M., Storb, R., Witherspoon, R. P., Weiden, P. L., Stewart, P., Sanders, J., Meyers, J. D., Martin, P. J., Doney, K. C., Deeg, H. J., Clift, R. A., Buckner, C. D., Appelbaum, F. R., Thomas, E. D. Second marrow infusion for poor graft function after allogeneic marrow transplantation. *Bone Marrow Transplant. 1,* 21-30 (1986).

17
Conditions Affecting the Growth of Hemopoietic Progenitors After Bone Marrow Transplantation

HANS A. MESSNER AND KAZUO YAMASAKI
Ontario Cancer Institute, University of Toronto, Toronto, Ontario, Canada

I. INTRODUCTION

Bone marrow transplantation is used therapeutically with curative intent in patients with hemopoietic deficiency disorders, hemopoietic malignancies, and a series of genetic disorders. In addition to its clinical usefulness, the procedure has provided the opportunity to characterize cell populations of donor origin in recipients of bone marrow transplants. In addition to myeloid and lymphoid cell populations, these may include osteoclasts (1,2), Kupffer cells (3), Langerhans cells (4), fibroblast cell populations (5), and some stromal cell components as shown in long-term bone marrow cultures (6). The profound changes associated with bone marrow transplantation are particularly apparent in patients with osteopetrosis (7) or myelofibrosis (8,9), in whom the typical dense fibrotic tissue that occupies the bone marrow space will be completely restructured and replaced with normal hemopoietic cells (Fig. 1). In spite of these favorable changes, bone marrow transplant recipients often remain unable to respond adequately to the increased hemopoietic demands that may be posed by severe infections, suggesting that complete normalization of hemopoiesis may not occur.

II. CHARACTERIZATION OF HEMOPOIESIS AFTER BONE MARROW TRANSPLANTATION

Bone marrow transplant recipients that reestablish hemopoiesis successfully and survive the early posttransplant period are usually able to produce peripheral blood cells in normal or near-normal quantities under steady-state conditions. Blood cells are usually of donor origin. However, some investigators have reported

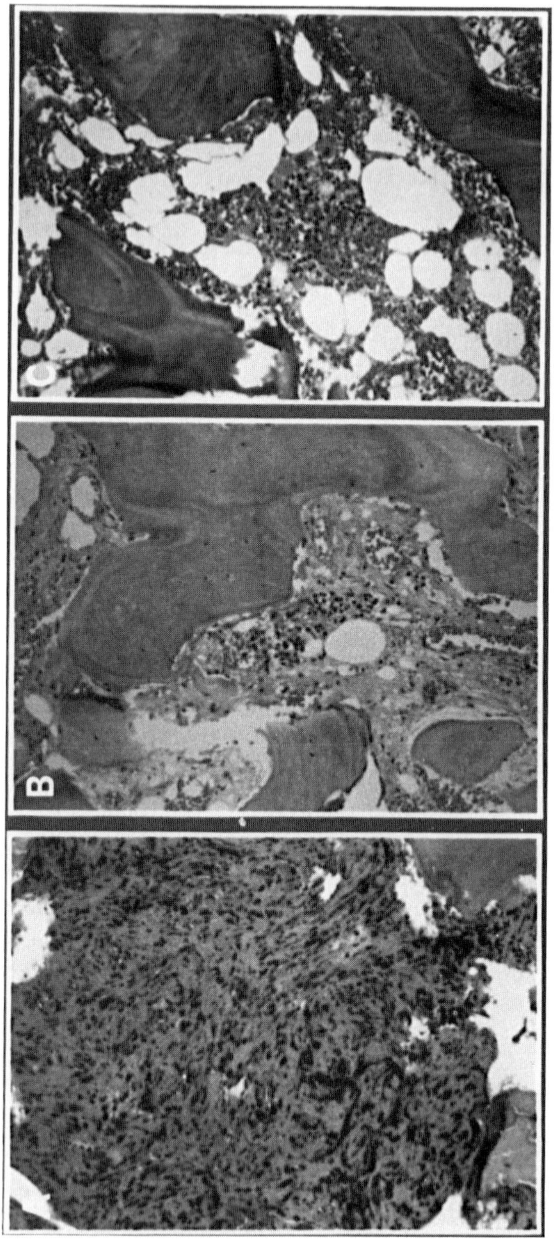

Figure 1 (A) Bone marrow biopsy derived from a patient with severe myelofibrosis before bone marrow transplantation. (B, C) Bone marrow biopsies of the same patient obtained 4 weeks and 5 months, respectively, after transplantation.

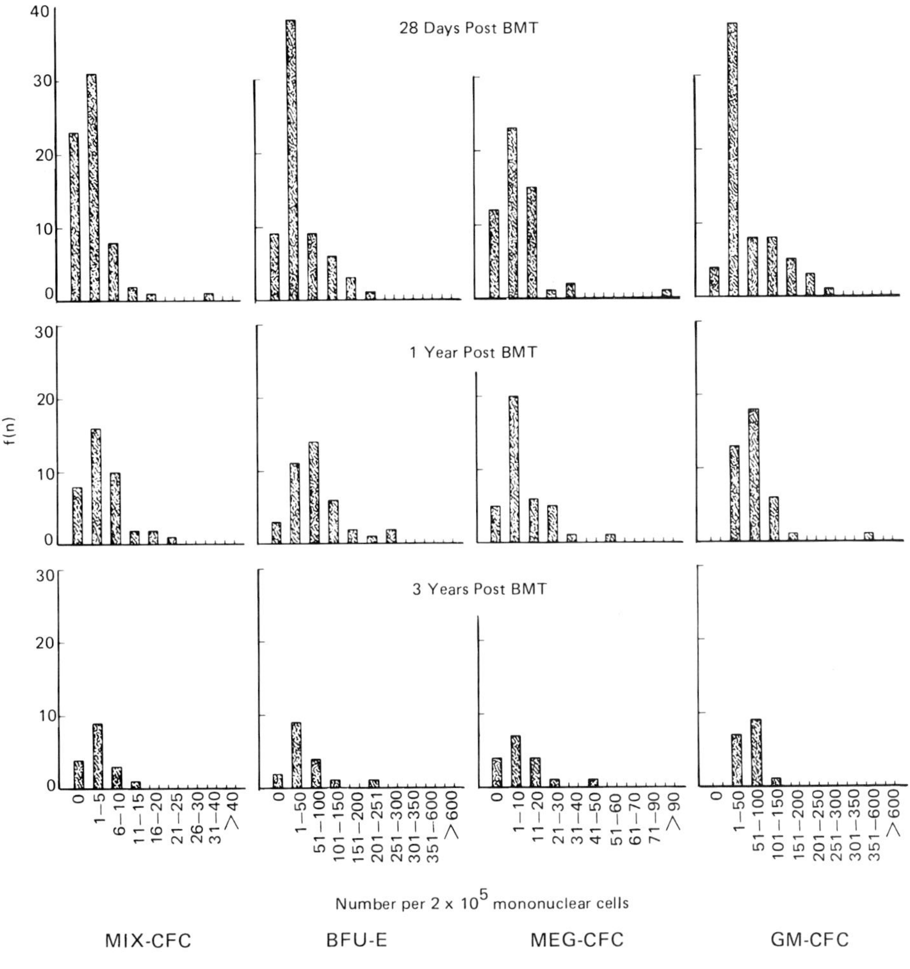

Figure 2 Frequency distribution profiles of Mix-CFC, BFU-E, Meg-CFC, and GM-CFC in bone marrow transplant recipients 28 days, 1 year, and 3 years, respectively, after transplantation.

the coexistence of donor- and host-derived cells, thus demonstrating the development of mixed hemopoietic chimeras (10-12).

In contrast to peripheral blood cells, clonogenic progenitors usually do not return to normal values even 3-5 years after transplantation (13,14). Our own data for multipotent progenitors (Mix-CFC) and precursors committed to erythropoiesis (BFU-E), megakaryocytopoiesis (Meg-CFC) and granulocyte-macrophage production (GM-CFC) are depicted in Figure 2. The distribution profiles obtained 28 days, 1 year, and 3 years after transplantation are essentially identical

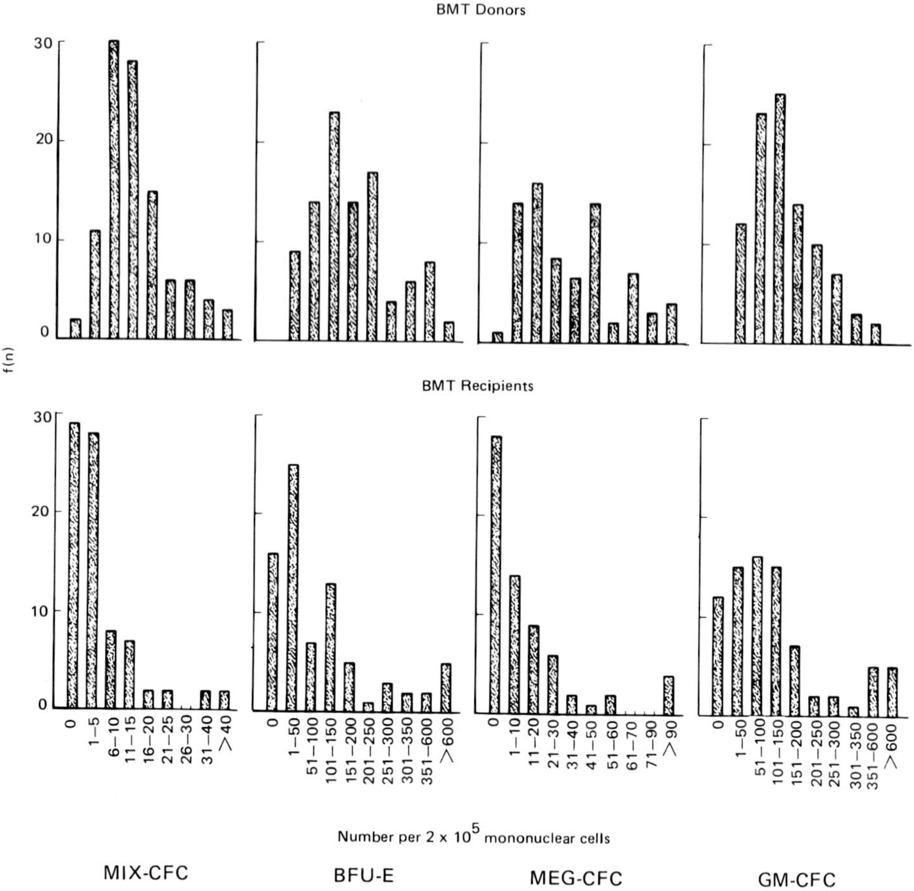

Figure 3 Frequency distribution profiles of Mix-CFC, BFU-E, Meg-CFC, and GM-CFC in normal bone marrow transplant donors and bone marrow transplant recipients before administration of the preparative chemoradiotherapy.

and show a shift toward lower values compared to the normal bone marrow donor population. The profiles are consistent with patterns observed in transplant recipients before administration of their preparative regimen (Fig. 3, lower panels). The observed frequencies of BFU-E and GM-CFC are similar to those in studies by other investigators (15,16).

In spite of normal peripheral blood counts, a large proportion of clonogenic progenitors continue to cycle as determined by tritiated thymidine suicide studies (14,17). This observation is consistent with the view that only a few enter a resting state. The reason for this marginal reserve of clonogenic progenitors after transplantation is currently not understood. One may speculate about the contribution to engraftment made by quantity and quality of the donor-derived transplant inoculum, and about conditions within the transplant recipient, which may prohibit complete normalization.

III. INFLUENCE OF THE BONE MARROW TRANSPLANT INOCULUM

It is common practice to transfuse approximately 3×10^8 nucleated cells per kilogram body weight of the recipient. The total number of nucleated cells may vary from 1×10^{10} to 4×10^{10} nucleated cells when individual transplants are evaluated. This number approximates only 3-10% of the total number of nucleated bone marrow cells of a normal individual. Transplant inocula contain varying numbers of pluripotent and committed hemopoietic progenitors.

In an analysis on 102 consecutive bone marrow transplants we have quantitated the total number of nucleated cells and clonogenic precursors to examine the influence of these cell populations on survival and time to engraftment (14). For this study, the latter was defined as the interval that had elapsed from transplantation to the time when more than 1500 granulocytes, 50,000 platelets, and 50,000 reticulocytes per cubic millimeter of peripheral blood were sustained without transfusions. Time to engraftment in this study was influenced neither by the total number of transplanted cells nor by the total number of clonogenic precursors. Survival was also not dependent on the frequency of clonogenic cells in the transplant inoculum. In contrast, the total number of nucleated cells transplanted correlated with survival. That is, patients who had received a larger number of nucleated cells had a higher probability of surviving. This observation confirmed previous results obtained from patients transplanted for severe aplastic anemia (18).

These results raised the question of whether currently available assays for clonogenic hemopoietic progenitors are able to accurately detect and measure cell populations that are responsible for engraftment. Alternatively, one may postulate that engraftment is not only a function of proliferative precursors as measured in these assays, but also a process that requires the functional unit of proliferating and auxiliary cells within the transplant inoculum. This view is supported by more recent data that T-cell-depleted bone marrow samples are associated with a significantly higher frequency of engraftment failures (19,20).

One may also consider the possibility that the relatively small numbers of transplanted cells are insufficient to establish a normal bone marrow function with adequate reserve. Animal experiments have clearly demonstrated that hemopoiesis may be restored in a lethally irradiated animal by as little as 10^5 nucleated marrow cells (21). However, it requires the transfusion of at least 5×10^7 nucleated bone marrow cells to render these animals fit to serve as secondary bone marrow donors (22).

Table 1 Clonogenic Progenitors in Bone Marrow Transplant Recipients Receiving More Than 3×10^8 Nucleated Cells/kg

Patient no.	Total number of cells transplanted	Days posttransplant	Number of colonies			
			Mix-CFC	BFU-E	Meg-CFC	GM-CFC
145	2.3×10^{10}	28	12	203	12	9
147	3.3×10^{10}	14	10	133	6	72
		28	16	147	9	57
148	3.3×10^{10}	14	9	10	3	35
		28	6	46	2	34
149	4.2×10^{10}	14	1	4	1	13
150	4.0×10^{10}	14	21	236	112	163

In a preliminary study we have attempted to transplant a larger than usual number of nucleated cells. The frequency of clonogenic cells observed early after transplantation in four of the five recipients was significantly higher than previously observed. The data approached normal values (Table 1). These studies require confirmation on a larger number of transplants to provide a sufficient base for survival studies.

IV. INFLUENCE OF HOST PARAMETERS

Bone marrow transplants are performed for a variety of hemopoietic disorders. Some of these, such as aplastic anemia, are characterized by reduced bone marrow function, as identified by low peripheral blood counts and usually absent clonogenic cells. Patients with hemopoietic malignancies at presentation and in relapse demonstrate the predominance of malignant cell populations, while normal precursors are usually severely reduced or not observed. The apparent reduction may result from a dilution of normal clonogenic progenitors by cells belonging to the malignant clone. Alternatively, the presence of malignant cells may actively suppress or eliminate normal hemopoietic progenitors. This phenomenon is best demonstrated in patients with chronic myeloid leukemia where members of the Philadelphia chromosome positive clone predominate. The reestablishment of polyclonal, Philadelphia chromosome negative hemopoiesis in long-term bone marrow cultures supports the concept of a reversible suppression (23,24). Besides these disease-related mechanisms, one also has to consider the influence of chemotherapy on hemopoietic precursors (see Chapters 3 and 4).

We have extensively examined the bone marrow of prospective transplant recipients before administration of the preparative regimen. As stated above, we observed that multi- and single-lineage precursors are reduced in frequency compared to the normal donor population (Fig. 3, lower panels).

We asked the question, Can the frequency of clonogenic precursors observed before the transplantation predict the clinical outcome of the transplant using time to engraftment and survival as parameters? The analysis yielded a significant correlation between the frequency of Meg-CFC and time of engraftment (14). Patients with higher numbers of Meg-CFCs engrafted faster than patients with lower numbers. The other clonogenic parameters did not contribute to the time of engraftment. None of the measured clonogenic cells were correlated with survival. The association between Meg-CFC and time to engraftment may reflect in vivo conditions that influence the redevelopment of this particularly fastidious cell lineage. The culture data certainly support the clinical observation that platelet recovery is more frequently a problem than the return of the other lineages.

V. SUPPORT OF MEGAKARYOCYTE GROWTH IN CULTURE

The documented association of Meg-CFC and time to engraftment is of interest because it may serve as a readout system for support of megakaryocyte growth in vivo. In our hands Meg-CFC colony growth is best supported by human plasma and a source of exogenous megakaryocyte colony-stimulating activity (Meg-CSA) (25,26). Normal human plasma does not usually promote the growth of megakaryocyte colonies but will support their formation in the presence of Meg-CSA. This activity is found in medium conditioned by phytohemagglutinin-stimulated leukocytes (PHA-LCM) (25). More recently, recombinant human granulocyte-macrophage colony-stimulating factor (GM-CSF) (27-30) and gibbon interleukin-3 (IL-3) were found to contain these megakaryocyte growth-promoting activities (31-33).

We asked whether or not this support of megakaryocyte colony growth may be altered in patients undergoing bone marrow transplantation. Plasma was therefore collected before administration of the preparative regimen and serially after transplantation. Each plasma sample was tested on normal, nonadherent target cells either alone or in conjunction with PHA-LCM as a source of Meg-CSA. The activities were compared to normal plasma. Results obtained on five patients are listed in Table 2. The growth-supporting activity of plasma derived from bone marrow transplant recipients prior to administration of the preparative regimen was significantly reduced in comparison to normal control plasma. One of the plasma samples gave rise to a small number of megakaryocyte colonies without addition of PHA-LCM.

A number of changes take place after transplantation with respect to both growth-supporting and growth-promoting activities for megakaryocyte progenitors. Plasma samples obtained 14 and 28 days after transplantation will usually not only support but also promote colony formation in the absence of PHA-LCM.

Table 2 Activities Supporting and Promoting Megakaryocyte Colony Growth in Plasma Samples of Bone Marrow Transplant Recipients

	Number of Meg-CFC (% control)[a]									
	Pretransplant		Day 14		Day 28		Day 60		1 year	
Patient no.	0	+	0	+	0	+	0	+	0	+
91	0	14	185	171	57	186	–[b]	–[b]	0	80
94	0	45	68	72	63	77	0	62	0	86
97	12	32	65	78	56	79	0	0	18	194
152	0	17	23	113	43	93	1	13	–[b]	–[b]
154	0	47	24	95	14	170	0	53	–[b]	–[b]

[a]0, Without PHA-LCM; +, with 10% PHA-LCM. The data expressed as percentage of colony numbers observed with normal plasma and PHA-LCM.
[b]Not available.

Addition of PHA-LCM may augment colony formation in samples derived from some patients. This release of Meg-CSA-like substances into the plasma and the improvement of growth-supporting activities is only transient and may return to pretransplant values by day 60. Long-term observation of some of these patients suggests a gradual return of the growth-supporting activities to near normal values by 1 year. The physiology of this seemingly complex process is not understood, and little is known about the source of these growth-supporting and -promoting activities. One may again speculate that these are associated with auxiliary cell populations such as T lymphocytes, monocytes, and stromal cells of either host or donor origin. This question may be studied in the future by comparing the activities in patients that have received unmanipulated grafts to those in patients who were transplanted with T-cell-depleted bone marrow. Furthermore, the availability of molecular probes for hemopoietic growth factors will permit a detailed characterization of cell populations that are involved in their production.

These studies will be of particular significance for approaches to evaluate the role of stromal cells and determine whether these remain of host origin or are eventually replaced by donor cells. It can be demonstrated that these stromal elements undergo a dynamic reconstruction process similar to that of hemopoietic cells, since a significant population of precursors of stromal fibroblasts appears to cycle after transplantation (34).

VI. SUMMARY

The reestablishment of hemopoiesis after bone marrow transplantation is a complex procedure that involves donor and host elements. Our culture studies have demonstrated that hemopoiesis of transplant recipients may already be altered by the underlying disorder or the administered therapy. Reestablishment of hemopoiesis after engraftment appears to be suboptimal with respect to the frequency of hemopoietic precursors. These are significantly reduced in number and appear to proliferate rapidly as indicated by the high proportion in DNA synthesis. In addition, significant changes can be identified in bone marrow transplant recipients with respect to the release of factors that may support and promote growth of hemopoietic precursors. Their role in the engraftment process will have to be clearly identified, since potential factor deficiencies may be corrected in the near future by administration of recombinant growth factors.

REFERENCES

1. Ash, P., Loutit, J. F., Townsend, K. M. S. Osteoclasts derived from haematopoietic stem cells. *Nature 283,* 669-670 (1980).
2. Coccia, P. F. Cells that resorb bone. *New Engl. J. Med. 310,* 456-457 (1984).
3. Gale, R. P., Sparkes, R. S., Golde, D. W. Bone marrow origin of hepatic macrophages (Kupffer cells) in humans. *Science 201,* 937-938 (1978).
4. Katz, S. I., Tamaki, K., Sachs, D. H. Epidermal Langerhans cells are derived from cells originating in bone marrow. *Nature 282,* 324-326 (1979).
5. Piersma, A. H., Brockbank, K. G. M., Ploemacher, R. E., Ottenheim, C. P. E. Recovery of hemopoietic stromal progenitor cells after lethal total-body irradiation and bone marrow transplantation in mice. *Transplantation 40,* 198-201 (1985).
6. Keating, A., Singer, J. W., Killen, P. D., Striker, G. E., Salo, A. C., Sanders, J., Fialkow, P. J. Donor origin of the in vitro haematopoietic microenvironment after marrow transplantation in man. *Nature 298,* 280-283 (1982).
7. Coccia, P. F., Krivit, W., Cervenka, J., Clawson, C., Kersey, J. H., Kim, T. H., Nesbit, M. E., Ramsay, N. K. C., Warkentin, P. I., Teitelbaum, S. L., Kahn, A. J., Brown, D. M. Successful bone marrow transplantation for infantile malignant osteopetrosis. *New Engl. J. Med. 302,* 701-708 (1980).
8. Wolf, J. L., Spruce, W. E., Bearman, R. M., Forman, S. J., Scott, E. P., Fahey, J. L., Farbstein, M. J., Rappaport, H., Blume, K. G. Reversal of acute ("malignant") myeloclerosis by allogenic bone marrow transplantation. *Blood 59,* 191-193 (1982).
9. Mehta, A. B., Baughan, A. S. J., Catovsky, D., Goldman, J. M., Johnson, S. A., Galton, D. A. G. Reversal of marrow fibrosis in acute megakaryoblastic leukemia after remission-induction and consolidation chemotherapy followed by bone marrow transplantation. *Brit. J. Haematol. 53,* 445-449 (1983).

10. Branch, D. R., Gallagher, M. T., Forman, S. J., Winkler, K. J., Petz, L. D., Blume, K. G. Endogenous stem cell repopulation resulting in mixed hematopoietic chimerism following total body irradiation and marrow transplantation for acute leukemia. *Transplantation 34,* 226-228 (1982).
11. Hill, R. S., Peterson, F. B., Storb, R., Appelbaum, F. R., Doney, K., Dahlberg, S., Ramberg, R., Thomas, E. D. Mixed hematologic chimerism after allogenic marrow transplantation for severe aplastic anemia is associated with a higher risk of graft rejection and a lessened incidence of acute graft-versus-host disease. *Blood 67,* 811-816 (1986).
12. Petz, L. D., Yam, P., Wallace, R. B., Stock, A. D., de Lange, G., Knowlton, R. G., Brown, V. A., Donis-Keller, H., Forman, S. J., Blume, K. G. Mixed hematopoietic chimerism following bone marrow transplantation for hematologic malignancies. in press.
13. Messner, H. A. Hemopoietic precursors in human bone marrow transplantation. *Int. J. Cell Cloning 4* (*Suppl. 1*), 11-18 (1986).
14. Messner, H. A., Curtis, J. E., Minden, M. D., Tritchler, D., Lockwood, G., Takahashi, T., Lepine, J., Jamal, N., Tweeddale, M., Wandl, U. Clonogenic hemopoietic precursors in bone marrow transplantation. *Blood 70,* 1425-1432 (1987).
15. Li, S., Champlin, R., Fitchen, J. H., Gale, R. P. Abnormalities of myeloid progenitor cells after "successful" bone marrow transplantation. *J. Clin. Invest. 75,* 234-241 (1985).
16. Arnold, R., Schmeiser, T., Heit, W., Frickhofen, N., Pabst, G., Heimpel, H., Kubanek, B. Hemopoietic reconstitution after bone marrow transplantation. *Exp. Hematol. 14,* 271-277 (1986).
17. Messner, H. A. Human stem cells in culture. *Clin. Haematol. 13,* 393-404 (1984).
18. Storb, R., Prentice, R. L., Thomas, E. D. Marrow transplantation for treatment of aplastic anemia—an analysis of factors associated with graft rejection. *New Engl. J. Med. 296,* 61-66 (1977).
19. Martin, P. J., Hansen, J. A., Buckner, C. D., Sanders, J. E., Deeg, H. J., Stewart, P., Appelbaum, F. R., Clift, R., Fefer, A., Witherspoon, R. P., Kennedy, M. S., Sullivan, K. M., Flournoy, N., Storb, R., Thomas, E. D. Effects of in-vitro depletion of T-cells in HLA-identical allogeneic marrow grafts. *Blood 66,* 664-672 (1985).
20. Mitsuyasu, R. T., Champlin, R. E., Gale, R. P., Ho, W. G., Lenarsky, C., Winston, D., Selch, M., Elashoff, R., Giorgi, J. V., Wells, J., Tevasaki, P., Billing, R., Feig, S. Treatment of donor bone marrow with monoclonal anti-T-cell antibody and complement for the prevention of graft-versus-host disease. *Ann. Intern. Med. 105,* 20-26 (1986).
21. Boggs, D. R., Boggs, S. S., Saxe, D. F., Gress, L. A., Canfield, D. R. Hematopoietic stem cells with high proliferative potential—assay of their concentration in marrow by the frequency and duration of cure of w/w^v mice. *J. Clin. Invest. 70,* 242-253 (1982).

22. Harrison, D. E., Astle, C. M. Loss of stem cell repopulating ability upon transplantation—effects of donor age, cell number, and transplantation procedure. *J. Exp. Med. 156,* 1767-1779 (1982).
23. Coulombel, L., Kalousek, D. K., Eaves, C. J., Gupta, C. M., Eaves, A. G. Long-term marrow culture reveals chromsomally normal hematopoietic progenitor cells in patients with Philadelphia chromosome-positive chronic myelogenous leukemia. *New Engl. J. Med. 308,* 1493-1498 (1983).
24. Dube, I. D., Arlin, Z. A., Kalousek, D. K., Eaves, C. J., Eaves, A. C. Non-clonal hemopoietic progenitor cells detected in long-term marrow cultures from a Turner syndrome mosaic with chronic myeloid leukemia. *Blood 64,* 1284-1287 (1984).
25. Messner, H. A., Jamal, N., Izaguirre, C. The growth of large megakaryocyte colonies from human bone marrow. *J. Cell. Physiol. Suppl. 1,* 45-51 (1982).
26. Solberg, L. A., Jamal, N., Messner, H. A. Characterization of human megakaryocytic colony formation in human plasma. *J. Cell. Physiol. 124,* 67-74 (1985).
27. Kaushansky, K., O'Hara, P. J., Berkner, K., Segal, G. M., Hagen, F. S., Adamson, J. W. Genomic cloning, characterization, and multilineage growth-promoting activity of human granulocyte-macrophage colony-stimulating factor. *Proc. Natl. Acad. Sci. USA 83,* 3101-3105 (1986).
28. Emerson, S. G., Sieff, C. A., Wang, E. A., Wong, G. G., Clark, S. C., Nathan, D. G. Purification of fetal hematopoietic progenitors and demonstration of recombinant multipotential colony-stimulating activity. *J. Clin. Invest. 76,* 1286-1290 (1985).
29. Sieff, C. A., Emerson, S. G., Donahue, R. E., Nathan, D. G., Wang, E. A., Wong, G. G., Clark, S. C. Human recombinant granulocyte-macrophage colony-stimulating factor: a multilineage hematopoietin. *Science 230,* 1171-1173 (1985).
30. Metcalf, D., Begley, C. G., Johnson, G. R., Nicola, N. A., Vadas, M. A., Lopez, A. F., Williamson, D. J., Wong, G. G., Clark, S. C., Wang, E. A. Biologic properites in vitro of a recombinant human granulocyte-macrophage colony stimulating factor. *Blood 67,* 37-45 (1986).
31. Messner, H. A., Yamasaki, K., Jamal, N., Minden, M. M., Yang, Y. C., Wong, G. G., Clark, S. C. Growth of human hemopoietic colonies in response to recombinant gibbon interleukin 3 (IL 3) in comparison with human recombinant granulocyte (G-CSF) and granulocyte-macrophage colony stimulating factor (GM-CSF). *PNAS 84,* 6765-6769 (1987).
32. Sieff, C. A., Neimeyer, C. M., Nathan, D. G., Ekern, S., Bieber, F. R., Yang, Y. C., Wong, G. G., Clark, S. C. Stimulation of human hematopoietic colony formation by recombinant gibbon multi-colony-stimulating factor or interleukin 3. Submitted for publication.
33. Leary, A. G., Yang, Y. C., Clark, S. C., Gasson, J. C., Golde, D. W., Ogawa, M. Recombinant gibbon interleukin-3 (IL-3) supports formation of human multilineage colonies and blast cell colonies in culture: comparison with re-

combinant human granulocyte-macrophage colony-stimulating factor (GM-CSF). *Blood 70,* 1343-1348 (1987).
34. Da, W. M., Ma, D. D. F., Biggs, J. C. Studies of hemopoietic stromal fibroblastic colonies in patients undergoing bone marrow transplantation. *Exp. Hematol. 14,* 266-270 (1986).

18

Recent Advances in the Knowledge of the Hemopoietic System

Possible Ways of Correcting Long-Term Damage

T. MICHAEL DEXTER
Paterson Institute for Cancer Research, Christie Hospital and Holt Radium Institute, Manchester, England

I. INTRODUCTION

A major problem in treating malignant disease with agents such as radiation or chemicals is that the cytotoxic effects are not usually restricted to the tumor cells. Both normal and malignant cells are killed. This results in short-term damage to the hemopoietic system (with obvious clinical manifestations) and may also result in longer-term effects as a result of pathological changes in various body systems that are not repaired, or corrected, by the normal cellular and humoral regulatory processes. By its nature, long-term damage is sometimes difficult to detect at the gross cellular level, and the true extent of damage becomes apparent only when, months or years following treatment, the persisting lesions lead to clinical conditions requiring treatment. The problem of "detection and nature" of long-term damage is, of course, a main focus of this book and is more easily understood when the structure of regenerating tissue systems is examined in detail.

In the gut, skin, and hemopoietic system—which are the major systems where both short- and long-term effects are seen following treatment with cytotoxic agents but not the only ones—all the mature cells are continually being generated from a small population of stem cells (1). These stem cells can proliferate to form more stem cells (equal to renewal of the stem cell system) or differentiate to produce progeny, which undergo further proliferation and maturation to produce the functional end cells. In the process of this development, the number of cells is tremendously amplified; consider, for example, that probably one or two hemopoietic stem cells are sufficient to regenerate both the entire hemopoietic stem cell and the mature cell systems of a mouse (2,2a). Obviously, the system must be sufficiently flexible to allow production of one or the other cell lineages as appropriate (for example, extra erythrocytes in hypoxic conditions). But homeostatic mechanisms must also operate to maintain a fairly constant ratio between the various compartments such that, in the normal steady state, a balance is maintained among the stem cells, their differentiated progeny, and the mature cells (3). Clearly, if all of the stem cells were destroyed, the system would rapidly fail as the differentiated cells worked their way through the different compartments. However, if only a proportion of the stem cells are destroyed, then two scenarios are possible. In the ideal situation, the surviving stem cells would undergo renewal to produce more stem cells, and homeostasis would be reestablished. But in less favorable circumstances and for reasons discussed later, recovery of the stem cell system to normal levels may not be possible. However, a persistent depletion of stem cells may not necessarily manifest itself at the gross level, i.e., at the level of the mature cells, since the intrinsic proliferation ability of the differentiating cells may well be sufficient to compensate for the stem cell depletion. In this case, therefore, obvious pathological changes may not be seen; at the functional level the system would appear normal. Consider, however, the proliferative stress now being placed upon the system not only at the stem cell level (to produce more differentiated progeny) but also at the level of the committed progenitor cells themselves (to produce the functional end cells). This extra proliferative demand may well lead to the exhaustion of stem cells or the generation of mistakes during DNA replication and the consequent emergence of abnormal clones, perhaps themselves malignant, or the clinical effects of long-term damage.

Clearly, to understand the nature and extent of damage demands a knowledge of the fine structure of the system—of the different cell compartments and the cells and cell-derived products that mediate their proliferation and development. These aspects have all been discussed in previous chapters, and what is apparent is that symptomatic clinical evidence of damage may reflect damage either to the stem cell compartment or to the environmental milieu that controls their proliferation and differentiation, or to a combination of both. This knowledge is important, since it determines, to a large extent, our approach to the problem and possible modes of prevention or treatment of such damage.

II. DEVELOPMENT OF LINEAGE- OR STAGE-SPECIFIC CYTOTOXIC AGENTS

From the previous discussion, it is clear that the development of new forms of chemotherapy are required: drugs that demonstrate a much greater selective effect upon the malignant cells. The problem here, of course, is that research over several decades has shown no fundamental and consistent difference between normal cells and tumor cells, particularly a difference that can be exploited at the therapeutic level. One reason for this is that the differences between normal and malignant cells are likely to be very subtle, as indicated by the finding that a single point mutation is sufficient to convert a normal "regulatory" protein (produced by a cellular protooncogene) into a protein with aberrant function and transforming ability (4,5). Such differences are going to be difficult to exploit.

However, an alternative approach is to design drugs that are targeted to or are specific for a particular stage of normal cell development. At first sight, this approach would appear to be unproductive, since the emphasis lies in killing *normal* cells. But, clearly, many differences exist between a granulocyte-macrophage progenitor and an erythroid progenitor cell, and similarly, between erythroid progenitor cells and progenitor cells of the T or B cell lineages. Obviously, the development of in vitro culture systems and clonal assays for these various cell populations —as well as the various growth stimuli required for their development—mean that mechanistic studies can now be performed on how these cells differ from one another. Of particular importance, of course, is to determine how they differ from stem cells. With an understanding of how these cells differ, it may well be possible to design agents that show a much greater bias toward a particular subpopulation of hemopoietic cells. Since many leukemias and lymphomas are themselves also lineage-restricted, that is, they are comparable in many ways to the normal committed progenitor cells, agents that preferentially kill the corresponding normal cells may be expected to have a preferential cytotoxic effect also on the tumor cells. The objective, then, is to spare the normal stem cells. Obviously, in the case of these leukemias and other forms of hematological disease that have a stem cell origin, alternative strategies must be considered; these will be discussed later.

Several agents that show a selectivity toward subpopulations of normal hemopoietic cells are currently under investigation in our laboratory. One of them, isopropyl methane sulfanate (IMS), has been shown to be selectively toxic to progenitor cells and a large proportion of multipotential stem cells (6). However, this agent spares the most primitive stem cells capable of extensive self-renewal, and complete regeneration of the hemopoietic system occurs following treatment. The efficacy of this agent in the treatment of hematological malignancies is presently being explored in experimental animal systems. However, it is noteworthy that IMS is a member of a homologous series, one of which, methyl dimethane sulfanate (MDMS), is already undergoing phase I clinical trials. Significantly, MDMS does *not* show the selective toxicity on the hemopoietic system that is demonstrated by IMS—showing that structurally similar members of the same chemical series (differing in chain length or end groups) may differ markedly in their biological effects. This presumably represents differences not only in their chemical structure and biological targets, but also in the nature of the target cells themselves. One outcome of these studies is to emphasize the difficulties faced in conventional screening of potentially useful antineoplastic agents.

It is no longer sufficient simply to look for damage to the normal system; rather, the nature of this damage needs to be determined (whether or not there has been a selective effect upon a subpopulation of the normal cells) and the longer-term outcome of the response must be examined.

Obviously, this is a tremendous challenge, and probably one that cannot readily be met from existing resources, since it involves such a diverse number of screening tests. However, it almost certainly means that a large number of potentially very useful drugs have been ignored because the biological screening was not adequate—in other words, the right predictive tests were not done. This, of course, is bound to occur frequently when drugs are screened on a random basis.

But, as pointed out previously, the problems inherent in screening drugs on a random basis for their tumoricidal activity may be largely overcome if more emphasis is placed on screening them for their effects on *normal* cell systems, and out of this may evolve a new generation of useful drugs as well as a clearer understanding of biochemical processes in normal tissue development.

An example of this has emerged from recent studies looking at signal transduction mechanisms in hemopoietic cells. As described in Chapter 1, the development of hemopoietic cells in vitro requires the continuous presence of growth factors. Some of these growth factors (an example being murine interleukin-3, IL-3) influence the proliferation and development of multipotent stem cells as well as the myeloid committed progenitor cells (7). Other growth factors are much more restricted in their biological activities and target cells; an example is macrophage colony-stimulating factor (M-CSF or CSF-1), which promotes only the growth of progenitor and precursor cells in the macrophage lineage (8). In all cases, the responses of these cells are elicited by the binding of the growth factor to a specific receptor present on the target cells, as a result of which a signal is transduced within the cell, which then activates the appropriate response. Thus the outcome of a response is determined by the growth factors present, whether or not receptors are expressed on the target cells, the biochemical events that are promoted by such binding, and the effects of this on the way in which different cells can respond in different ways to the same growth factor; i.e., a macrophage progenitor cell can respond to CSF-1 by undergoing proliferation and differentiation, while in a mature macrophage, CSF-1 simply activates the function (e.g., increased phagocytic activity) of the cell (9,10). In an attempt to dissect how these responses are elicited, we have been looking at the effects of agents that may interfere with the way in which the growth factor-receptor binding signal is transduced into the cell.

Many signal transduction mechanisms involve a guanine-nucleotide (GTP) binding protein (G protein), which couples the receptor to an effector molecule (a signal protein), an example being the adenylcyclase system (11). Here, modulation of the function of the G protein is determined by the binding of GTP and its subsequent hydrolysis to GDP as a result of the intrinsic GTPase activity of the G protein. It has been known for some time that the function of G proteins can be dramatically influenced by ADP ribosylation (12), which apparently inhibits the GTPase activity of the protein. Examples of this are seen in the adenylcyclase system upon treatment with cholera toxin or pertussis toxin. Recent work also suggests a role for a function of ADP ribosylation of proteins in normal cells in the absence of treatment with toxins (13,14). These data led us to examine the response of cells to various hemopoietic cell growth stimuli in the presence of agents that are known to modify mono-ADP ribosylation of proteins.

The effects were dramatic: several compounds were found that demonstrated a marked selective effect upon hemopoietic cell development. In particular, treatment of long-term marrow cultures (which represent an in vitro system analogous with hemopoiesis in vivo, vis-à-vis stromal cell-hemopoietic cell interactions) with these compounds led to a marked decrease in the numbers of mature myeloid cells and committed myeloid progenitor cells, while sparing the multipotent stem cells (15). Apparently, these modifiers of ADP-ribosylation could block the transition (differentiation?) from multipotent stem cells to committed progenitor cells in a nontoxic, dose-dependent, and reversible manner. The differential response to these agents seen in multipotent stem cells as opposed to committed progenitor cells is presumably a reflection of intrinsic metabolic differences in these cell populations. What does this mean therapeutically? This result has now led us to examine the effects of such compounds on the growth of leukemic cells, since, as discussed earlier, many leukemias may well reflect an abnormal proliferation of committed progenitor cells rather than multipotent stem cells. The leukemia examined was the WEHI-3B myelomonocytic leukemia cell line.

The WEHI-3B cells were chosen because (1) they can be readily grown in vitro, allowing quantitative clonal assays to be performed; (2) when injected in vivo they rapidly proliferate and kill the recipient mice within a few weeks; and (3) as far as is known, they represent "committed" myelomonocytic cells, probably related to the normal granulocyte-macrophage progenitor cells. Thus, the question examined was whether the modifiers of ADP-ribosylation—shown to be very effective inhibitors of the development and growth of normal myeloid progenitor cells—would have a similar inhibitory effect upon the leukemic cells in the absence of significant stem cell toxocity. Obviously, to approach this problem requires a system, preferentially in vitro, in which the interactions between normal and leukemic hemopoietic cells can be monitored. In this respect, the long-term marrow cultures are suitable vehicles for such studies (16).

In these long-term cultures, normal hemopoiesis can be maintained for many months (16). When the cultures were inoculated with WEHI-3B cells, the leukemic cells infiltrated the marrow stroma and underwent rapid proliferation. A result of this was that normal hemopoiesis diminished to undetectable levels; the situation was therefore analogous to the growth of leukemic cells in vivo (Fig. 1). Significantly, treatment of such cultures, once weekly for 3 weeks, with

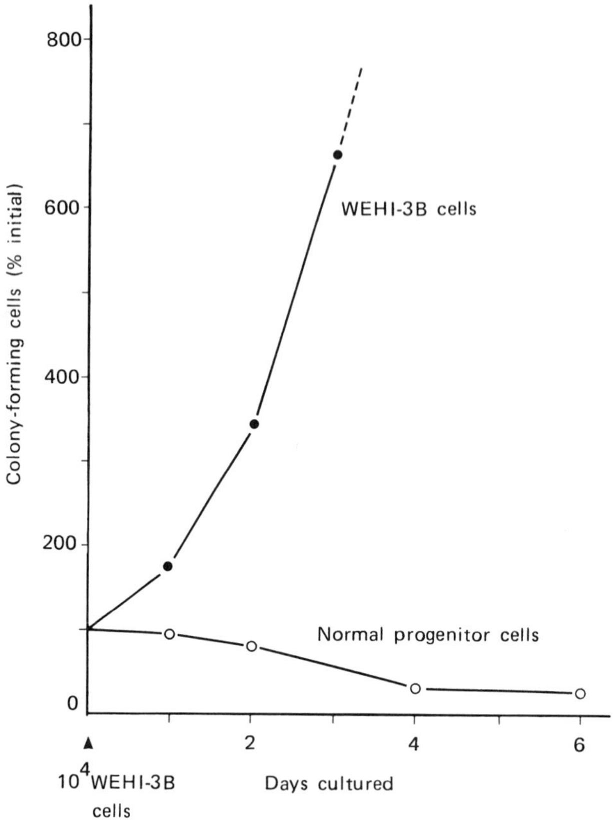

Figure 1 Growth of WEHI-3B cells in long-term marrow cultures. Cultures were established for 3 weeks (16) prior to inoculation with 10^4 WEHI-3B myelomonocytic leukemia cells. Subsequently, the numbers of clonogenic leukemic cells and normal progenitor cells were assessed on a daily basis.

compound CC15905A (one of the ADP-ribosylation modifiers discussed earlier) led to a rapid fall in the number of clonogenic WEHI-3B leukemic cells, while at the same time the number of normal multipotent stem cells was maintained at high levels (Fig. 2). Upon cessation of treatment, normal hemopoiesis recovered to untreated control levels, but there was no evidence for reemergence of the leukemic cells. The leukemia had been effectively cured in vitro. Indeed, when cells from long-term cultures (several weeks after treatment) were injected into mice, no leukemias subsequently developed. Since the in vivo assay is capable of detecting as few as 10 leukemic cells, these data strongly suggest that the WEHI-3 leukemic cells had been ablated in culture as a result of treatment. Obviously,

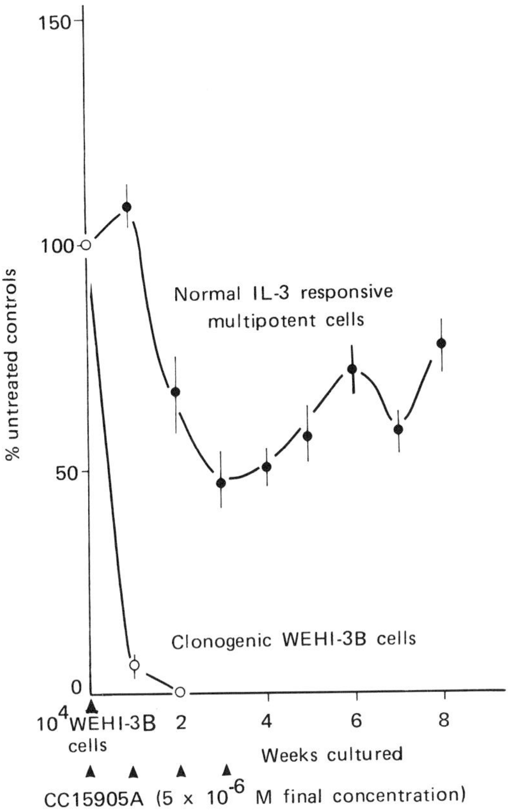

Figure 2 Effect of CC1 5905A on growth of WEHI-3B cells in long-term marrow cultures. Cultures established as in Figure 1 were treated at daily intervals with 5 X 10^{-6} M (final concentration) of Glaxo compound CC15905A, and the numbers of clonogenic leukemic cells and normal progenitor cells were assessed on a daily basis.

studies in vivo are now urgently required to test the efficacy of these compounds in alleviating or curing leukemic disease. However, what the studies do stress is that the concept underlying the basis of this work is essentially correct, i.e., that an understanding of the nature of normal cell populations (and their response to chemicals) may well suggest a significant approach for designing agents that are able to kill the corresponding tumor cells. As also stressed previously, this work is based on protection of the normal stem cells, which then provide the pool of cells to regenerate the damaged normal tissue. Another important point can now be discussed: Are there ways in which the growth of the normal cells can be further encouraged to minimize the extent and duration of the damage?

III. BIOLOGICAL RESPONSE MODIFIERS: THEIR ROLE IN TREATMENT

Growth factors are required to sustain survival, proliferation, and development of hemopoietic cells in vitro. While the exact role of many of these growth factors in vivo still remains to be determined, it is likely that they have a powerful part to play in the regulation of hemopoiesis—either in the normal steady state or in emergency situations (e.g., bacterial infections, hemorrhage) requiring rapid activation or regeneration of specific cell types. Indeed, it is likely that some, or all, of these growth factors are produced by regulatory cells in the bone marrow and other sites of hemopoiesis and exert their effects locally, probably involving cell-cell interactions (17).

In vivo analysis of the potential therapeutic applications of such growth factors was limited by the small amounts of material available. However, most of the growth factors have now been purified to homogeneity and molecularly cloned in suitable expression vectors (Table 1) (7-10, 18-37). As a result of this, of course, large amounts of material are now available for use in an in vivo analysis of their effects. Two points have emerged: First, the growth factors do exert effects upon hemopoiesis when administered in vivo, and second, the effects elicited are sometimes surprising and were not immediately predicted from the in vitro data.

Murine interleukin-3 (IL-3) is a lineage-indifferent growth factor which, in vitro, stimulates proliferation and differentiation of stem cells as well as granulocyte-macrophage, eosinophil, megakaryocyte, erythroid, and mast cell precursors. Although IL-3 is produced as a "lymphokine" from activated T cells, it has so far been difficult to detect this growth factor in vivo, even in mice undergoing a panlymphocytic response to antigen. However, injection of recombinant IL-3 in vivo into normal mice leads to a marked stimulation of hemopoiesis, particularly in the spleen, where multipotent stem cells and myeloid progenitor cells can reach levels 10-20-fold those found in untreated mice. Significantly, there is little effect upon circulating blood leukocyte levels. The recent molecular cloning of the human IL-3 gene should facilitate clinical studies with this important growth factor.

Granulocyte-macrophage colony-stimulating factor (GM-CSF) is somewhat more restricted than IL-3 in its target cells. In vitro, it stimulates proliferation of some (but not all) multipotent stem cells and acts as a proliferative and developmental stimulus for granulocyte-macrophage and eosinophil progenitor cells. Some recent evidence indicates that GM-CSF can stimulate erythroid and megakaryocyte progenitors also. Of some interest is that the gene for GM-CSF has been cloned from both mouse and human cells, and extensive homology is found. This evolutionary conservation suggests an important role for this growth factor in development. Injection of GM-CSF into normal mice has effects that are remarkably similar to those seen following injection of IL-3: a marked stimulation of hemopoiesis, particularly in the spleen. But perhaps more significant were the effects found on treatment of monkeys with human recombinant GM-CSF. In

Table 1 Growth Factors in Myelopoiesis

Growth factor[a]	Synonym	Species	Target cells[b] CFU-S	Mix-CFC	GM-CFC	BFU-E	Eo-CFC	Meg-CFC	Mast cells	CFU-E	Mature myeloid cells
IL-3	Multi-CSF	Mouse	+	+	+	+	+	+	+	±	+
	HCGF	Human	Not sufficient data								
	BPA	Gibbon									
GM-CSF	MGI-GM	Mouse, Human	–	+	+	+	+	+	–	–	+
G-CSF	MGI-G	Mouse	–	–	+(G)	–	–	–	–	–	+
	Pluripoietin	Human	N/A	(+)	+(G)	(+)	(+)	(+)	–	–	+
M-CSF	MGI-M	Mouse	–	–	+(M)	–	–	–	–	–	+
	CSF-1	Human									
Eo-DF	IL-4	Mouse	–	–	–	–	+	–	–	–	+
Erythropoietin		Human, Monkey, Mouse	N/A	–	–	–	–	–	–	+	–

[a]These growth factors have all been molecularly cloned, from at least one species.

[b]–, No reported effect; +, direct stimulation; (+), indirect stimulation. G, Granulocyte; M, macrophage; N/A, not applicable. CFU-S, Murine spleen colony-forming cells; Mix-CFC, colony-forming cell, mixed, i.e., multipotent in vitro colony-forming cell; BFU-E, erythroid burst-forming unit; Eo-CFC, eosinophil colony-forming cell; Meg-CFC, megakaryocyte colony-forming cell; CFU-E, erythroid colony-forming cell.

See Refs. 7-10 and 18-37.

this case, administration of the growth factor induced a dramatic increase in blood leukocyte levels. All circulating blood components (including lymphocytes) increased in numbers to about 10 times their normal level. Of great interest also is that a monkey suffering from a viral-induced pancytopenia was also treated with GM-CSF. In this case, the aplasia rapidly resolved and blood leukocyte levels returned to values in excess of normal, at least in the short term. Obviously, these data need to be confirmed and the longer-term effect of treatment with GM-CSF examined. However, the results are certainly encouraging, and their wider significance will be discussed later.

Equally encouraging were the results found with pluripoietin (or granulocyte colony-stimulating factor, G-CSF). Again, both the murine and the human gene have been cloned, and the extensive homology indicates a wide degree of evolutionary conservation. Also, unlike IL-3 and GM-CSF, the G-CSF is not so species-restricted; the recombinant human G-CSF is as effective on murine cells as the murine G-CSF. (Note, however, that in common with many other biological regulatory molecules, this works only one way; i.e., human is active on mouse, but mouse material is inactive on human cells.) G-CSF, in vitro, can directly stimulate GM-CFCs to proliferate and develop into mature neutrophils. Indirectly, however, the G-CSF can also stimulate proliferation and development of multipotent stem cells and other myeloid progenitor cells, presumably by stimulating the production of other regulatory molecules by accessory cells present in the target cell population. When recombinant G-CSF is injected into normal mice, it dramatically stimulates hemopoiesis. As with IL-3 and GM-CSF, the major effect is in the spleen. But, unlike IL-3 and GM-CSF, G-CSF treatment of mice can induce a large increase in circulating leukocyte levels and (although the stimulatory effect is again most apparent in the spleen) an overall increase in the total body number of multipotent stem cells. Also highly significant is the report that G-CSF can prevent the postchemotherapeutic nadir in circulating leukocyte levels seen after in vivo treatment with cyclophosphamide. The significance of this will be discussed later.

Other growth factors that have been cloned include eosinophil-stimulating factor, B-cell-stimulating molecules, the various lymphokines involved in T cell activation (Il-I and IL-2), and erythropoietin. The latter, in particular, will be a powerful tool for stimulating erythropoiesis in vivo.

What are the therapeutic implications of this work? There are several points worth considering. First, a major problem following administration of cytotoxic agents is the induced short-term damage, which is reflected in a profound decrease in circulating leukocyte levels. This makes the patient particularly prone to opportunistic infections and is a frequent reason for curtailing therapy before an adequate therapeutic response has been obtained. Two possible approaches (not mutually exclusive) for alleviating this problem are (1) to increase the size of the hemopoietic system prior to therapy, i.e., to convert yellow marrow to actively hemopoietic red marrow; and (2) to hasten recovery of circulating leukocytes by recruiting more cells into the maturing cell compartments. The growth factors described, GM-CSF and G-CSF, seem to be particularly useful in these respects, and the preliminary in vivo data discussed here are certainly encouraging.

It is possible, of course, that alleviation of the short-term effects seen following treatment with cytotoxic agents may decrease the magnitude of the long-term effects. For example, if the long-term damage arises as a consequence of extra proliferative stress being placed on the few surviving stem cells, then increasing their number prior to treatment may reduce some of this stress and thus maintain the proliferative integrity of the stem cell pool. If, on the other hand, the longer-term effects of cytotoxic treatment represent the expression of damage to the regulatory cells (the marrow stroma and/or lymphocytes, which themselves produce many of the growth factors), then it is difficult to see how administration of hemopoietic stimulatory molecules prior to or during cytotoxic treatment will counteract this effect. In this case, however, what becomes important is to assess the *nature* of these changes—the target cells affected and perturbations in the regulatory molecules that they produce. Knowing this, it may then be possible to perform "replacement" therapy, using either the cells themselves or the growth factors they produce.

Naturally, if the longer-term effects are due to damage to the stem cells themselves, the possibilities for therapy are much reduced. Even here, however, some therapeutic approaches are possible. For example, we have recently shown that hemopoietic cells can be successfully cultured in vitro and used to reconstitute hemopoiesis in patients, i.e., to perform an autologous marrow transplant (38). In particular, we and others have shown that in vitro culture conditions that are optimal for the growth of normal stem cells can suppress the growth of leukemic cells, which means that in vitro culture can be effectively used (at least in some myeloid leukemias) to purge marrow of abnormal cells (39,40). Perhaps eventually it may be possible to perform such protocols using marrow from patients suffering the long-term effects of damage by cytotoxic agents. Certainly, it is unlikely that all the stem cells from such patients have been damaged by the treatment, and if the normal (undamaged) stem cells can be encouraged to grow in vitro, then perhaps they could be given back to the patient to alleviate the hematological symptoms.

Obviously, much of this is speculative at present. However, it is clear that rapid progress has been made in recent years in understanding the nature of regenerating systems and the various factors that control the proliferation, development, and behavior of the cells. There is little doubt that this "new biology" will have an equally dramatic impact in the clinic.

ACKNOWLEDGMENTS

I thank the Cancer Research Campaign (U.K.) for supporting this research. Thanks are also due to the numerous colleagues who have contributed to discussions and to Dr. J. Martinez for allowing me to publish our observations shown in Figures 1 and 2.

REFERENCES

1. Lord, B. I., Potten, C. S., Cole, R. J. *Stem cells and tissue homeostasis.* Cambridge University Press, Cambridge, England, 368 pp. (1978).
2. Boggs, D. R., Boggs, S. S., Saxe, D. F., Gress, L. A., Garfield, D. R. Hematopoietic stem cells with high proliferation potential. Assay of their concentration in marrow by the frequency and duration of cure of W/W^v mice. *J. Clin. Invest. 70,* 243-247 (1982).

2a. Golde, D. W., Takaku, F. *Hematopoietic stem cells,* Marcel Dekker, New York and Basel (1985).

3. Dexter, T. M., Spooncer, E., Schofield, R., Lord, B. I., Simmons, P. Haemopoietic stem cells and the problem of self-renewal. *Blood Cells 10,* 315-339 (1984).
4. Tabin, C. J., Bradley, S. M., Baigmann, C. I., Weinberg, R. A., Papageorge, A. G., Scolnick, G. M., Lowy, D. R., Chang, E. H. Mechanism of activation of a human oncogene. *Nature 300,* 143-149 (1982).
5. Reddy, E. P., Reynolds, R. K., Santos, E., Barbacid, M. A point mutation is responsible for the acquisition of transforming properties by the T24 human bladder carcinoma oncogene. *Nature 300,* 149-150 (1982).
6. Schofield, R., Lajtha, L. G. Effects of isopropylmethane sulphonate on haemopoietic colony-forming units. *Brit. J. Haematol. 25,* 195-202 (1973).
7. Hapel, A. J., Fung, M. C., Johnson, R. M., Young, I. G., Johnson, G., Metcalf, D. Biologic properties of molecularly cloned and expressed murine interleukin-3. *Blood 65,* 1453-1459 (1985).
8. Das, S. K., Stanley, E. R. Structure-function studies of a colony stimulating factor (CSF-1). *J. Biol. Chem. 257,* 13679-13684 (1982).
9. Metcalf, D. The granulocyte-macrophage colony stimulating factors. *Science 229,* 16-22 (1985).
10. Metcalf, D. The molecular biology and functions of the granulocyte-macrophage-colony stimulating factors. *Blood 67,* 257-267 (1986).
11. Gilman, A. G. G proteins and dual control of adenylate cyclase. *Cell 36,* 577 (1984).
12. Schleijer, L. S., Kahn, R. A., Hanski, E., Northup, J. K., Sternweis, P. C., Gilman, A. G. Requirements for cholera-toxin dependent ADP-ribosylation of the purified regulatory component of adenylate cyclase. *J. Biol. Chem. 257,* 20-27 (1982).
13. Oka, J., Heda, E., Hayaishi, O., Komura, H., Nakanishi, K. ADP-ribosyl protein lyase. Purification, properties and identification of the product. *J. Biol. Chem. 259,* 986-996 (1984).
14. Rsai, S., Adamik, R., Moss, J., Vaughan, M., Maune, V., Kung, H. Effects of phospholipids and ADP-ribosylation on GTP hydrolysis by *E. coli*-synthesised Ha-ras oncogene p21. *Proc. Natl. Acad. Sci. USA 82,* 8310-8314 (1985).
15. Dexter, T. M., Whetton, A. D., Heyworth, C. M. Inhibitors of choleratoxin-induced adenosine diphosphate ribosylation of membrane associated proteins can block stem cell differentiation. *Blood 65,* 1544-1548 (1985).

16. Dexter, T. M., Spooncer, E., Simmons, P., Allen, T. D. Long-term marrow cultures: an overview of techniques and experience. In: *Long-term bone marrow cultures.* Wright, D. G., Greenberger, J. S. (Eds.). Liss, New York, pp. 57-96 (1984).
17. Dexter, T. M., Spooncer, E., Toksoz, D., Lajtha, L. G. The role of cells and their products in the regulation of *in vitro* stem cell proliferation and granulocyte development. *J. Supramol. Struct. 13,* 513-524 (1980).
18. Burgess, A. W., Nicola, N. A. *Growth factors and stem cells.* Academic Press, London, 355 pp. (1983).
19. Donahue, R. E., Wang, E. A., Stone, D. K., Kamen, R., Wong, G. G., et al. Stimulation of haematopoiesis in primates by continuous infusion of recombinant human GM-CSF. *Nature 321,* 874-875 (1986).
20. Gabrilove, J. L., Welte, K., Harris, P., Platzer, E., Lu, L., et al. Pluripoietin alpha: a second hematopoietic colony stimulating factor produced by the human bladder carcinoma cell line 5637. *Proc. Natl. Acad. Sci. USA 83,* 2478-2482 (1986).
21. Gough, N. M., Gough, J., Metcalf, D., Kelso, A., Grail, A., et al. Molecular cloning of cDNA encoding a murine haemopoietic growth regulator granulocyte/macrophage colony stimulating factor. *Nature 309,* 763-767 (1984).
22. Jacobs, K., Shoemaker, C., Rudersdorf, R., Neill, S. D., Kaufman, R. J., et al. Isolation and characterisation of genomic and cDNA clones of human erythropoietin. *Nature 313,* 806-810 (1985).
23. Kawasaki, E. S., Ladner, M. B., Wang, A. M., van Arsdell, J., Waffen, M. K., et al. Molecular cloning of a complementary DNA encoding human macrophage-specific colony-stimulating factor (CSF-1). *Science 230,* 291-296 (1985).
24. Kindler, V., Thorens, B., de Kossodo, S., Allet, B., Eliason, J. F. Stimulation of hematopoiesis *in vivo* by recombinant bacterial murine interleukin 3. *Proc. Natl. Acad. Sci. USA 83,* 1001-1005 (1986).
25. Lang, R. A., Metcalf, D., Gough, N. M., Dunn, A. R., Gonda, T. J. Expression of a hemopoietic growth factor cDNA in a factor dependent cell line results in autonomous growth and tumorigenicity. *Cell 43,* 531-542 (1985).
26. Lord, B. I., Molineux, G., Testa, N. G., Kelly, M., Spooncer, E., Dexter, T. M. The kinetic response of haemopoietic precursor cells, *in vivo,* to highly purified recombinant interleukin-3. *Lymphokine Res. 5,* 97-104 (1986).
27. Metcalf, D., Begley, C. G., Nicola, N. A., Lopez, A. F., Williamson, D. J. Effects of purified bacterially synthesised murine multi-CSF (IL-3) on hematopoiesis in normal adult mice. *Blood 68,* 46-57 (1986).
28. Nicola, N. A., Begley, C. G., Metcalf, D. Identification of the murine analogue of a regulator that induces differentiation in murine leukaemic cells. *Nature 314,* 625-628 (1985).
29. Nicola, N. A., Metcalf, D. Binding of ^{125}I-labelled granulocyte colony-stimulating factor to normal murine hemopoietic cells. *J. Cell. Physiol. 124,* 313-321 (1985).

30. Nicola, N. A., Metcalf, D., Matsumoto, M., Johnson, G. R. Purification of a factor inducing differentiation in murine myelomonocytic leukaemia cells. *J. Biol. Chem. 258,* 9017-9023 (1983).
31. O'Garra, A., Warran, D. J., Holman, M., Popham, A. M., Sanderson, C. J. Interleukin 4 (B-cell growth factor II/eosinophil differentiation factor) is a mitogen and differentiation factor for preactivated murine B lymphocytes. *Proc. Natl. Acad. Sci. USA 831,* 5228-5232 (1986).
32. Park, L. S., Friend, D., Gillis, S., Urdal, D. L. Characterisation of the cell surface receptor for human granulocyte-macrophage colony-stimulating factor. *J. Exp. Med. 164,* 251-262 (1986).
33. Sachs, L. Normal development programmes in myeloid leukaemia: regulatory proteins in the control of growth and differentiation. *Cancer Surv. 1,* 321-342 (1982).
34. Souza, L. M., Boone, T. C., Gabrilove, J., Lai, P. H., Zsebo, K. M., et al. Recombinant human granulocyte colony-stimulating factor: effects on normal and leukemic myeloid cells. *Science 232,* 61-65 (1986).
35. Stanley, E. R., Bartocci, D. P., Rosendaal, M., Bradley, T. R. Regulation of very primitive multipotent hemopoietic cells by hemopoietin-1. *Cell 45,* 667-674 (1986).
36. Whetton, A. D., Dexter, T. M. Haemopoietic growth factors. *Trends Biochem. Sci. 11,* 207-211 (1986).
37. Yang, Y.-C., Ciarletta, A. B., Temple, P. A., Chung, M. P., Kovacic, S., et al. Human IL-3 (multi-CSF): identification by expression cloning of a novel hematopoietic growth factor related to murine IL-3. *Cell 47,* 3-10 (1986).
38. Chang, J., Morgenstern, G., Deakin, D., Testa, N. G., Coutinho, L., Scarffe, J. H., Harrison, C., Dexter, T. M. Reconstitution of haemopoietic system with autologous marrow taken during relapse of acute myeloblastic leukaemia and grown in long-term culture. *Lancet 1,* 294-295 (1986).
39. Coulumbel, L., Kalousek, D. K., Eaves, C. S., Gupta, C. M., Eaves, A. C. Long-term marrow culture reveals chromosomally normal hemopoietic progenitor cells in patients with Ph-positive chronic myelogenous leukemia. *New Engl. J. Med. 306,* 1493-1498 (1983).
40. Eaves, C., Coulumbel, L., Dube, I., Kalousek, J., Cashman, J., Eaves, A. C. Maintenance of normal and abnormal hemopoietic cell population in long-term cultures of CML and AML marrow cells. In: *Hematopoietic stem cell physiology.* Cronkite, E. P., Dainiak, N., McCaffrey, R. P., Palek, J., Quesenberry, P. J. (Eds.). Liss, New York, pp. 403-413 (1985).

19

Bone Marrow Function
Recent Progress and Future Directions

NYDIA G. TESTA
Paterson Institute for Cancer Research, Christie Hospital and Holt Radium Institute, Manchester, England

ROBERT PETER GALE
University of California—Los Angeles School of Medicine, Los Angeles, California

I. GROWTH REGULATORS: FACTORS AND CELLS

The major recent advance in our knowledge of the hemopoietic system has been the description, characterization, and isolation of hemopoietic growth factors. Demonstration of effects of molecularly cloned hemopoietic growth factors in animals has led to clinical trials of GM-CSF and G-CSF. These are in progress. Possible uses include attempts to decrease the period of neutropenia following chemotherapy or to accelerate recovery of hemopoiesis after bone marrow transplantation. However, since the most striking effect is likely to be an increase in the number of mature granulocytes in the circulation, it is not yet clear whether these factors will affect long-term hemopoietic damage induced by chemotherapy or correct the anomalies that may be observed after transplantation. The reason long-term effects might not be ameliorated is that this damage is characterized by alterations in stem cells and progenitor cells rather than by subnormal production of mature cells. Compensatory mechanisms, which include expansion of the active bone marrow space, increased cycling of stem cells and progenitor cells, and shortening of cell cycle times, may lead to normal or near normal numbers of mature cells in peripheral blood.

However, it is possible that alterations in the production of growth factors may affect long-term hemopoiesis via the regulatory cellular networks in the bone marrow. Such alterations have been documented following cytotoxic chemotherapy and bone marrow transplantation and are reviewed in the preceding chapters. Some subjects worthy of further study are listed in Table 1.

In what ways are stromal elements of the bone marrow damaged by the pretransplant conditioning regime, by prior treatment, or by the nature of the under-

Table 1 Studies Relevant to the Better Definition of Long-Term Bone Marrow Damage

1. Further characterization of the regulatory cell populations and their interrelationships.
2. Type and level of growth factors produced in the bone marrow. How well do the networks regulating their production operate?
3. Fuller characterization of the action of growth factors (direct and indirect effects).
4. Life span and turnover of stromal cells in normal steady state and after cytotoxic injury. Production of extracellular matrix.
5. Transplantability (or lack of transplantability) of components of the regulatory stroma (lodging in the bone marrow, regeneration, function).

lying disease? It is known that although some stromal populations, like CFU-F, respond to cytotoxic damage by increased proliferation, their numbers may remain subnormal for long periods or perhaps permanently. No clear data have yet emerged on the extent of regeneration of other cellular elements such as vascular endothelium. For example, doses of radiation that abolish completely the regeneration of the capillary bed are only about two times higher than the doses used prior to bone marrow transplantation. It is therefore logical to expect that endothelial cell populations may be impaired by therapeutic regimens. Impairment to various stromal cell populations has been documented using experimental functional tests of the bone marrow microenvironment such as hemopoiesis in ectopic bone marrow implants in vivo or in long-term bone marrow cultures.

If host stromal cell populations are permanently damaged, their functions may become subnormal only following a long time after the injury when slowly turning over populations are sufficiently depleted.

The question arises as to whether deficient stromal populations can be corrected by transplantation. Although some data indicate that this is possible, recent information, reviewed in this book, disputes that assertion. Furthermore, it is known that fibroblastoid cells, possibly the best studied component of the bone marrow stroma, are not transplantable. A second consideration is that even if stromal elements were transplantable there is no evidence that they proliferate and become a *functional* component of the bone marrow environment. One interesting possibility is that, in cases of aplastic anemia caused by defects in the bone marrow microenvironment the disease may be corrected by (in situ?) transplantation of selected stromal populations. The anemic Sl/Sl^d mutant mouse is an ideal model supporting this hypothesis. Considerable data indicate that this anemia can be corrected by transplantation of normal hemopoietic tissue, but only if the structure of the tissue is not disrupted; the defect is not corrected by intravenous infusion of bone marrow.

Other cell populations relevant to the regulation of hemopoiesis belong to the immune system, including T cells and NK cells. The former are the predominant source of some hemopoietic growth factors. In this context, the late hemopoietic failure seen in patients transplanted with T-cell-depleted bone marrow is of concern.

II. IMMUNOLOGICAL ALTERATIONS

Although one immediate effect of cytotoxic drugs and radiation is on the myeloid system, the lymphoid compartment is also affected. The frequency and type of alterations in the immune system vary greatly in different malignancies and in different stages of the same malignancy. They are also related to other factors, such as age. Combined modality treatment, including biological molecules such as interferon, makes interpretation of the etiology of immune alterations difficult. However, following treatment, a tendency toward normalization of the mature cells and their products is observed, even if sometimes with alterations in more immature populations. Alterations in numbers, subtypes, and function of T cells, which may last years after cessation of therapy, have been documented and reviewed in this book. Implications of those alterations for immune surveillance and the development of secondary tumors are a matter of controversy.

III. SECONDARY MALIGNANCIES

Studies of chromosome abnormalities after therapeutic, occupational, environmental, or accidental exposure to radiation or drugs indicate an increased frequency of aberrations in exposed populations.

However, prospective studies using sensitive modern techniques of cytogenetics combined with molecular biology are needed. In particular, the relevance of chromosome aberrations in lymphocytes to those in bone marrow cells or in cells of other tissues that are most likely to develop tumors require further study.

Of special interest to hematologists and oncologists is the possibility of rearrangements or breaks that may interfere with regulatory regions or genes related to hemopoiesis. In this context, the cluster of regulatory genes located on chromosome 5 (IL-3, GM-CSF, M-CSF, and the receptor for M-CSF) are of particular interest.

IV. NEW THERAPEUTIC APPROACHES

As indicated, the use of GM-CSF or related molecules immediately preceding, during, or following cytotoxic chemotherapy or radiation is likely to ameliorate

Table 2 New Therapeutic Approaches

1.	Protection of stem cells with specific proliferation inhibitors
2.	Selection of drugs that selectively spare the stem cell populations
3.	Antibody targeting of malignant cells
4.	New systems of drug delivery

the acute effects of these agents. Whether they will prevent or correct the long-term effects of these agents is debatable. However, other approaches to therapy are being explored (Table 2). In the near future it may be possible to protect stem cells during cytotoxic treatment by blocking their entry into active proliferation by use of inhibitors specific for stem cells. It is also possible to use drugs that act selectively on some hemopoietic populations and that damage stem or regulatory cells to a lesser extent than more mature populations. Examples reviewed in the preceding chapters are cyclophosphamide and its derivatives. Ideally, drug combinations should be selected not only because of their antitumor effect, but also because of their capacity to spare stem cells or regulatory stromal cell populations. New therapeutic approaches that aim to deliver drugs to specific targets are being explored; if successful, they may overcome the problem of bone marrow toxicity.

Index

D

E

F

G

H

I

K